BODY IMAGE

BODY IMAGE

A Handbook of Theory, Research, and Clinical Practice

Edited by
Thomas F. Cash
Thomas Pruzinsky

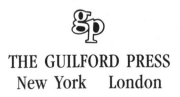

THE GUILFORD PRESS
New York   London

© 2002 The Guilford Press; Preface to the Paperback Edition © 2004
A Division of Guilford Publications, Inc.
72 Spring Street, New York, NY 10012
www.guilford.com

Chapters 4 and 52 © 2002 David W. Krueger

Paperback edition 2004

Printed in the United States of America

This book is printed on acid-free paper.

Last digit is print number: 9 8 7 6 5 4 3

Library of Congress Cataloging-in-Publication Data

Body image: a handbook of theory, research, and clinical practice / edited by
    Thomas F. Cash, Thomas Pruzinsky.
        p.   cm.
    Includes bibliographical references and index.
        ISBN 1-57230-777-3 (hc.)   ISBN 1-59385-015-8 (pbk.)
        1. Body image.   I. Cash, Thomas F.   II. Pruzinsky, Thomas.
BF697.5.B63 B617 2002
306.4—dc21

                                               2002006334

About the Editors

Thomas F. Cash, PhD, is Professor of Psychology at Old Dominion University in Norfolk, Virginia. During the past 30 years, he has published over 150 scientific articles and chapters on the psychology of physical appearance. His works span a range of topics—body image development, assessment and treatment, eating disorders, obesity, appearance stereotyping and discrimination, appearance-altering medical conditions, cosmetic surgery, and body image quality of life. Dr. Cash has developed an empirically supported program to help people have a more positive body image, available as *The Body Image Workbook: An 8-Step Program for Learning to Like Your Looks*. He has served on the editorial boards of several professional journals and is currently founding a new international journal of body image scholarship. His website is located at *www.body-images.com*.

Thomas Pruzinsky, PhD, is Professor of Psychology at Quinnipiac University and Adjunct Assistant Professor in the Department of Plastic Surgery at the New York University School of Medicine. His research and clinical interests focus on the psychological aspects of plastic and reconstructive surgery. He is particularly interested in long-term body image adaptation to acquired and congenital facial disfigurement and has published numerous articles and chapters on these topics. A previous visiting professor at the Yale University Medical School Division of Plastic Surgery, he continues to collaborate with his colleagues at Yale on research projects evaluating body image adaptation in cosmetic and reconstructive surgery. He also has served as a manuscript reviewer for *Plastic and Reconstructive Surgery, Health Psychology,* and *Cleft Palate–Craniofacial Journal*.

Contributors

Liana Abascal, MA, was originally trained as a computer scientist but is now a research coordinator in the Department of Psychiatry and Behavioral Sciences at Stanford University. She applies her analytical background in coordinating longitudinal research to the prevention of eating disorders.

Diann M. Ackard, PhD, is a clinical psychologist in private practice in Minneapolis, Minnesota. Her research interests include the association between disordered eating, body image, and physical and sexual abuse among adolescents and adults, indicators of positive treatment outcome from eating disorders, and body image development among youth.

Andrea Allen, PhD, a clinical and social psychologist, is Assistant Professor in the Compulsive, Impulsive and Anxiety Disorders Program, Department of Psychiatry, Mount Sinai School of Medicine in New York City. Her research interests are focused on understanding the etiology, neurobiology, and treatment of obsessive–compulsive spectrum disorders, especially body dysmorphic disorder.

Madeline Altabe, PhD, is Assistant Professor at the Florida School of Professional Psychology at Argosy University–Tampa, and in private clinical practice in Tampa, Florida. Her clinical and research interests include cognitive factors and multicultural issues in body image and eating disorders.

Arnold E. Andersen, MD, is Professor of Psychiatry at the University of Iowa College of Medicine. His research interests include diagnosis and treatment of eating disorders, medical complications of eating disorders, males with eating disorders, eating behavior in eating disorders, developmental aspects of eating disorders, and developing statewide programs for diagnosis and treatment of eating disorders by primary care physicians.

Jay M. Behel, PhD, is a clinical psychologist with Rehabilitation Associates of the Midwest. His clinical interests include chronic pain, cardiac psychology and posttraumatic stress disorder. Previous research has included investigations of posttraumatic adjustment in survivors of rape and perceived vulnerability in individuals with amputations.

Marion A. Bilich, PhD, is a licensed psychologist in private practice in Long Island, New York. Her professional interests and publications include work on weight loss and compulsive eating.

Kelly D. Brownell, PhD, is a clinical psychologist, Professor of Psychology, Epidemiology and Public Health, and Director of the Yale Center for Eating and Weight Disorders at Yale University in New Haven, Connecticut. His research interests pertain to the social causes and remedies of obesity stigma, as well as public policy as a means for improving diet and physical activity at the national level.

Thomas F. Cash, PhD. See "About the Editors."

Angela A. Celio, MA, is a doctoral student in the San Diego State University and University of California, San Diego, Joint Doctoral Program in Clinical Psychology. Her research interests include prevention and treatment of eating disorders, development and evaluation of Internet-delivered interventions, and treatment of childhood obesity.

Elizabeth Chapman, PhD, is a Research Associate in the Centre for Family Research, University of Cambridge, United Kingdom, currently holding a Wellcome Trust Postdoctoral Fellowship in Biomedical Ethics. Her research interests focus on how the body is experienced in different illness and health contexts, with investigations of HIV, genetic conditions, and transplantation.

Caroline Davis, PhD, is a health psychologist and Professor in the Department of Kinesiology and Health Science at York University in Toronto, Canada. She is also a Research Scientist in the Department of Psychiatry, Faculty of Medicine, at the University of Toronto. Her research interests focus on eating disorders and other addictive behaviors, including the role of exercise and sports in the development of weight and body image concerns.

Patricia Fallon, PhD, is a psychologist in private practice and on the clinical faculty at the University of Washington in Seattle. She has authored various books and articles on eating disorders, and her particular interests include trauma, family therapy, and feminist theory. She is also the President of the Academy for Eating Disorders for 2002–2003.

Emily C. Fleming, BA, is a doctoral student in the Virginia Consortium Program in Clinical Psychology in Norfolk, Virginia. Her research interests include the impact of body image on quality of life and positive body image.

Gary D. Foster, PhD, is Associate Professor and Clinical Director at the Weight and Eating Disorders Program in the Department of Psychiatry at the University of Pennsylvania School of Medicine in Philadelphia, Pennsylvania. His research interests pertain to the biological and behavioral aspects of obesity and weight loss.

Debra L. Franko, PhD, is Associate Professor of Counseling Psychology at Northeastern University in Boston, Massachusetts, and Assistant Professor of Psychology in the Department of Psychiatry at Harvard Medical School. She teaches and conducts research on the prevention of eating disorders.

Rick M. Gardner, PhD, is an experimental psychologist and Professor Emeritus in the Department of Psychology at the University of Colorado at Denver. His current research interests are the perceptual and attitudinal aspects of body image in children and in adults.

David M. Garner, PhD, is the Director of the River Centre Clinic in Ohio. He is Adjunct Professor at Bowling Green State University (Psychology) and the University of Toledo (Women's Studies). His research interests are in the areas of obesity and eating disorders, including assessment, diagnosis, treatment outcome, psychopathology, and the biology of weight regulation.

Jane Gilmour, PhD, DClinPsych, is a lecturer in clinical psychology at the Institute of Child Health, University College London. Her clinical and research interests include the psychosocial aspects of short stature and the neuropsychology of neurodevelopmental disorders.

Jessica L. Gokee, BA, is a doctoral student in the Clinical Psychology Program at the University of Central Florida in Orlando. Her research interests include eating expectancies and the role of social comparison in body image disturbance.

Angela S. Guarda, MD, is a psychiatrist and Assistant Professor in the Department of Psychiatry and Behavioral Sciences at Johns Hopkins University School of Medicine, where she is Director of the Eating Disorders Program. Her research interests include body image and women's mental health problems in the eating disorder population. Her clinical work focuses on the treatment of anorexia nervosa and bulimia.

Bert Hayslip, Jr., PhD, is a Regents Professor in Psychology at the University of North Texas and is Editor of *The International Journal of Aging and Human Development*. His research deals with cognitive processes in aging, interventions to enhance cognitive functioning in later life, personality–ability relationships in aged persons, grief and bereavement, death anxiety, and mental health and aging.

Leslie J. Heinberg, PhD, is a clinical psychologist and Assistant Professor in the Department of Psychiatry and Behavioral Sciences at Johns Hopkins University School of Medicine. Her research interests focus on the sociocultural aspects of body image, body image in medical populations, and cognitive-behavioral interventions for body image and eating disorders. Her clinical work includes cognitive-behavioral interventions for medical populations and eating disorders.

Eric Hollander, MD, is a psychiatrist and the Director of the Compulsive, Impulsive and Anxiety Disorders Program, the Director of Clinical Psychopharmacology, and Professor in the Department of Psychiatry, Mount Sinai School of Medicine in New York City. His research interests focus on obsessive–compulsive spectrum disorders, including body dysmorphic disorder, obsessive–compulsive disorder, autism, pathological gambling, and impulsive aggression.

Linda A. Jackson, PhD, is a social psychologist and Professor in the Department of Psychology at Michigan State University. She has published extensively on physical appearance and body image. Her current research interests focus on the social psychological causes and consequences of using information technology (e.g., the Internet) in the home and workplace.

Kathleen Y. Kawamura, PhD, is a graduate of the Clinical Psychology Program at the University of Massachusetts, Amherst. She is completing a postdoctoral fellowship in behavioral medicine at the Cambridge Health Alliance, an affiliate of Harvard Medical School. Her research interests are in the areas of both Asian American mental health and perfectionism.

Ann Kearney-Cooke, PhD, is Director of the Cincinnati Psychotherapy Institute. She is a distinguished scholar at the Partnership for Women's Health at Columbia University in New York, where she developed the Helping Girls Become Strong Women

Project. Her research interests pertain to understanding body image development and the treatment of body image disturbances and eating disorders.

Marcel Kinsbourne, MD, is a behavioral neurologist as well as an experimental psychologist and Professor of Psychology at the New School University in New York City. His research addresses a range of issues in normal and abnormal development (including ADHD and language disorders) as well as neuropsychological analysis of focal brain damage.

H. Asuman Kiyak, PhD, is Professor of Oral and Maxillofacial Surgery, Adjunct Professor of Psychology, and Director of the Institute on Aging at the University of Washington. Her research includes a focus on psychological responses to surgical and conventional orthodontics, informed consent for elective and dental procedures, and innovative health promotion methods for older adults. She received the Distinguished Scientist Award from the International Association of Dental Research in 2000.

John Y. M. Koo, MD, is Professor and Vice Chairman of the Department of Dermatology at the University of California San Francisco Medical Center. He is board certified in psychiatry and dermatology and is well published in psychodermatology.

David W. Krueger, MD, FAPA, is in the private practice of psychiatry and psychoanalysis in Houston, Texas, and is Clinical Professor of Psychiatry at Baylor College of Medicine. His professional interests and publications include developmental and clinical integration in disorders of the self.

Michael P. Levine, PhD, is Professor of Psychology at Kenyon College in Gambier, Ohio. His special interests are mass media and body image, and prevention of disordered eating. From 1993 to 2000, he was a volunteer trustee of Eating Disorders Awareness & Prevention, Inc. (now the National Eating Disorders Association).

Catherine M. Lichtenberger, BKin, is a graduate student studying health and exercise psychology in the Department of Kinesiology at McMaster University. Her research concerns body image and its relationship with both psychological and physiological well-being, and the relationship between exercise and body image among people with chronic disease and disability.

Kathleen A. Martin, PhD, is Assistant Professor of Health and Exercise Psychology in the Department of Kinesiology at McMaster University. Her research focuses on body image and other psychological factors related to exercise adoption and adherence, and the effects of exercise training on psychological well-being among people with disease and disability.

Patty E. Matz, PhD, is a fellow of psychology in psychiatry at the Cornell Cognitive Therapy Clinic, Weill Medical College of Cornell University, and Professional Associate (Psychology) at the New York Presbyterian Hospital in New York. Her research interests relate to cognitive-behavioral interventions for negative body image and obesity in overweight populations.

Nita Mary McKinley, PhD, is Assistant Professor in the Department of Interdisciplinary Arts and Sciences, University of Washington, Tacoma, where she teaches developmental psychology and psychology of women. Her research interests include women's body experience, women's and men's objectification of women, and women's resistance to objectification.

Keisha-Gaye N. O'Garo, BA, is a graduate student at the Florida School of Professional Psychology at Argosy University–Tampa. Her professional interests include multicultural issues in eating disorders.

Roberto Olivardia, PhD, is a clinical psychologist and clinical research fellow in the Department of Psychiatry at Harvard Medical School. He provides psychotherapy at McLean Hospital in Belmont, Massachusetts, specializing in body image disorders and men's issues. His research interests pertain to body image in boys and men.

Katharine A. Phillips, MD, is Associate Professor of Psychiatry at Brown University School of Medicine, as well as Director of the Body Image Program at Butler Hospital in Providence, Rhode Island. Her research focuses on the psychopathology, treatment, and other aspects of body dysmorphic disorder.

Thomas Pruzinsky, PhD. See "About the Editors."

Judith Ruskay Rabinor, PhD, is Director of the American Eating Disorder Center of Long Island, Consultant to The Renfrew Center Foundation, Instructor and Supervisor at The Center for Anorexia and Bulimia in New York City, and Associate Professor at the Derner Institute at Adelphi University in Garden City, New York. She has extensive interests in psychotherapy and the eating disorders.

Lisa M. Radika, PhD, is currently a postdoctoral fellow at the Veterans Administration Hospital in Dallas, Texas. Her clinical and research interests include personality assessment and neuropsychological assessment of adults; cognitive processes and aging; perceptions of elder abuse; and gerontological aspects of diagnosis, assessment, and treatment.

Marisa Reichmuth, BS, is currently enrolled in the University of Washington School of Dentistry, after having completed her undergraduate degree in psychology. She has worked as a research assistant on studies of children's perceptions of their needs for orthodontics and on a clinical trial to test low cost preventative regimens for older persons.

Esther D. Rothblum, PhD, is Professor of Psychology at the University of Vermont. Her research has focused on weight and employment discrimination; the stigma of body weight in the United States, Australia, and Africa; and social skills related to compensating for weight in the workplace. In 1992 she received the Distinguished Achievement Award from the National Association to Advance Fat Acceptance.

Nichola Rumsey, PhD, is a Reader in Health Psychology and Director of the Centre for Appearance and Disfigurement Research at the University of the West of England, Bristol, United Kingdom. Her research focuses on the psychological effects of disfigurement and on services for people with visible differences.

Bruce D. Rybarczyk, PhD, is a clinical psychologist and Associate Professor in the Departments of Psychology and Physical Medicine and Rehabilitation at Rush Medical College in Chicago. He is also a diplomate in rehabilitation psychology. His recent research interests focus on psychological interventions that enhance the quality of life of older adults with chronic illness.

David B. Sarwer, PhD, is Assistant Professor of Psychology in Psychiatry and Surgery at the University of Pennsylvania School of Medicine. He is a consultant at the Edwin and Fannie Gray Hall Center for Human Appearance at the University of Pennsylvania, where he conducts research on the psychological issues in plastic surgery. He is also Director of Education at the Weight and Eating Disorders Program at the University of Pennsylvania, where he has research and clinical interests in the treatment of obesity.

Marlene B. Schwartz, PhD, is a clinical psychologist and Codirector of the Yale Center for Eating and Weight Disorders at Yale University in New Haven, Connecticut. Her research interests address understanding the factors that lead to the development of eating disorders and obesity, and studying the treatment and prevention of these problems.

Karyn M. Skultety, MS, is a clinical psychology graduate student at the University of Massachusetts, Amherst. Her clinical and research interests pertain to older adults' utilization of psychological services and to identity and aging, particularly gender differences in identity processes and self-esteem.

Linda Smolak, PhD, is Professor of Psychology and Women's and Gender Studies at Kenyon College in Gambier, Ohio. Her research specialization is the developmental psychopathology of eating problems, particularly in terms of the special vulnerabilities of young girls.

Tiffany M. Stewart, MA, is a doctoral candidate in clinical psychology at Louisiana State University. Her research has emphasized the assessment and treatment of body image disturbances associated with eating disorders and obesity.

Eric Stice, PhD, is Associate Professor of Clinical Psychology at the University of Texas at Austin. His research interests focus on the etiology and prevention of eating pathology and substance abuse.

Melissa D. Strachan, PsyD, is a licensed clinical psychologist with a consultative body image practice in the St. Louis area. Her clinical and research interests include feminist perspectives on body image as well as the cognitive-behavioral treatment of body image difficulties.

Ruth H. Striegel-Moore, PhD, is a clinical psychologist and Professor of Psychology at Wesleyan University in Middletown, Connecticut. Her research focuses on risk factors for and prevention of body image and eating disturbances.

Stacey Tantleff-Dunn, PhD, is a clinical psychologist and Associate Professor in the Department of Psychology at the University of Central Florida in Orlando. Her research interests include appearance-related feedback and other interpersonal influences on body image, as well as cognitive processing models of body image disturbance.

C. Barr Taylor, MD, is Professor of Psychiatry at Stanford University School of Medicine, where he serves as Director of the Laboratory for the Study of Behavioral Medicine and Adult Psychiatry Residency Training Director. His research has focused on developing strategies for and evaluating innovative techniques for prevention of various disorders.

J. Kevin Thompson, PhD, is a clinical psychologist and Professor of Psychology in the Department of Psychology at the University of South Florida in Tampa, Florida. His current research interests are risk factors in the development and maintenance of body image disturbances.

Marika Tiggemann, PhD, is Associate Professor in the School of Psychology at Flinders University in South Australia. Her research interests cover women's health broadly, and in particular weight, dieting, and body image issues.

Steven M. Tovian, PhD, ABPP, is Director of Health Psychology and Chief Psychologist in the Department of Psychiatry and Behavioral Sciences at Evanston Northwestern Healthcare in Evanston, Illinois. He is also Associate Professor of Psychiatry and Behavioral Sciences at Northwestern University Medical School. His research interests include psychological assessment in medical settings and psychological interventions with urology and dermatology patients.

Patricia van den Berg, MA, is a doctoral student in clinical psychology at the University of South Florida in Tampa, Florida. Her current research interests are family, peer, and media influences on body image.

Patricia Westmoreland Corson, MD, is a resident physician in the Departments of Internal Medicine and Psychiatry at the University of Iowa College of Medicine. Her interests are in disorders that span the medicine–psychiatry spectrum, in particular eating disorders and the comorbidity of medical illnesses and affective disorders.

Susan Krauss Whitbourne, PhD, is Professor of Psychology at the University of Massachusetts, Amherst, and the author of several texts on psychology and aging. Her research interests are in identity and aging, with particular focus on physical and cognitive changes and their effects on the individual.

Craig A. White, ClinPsyD, is a clinical psychologist and clinical research fellow in the Department of Psychological Medicine, University of Glasgow, Scotland. His research interests are in the psychological aspects of oncology. He is a Founding Fellow of the Academy of Cognitive Therapy, Fellow of the Royal Society of Medicine, and Associate Fellow of the British Psychological Society.

Marney A. White, MA, is a doctoral candidate in clinical psychology at Louisiana State University. She has focused her research on the development of assessment inventories related to obesity and eating disorders and on sociocultural factors that determine eating disorders.

Michael W. Wiederman, PhD, is Associate Professor of Psychology in the Department of Human Relations at Columbia College in Columbia, South Carolina. He is an active member of the Society for the Scientific Study of Sexuality, and his research interests include gender, jealousy, and sexual behavior, attitudes, and beliefs.

Denise E. Wilfley, PhD, is the Director of the Center for Eating and Weight Disorders and Associate Professor in the San Diego State University and University of California, San Diego, Joint Doctoral Program in Clinical Psychology. Her research interests focus on causes, prevention, and treatment of eating disorders and obesity.

Donald A. Williamson, PhD, is Professor of Psychology at Louisiana State University and Chief of Health Psychology at Pennington Biomedical Research Center. His research interests pertain to body image, eating disorders, and obesity.

Andrew J. Winzelberg, PhD, is a researcher in the Department of Psychiatry and Behavioral Sciences at Stanford University. His research interests include the prevention of mental disorders, the use of computer technology in delivering prevention and treatment interventions, and stepped-care approaches to mental health treatment.

Jensen Yeung, MD, is a resident in dermatology at the University of Toronto in Canada. He completed his undergraduate degree in psychology and his MD degree at McMaster University. His current interests are in psychodermatology and quality-of-life measurements in dermatology.

Emily York-Crowe, BA, is a doctoral candidate in clinical psychology at Louisiana State University. Her research interests pertain to the development of innovative treatment approaches for eating disorders and obesity.

Marion F. Zabinski, MS, is a doctoral student in the San Diego State University (SDSU) and University of California, San Diego, Joint Doctoral Program in Clinical Psychology and the SDSU Graduate School of Public Health. Her research interests include eating disorder prevention, childhood obesity treatment, health promotion behaviors, and the development and evaluation of Internet-delivered interventions.

Preface to the Paperback Edition

Nearly 2 years have passed since our completion of the initial edition of this comprehensive volume. During this time, the field has continued to grow in the dissemination of empirical research on the multidimensional concept of body image and its applications. Our purpose then and now is to promote better understanding of the psychosocial meanings of human embodiment. The scholarly chapters in *Body Image: A Handbook of Theory, Research, and Clinical Practice* capture the rich diversity of body image in well-studied areas (i.e., eating disorders and obesity), as well as in areas that represent the new frontiers of the field (i.e., many medical specialties). We are pleased by the publication of very positive reviews of this work, a testimony to the expertise and insights of our knowledgeable contributors.

This *Handbook* was a catalyst for a new journal that began in 2004, *Body Image: An International Journal of Research* (*www.elsevier.com/locate/bodyimage*). Until now, body image scholarship has had no real "home." That is, the publication of important scientific advances of knowledge has been widely scattered across numerous disciplines and journals. One of us (Tom Cash) is the founding Editor-in-Chief of this new integrative, peer-reviewed scientific publication. The other (Tom Pruzinsky) is an Associate Editor. On the journal's Editorial Board are many of the experienced authors of chapters in this volume.

Our sincere hope is that this paperback edition of the *Handbook* will encourage even more students and professionals to learn about body image, conduct edifying research, and provide effective help to persons with body image challenges. After all, as we state in the final sentence of this volume, "the experience of embodiment is central to the quality of human life."

THOMAS F. CASH, PhD
THOMAS PRUZINSKY, PhD

important literature on eating disorders, obesity, and body dysmorphic disorder. You will see in the pages that follow that our esteemed contributors rose to the occasion with great competence, conscientiousness, and creativity. As editors, we made certain that chapters informatively cross-reference one another. As catalysts for further discovery, each chapter offers an annotated bibliography of "Informative Readings."

Body Image reviews sociocultural, neurocognitive, psychodynamic, cognitive-behavioral, information-processing, and feminist viewpoints. Our contributors discern the development of body image across the lifespan. They thoroughly examine body image experiences in relation to gender, sexual orientation, race/ethnicity, and important physical characteristics, including adiposity, muscularity, athleticism, and disfiguring congenital conditions. This book also explores often overlooked body image issues that arise in dermatology, plastic and reconstructive surgery, oncology, physical rehabilitation, obstetrics and gynecology, urology, endocrinology, and dentistry, as well as for individuals with HIV and AIDS.

Among the book's most practical contributions are its prescriptive reviews of body image assessments for children, adolescents, and adults. Equally useful are its evaluations of interventions for body image change, whether by modifications of the body or by psychological change. Experts address weight loss, fitness regimens, cosmetic surgery for "elective" appearance changes, reconstructive surgeries for congenital and acquired deformities, and psychopharmacological treatments. Psychosocial interventions encompass cognitive-behavioral, psychodynamic, and experiential approaches for treatment and psychoeducational and ecological activist approaches to prevention.

For seasoned and aspiring professionals, *Body Image* is a distinctively comprehensive, scientifically up-to-date, and clinically valuable resource, particularly for scientists and practitioners in psychology and mental health, as well as those in medical and allied health fields. Reflecting the rapidly expanding diversity of the field, this handbook is testimony to the integral importance of body image in the full range of human experience. Our most sincere hope is that this volume contributes, in science and clinical practice, to the alleviation of body image suffering and to a movement to promote body image acceptance.

In addition to the contributing authors, many people were vital in the production of this work. As always, The Guilford Press was a superlative publisher. Our editor Jim Nageotte provided thoughtful, patient, and constructive guidance throughout the project. The hard work of Kim Miller (marketing assistant), Anna Nelson (production editor), and Margaret Ryan (copy editor) was also essential to the fruition of this book.

Tom Cash voices special words of thanks to the following: I express sincere appreciation to my students and colleagues in the Department of Psychology at Old Dominion University, my home for 29 years. Throughout my career, the opportunity to teach, mentor, and collaborate with students has been tremendously fulfilling. I am grateful to my university for awarding me a research leave to devote the essential time and energy to this volume. I am appreciative as well of the beauty, inspiration, and solace of the Chesapeake Bay. Outside my window and steps from my home, she is always there to give me perspective. I am also grateful to Lynn Weiler for her loving support and the balance she gives to my life. Finally, I express my heartfelt and enduring thanks to my sons, Ben and T. C., who always enhance the meaning of my life. With my love, I dedicate this book to them and to my grandson, Thomas Hayden Cash.

Tom Pruzinsky expresses his own heartfelt acknowledgments: It is a great joy to put into words my gratitude to Ina Langman for giving me the opportunity to develop a clinical and research career focused on the psychological aspects of plastic surgery—and even more for gracing my wife and me with her friendship, humor, and wisdom. Milton Edgerton gave me (and scores of others) a once-in-a-lifetime education about the true meaning of being a physician and serving others. My deepest appreciation goes to Tom Borkovec for sharing his knowledge, his joy in learning, and his friendship. Quinnipiac University has been a generous source of research support, with especially wonderful colleagues. I have also been blessed by the immeasurable support of family members, especially my Aunt Irene and Uncle John Sulinsky. My gratitude goes to my wife, Rhonda, for sharing her life with me—nothing seems quite complete until it is shared with her. I dedicate this book to my parents, Agnes and Joseph Pruzinsky, to thank them for generously giving me the love and knowledge that allowed me to build a life filled with many blessings.

Finally, we thank one another, two Toms, for our enduring friendship and our shared belief that together we can make a difference.

THOMAS F. CASH, PhD
THOMAS PRUZINSKY, PhD

Contents

I

Conceptual Foundations

1

Understanding Body Images
Historical and Contemporary Perspectives

THOMAS PRUZINSKY
THOMAS F. CASH

Looking back over nearly a century of scholarly attempts to understand the profoundly human experience of embodiment that we call "body image," we find a very rich and inspiring history. From diverse vantage points, psychologists, physicians, and philosophers have theorized about the nature and significance of body image. Scientists have made systematic observations to test their ideas and discover the meanings of body image. Clinical practitioners have pursued remedies directed toward the body, the mind, or both to help people whose quality of life is diminished by their body image experiences.

This introductory chapter offers a historical and conceptual context for the volume by highlighting specific books that mark important milestones in body image scholarship, identifying and discussing core conceptual themes about body image that permeate past and current eras, and articulating contemporary perspectives on body image by summarizing the organization and contents of this handbook, which speak to its rationale and uniqueness.

MILESTONES IN BODY IMAGE SCHOLARSHIP

Pre-1990 Legacies

Understanding modern perspectives on body image requires insight into the long and rich lineage of the body image construct. In the single most informative historical review of body image, the late Seymour Fisher, in his

3

1990 chapter, reviews the origins of body image inquiry, which focused on neuropathological forms of body experience, with very limited consideration of psychological variables. Early "body image" research was dominated by investigation of the "body schema," a proposed neural mechanism whereby changes in body posture and movement were centrally coordinated.

Fisher further documents how Paul Schilder, who was trained as a neurologist, was "single-handedly" responsible for moving the study of body image beyond the exclusive domain of neuropathology. Indeed, he was "the first to devote entire volumes to the topic of body image" (p. 12). In his 1935/1950 *The Image and Appearance of the Human Body*, Schilder presciently argued for a biopsychosocial approach to body image, emphasizing the need to examine its neurological, psychological, and sociocultural elements. Insight into the multifaceted nature of body image allowed Schilder to foresee, as Fisher notes, "most of the modern lines of research dealing with body experience" (p. 12).

One of the most important body image scholars is Seymour Fisher, who, with his colleague Sidney Cleveland, published two editions of the text *Body Image and Personality* in 1958 and 1968. Their volumes reflect the then pervasive psychodynamic views of body image, especially Fisher's theory about "body image boundaries"; they reviewed empirical research on the "barrier" and "penetration" concepts, posited to reflect the strength or permeability of body boundaries. These investigations, with "normal" subjects as well as psychiatric and medical patients, almost invariably used projective methodologies. Similar topics are reprised and revised in Fisher's 1970 book, *Body Experience in Fantasy and Behavior*.

Fisher's 1986 two-volume opus, *Development and Structure of the Body Image*, is the apex of that portion of his career devoted to body image scholarship. This comprehensive review of research cites over 4,000 references, with more than 70 papers by Fisher and colleagues. The second volume analyzes and synthesizes data pertinent to Fisher's own concepts, including "body image boundary; assignment of meaning to specific body areas; general body awareness; and distortions in body perception" (p. xi). These works are arguably underappreciated as a resource for insights into body image functioning. Similarly, Fisher's 1989 volume, *Sexual Images of the Self: The Psychology of Erotic Sensations and Illusions*, seems overlooked as a rich source of thought about body image functioning in sexual experience.

One reasonable explanation for the relative neglect of Fisher's pioneering insights is that his work was eclipsed by the growing predominance of cognitive-behavioral approaches to body image, along with a waning reign of psychodynamic perspectives on body image (and in psychology, in general), and the growing disfavor of projective methodologies. However, relegating his contributions to the category of "historically significant" misses the breadth and depth of Seymour Fisher's understanding of body image. His insights are an antidote to a current view of body image in which investigation of eating disorders has become paradigmatic for body image research.

Franklin Shontz, in his 1969 *Perceptual and Cognitive Aspects of Body Experience* and in later writings, was a pioneer in directing body image research away from the domination of psychodynamic thinking. Shontz remarked (in our 1990 volume) that the shift from neurological to psychodynamic conceptions had removed "body" from body image. He also critically noted that Fisher's psychodynamic view of body image as "a projection screen for emotional learning and experience" served to eradicate the "image" from body image by operationally defining it as a manifestation of perceiving inkblots or other ambiguous stimuli. Shontz redressed these limitations in several ways as he argued for the study of multifaceted "body experience." He emphasized the use of diverse scientific methods and encouraged expansion and integration of theoretical developments, especially from field theory, Gestalt psychology, and cognitive theory. Shontz sought to put the body back into body image, partly by applying body image concepts to the study of physical disability. He endeavored to return the *image* to body image by articulating cognitive and perceptual dimensions of body experience. Today's students of body image, who assume that information-processing perspectives began in the past decade or two, would be well advised to visit Shontz's writings.

Although the study of body image has become less exclusively guided by the psychodynamic paradigm, we would be shortsighted to marginalize this viewpoint. David Krueger's 1989 volume, *Body Self and Psychological Self: Developmental and Clinical Integration in Disorders of the Self*, and his chapter in our 1990 volume both exemplify how modern psychodynamic thought can illuminate facets of body image functioning, including the seminal influences of interpersonal attachments and other developmental processes on body image formation. Krueger's clinical insight into neglected nuances of body image development and treatment refutes any notion that a psychodynamic view on body image is "dead" or only historically relevant.

The Decade of the 1990s

The 1990s constituted a pivotal era in the evolution of body image scholarship. Kevin Thompson's prolific contributions began with *Body Image Disturbance: Assessment and Treatment* in 1990 and continued with his 1996 edited book, *Body Image, Eating Disorders, and Obesity: An Integrative Guide for Assessment and Treatment*. Reflecting the burgeoning scientific and clinical interest in eating disorders and obesity, these works greatly enhanced our knowledge of the assessment and treatment of body image disorders. Mirroring the zeitgeist within the broader field of psychology, these contributions reflect the shift away from psychodynamic views of body image to cognitive-behavioral and feminist perspectives.

The 1990s represent a productive period of conceptual, psychometric, and psychotherapeutic developments. *Exacting Beauty: Theory, Assessment, and Treatment of Body Image Disturbance*, written in 1999 by Thompson, Heinberg, Altabe, and Tantleff-Dunn, provided a needed compilation and synthesis of the massive progress in body image research. A few years later, Thompson and Smolak edited a long-anticipated volume about body image in childhood and adolescence, *Body Image, Eating Disorders, and Obesity in Youth: Assessment, Prevention, and Treatment.*

Another edifying book of the decade is Linda Jackson's 1992 *Physical Appearance and Gender: Sociobiological and Sociocultural Perspectives*. In this comprehensive work, she uniquely integrates both body image research and the social–psychological literature on physical attractiveness in the context of gender, compares disparate theoretical views, and considers the implications of the conclusions.

The decade began with our own 1990 contribution, *Body Images: Development, Deviance, and Change*. We would like to believe that our volume was a catalyst in the recognition and refinement of the multidimensional nature of body image and its multidisciplinary relevance. In addition to reviewing thoroughly the empirical and clinical literatures on body image concepts, we sought to expand their application into areas of investigation previously inadequately explored—for example, disfigurement, disability and rehabilitation, and plastic and reconstructive surgery. This work led one of us (T.F.C.) to continue developing an empirically based program of body image treatment, resulting in publication of an audiocassette series for clinicians in 1991 and books for both practitioners and the public in 1995 and 1997.

BRIDGING HISTORICAL AND CONTEMPORARY PERSPECTIVES: ENDURING THEMES

A number of recurring themes provides a bridge between historical and contemporary body image perspectives. We will briefly discuss three of these: (1) a conviction that body image plays an integral role in understanding human experience, (2) recognition of the complexity of the body image construct, and (3) the dearth of empirical and theoretical integration within and across disciplines.

Body Image and Human Experience

Over the course of body image scholarship, body experience has been viewed as a fundamental construct for understanding human functioning. For example, Fisher states, "The inexhaustible list of behaviors that has turned out to be linked with measures in the body-experience domain documents the ubiquitous influence of body attitudes. Human identity cannot be separated from its somatic headquarters in the world" (1990, p. 18). This vital role of body image means that it has the potential to dramatically influence our quality of life. From early childhood on, body image affects our emotions, thoughts, and behaviors in everyday life. Perhaps most poignantly, body image influences our relationships—those that are public as well as the most intimate. If, as scientists and clinicians, we can appreciate the breadth and depth of body experiences, then we have the capacity to prevent and relieve the suffering of persons whose body images undermine the quality of their lives.

Complexity of Body Image

Body image scholars, past and present, increasingly agree that body image is a multidimensional phenomenon. It is far more complex than implied by Schilder's definition as "the picture of our own body which we form in our own mind" (1935/1950, p. 11). This complexity is partly due to terminological confusion—a consistent historical and contemporary problem in studying body image.

In the final section of our 1990 book, we observed that "despite its long history, the concept of body image has remained rather elusive, in part because it has meant different things to different scientists and practitioners" (p. 346). Similarly, in 1999 Thompson and colleagues noted that defining body image was "tricky" because "there are many other terms used to define the different components of body image, and in some cases researchers and clinicians use these terms interchangeably when perhaps they should not" (pp. 9–10). Aptly illustrating this point, they list 16 "definitions" of body image (weight satisfaction, size perception accuracy, body satisfaction, appearance satisfaction, appearance evaluation, appearance orientation, body esteem, body concern, body dysphoria, body dysmorphia, body schema, body percept, body distortion, body image, body image disturbance, and body image disorder; p. 10). The list could be even longer. However, in many instances, different terms are used as synonyms for some facet of body experience.

Terminology proliferates as body image research progresses. Some might argue that we have contributed to the confusion by using the plural version of the term *body images*, which we initiated in 1990. We agree that "body images" is mildly awkward and unconventional. However, our plural usage is intended to convey the construct's complexity and inherent multidimensionality—a reminder of Fisher's pronouncement that "there is no such entity as 'The Body Image' " (1990, p. 18). Ultimately, terminological lucidity can be attained by precisely defining conceptual referents within the context of the multidimensionality of body experience.

Lack of Theoretical and Empirical Integration

There has been little attempt to integrate the diverse lines of thinking and research on body image. Shontz and Fisher lamented this fact decades ago. Fisher notes that

> what particularly impresses me about the multiple branches of the current work dealing with body attitudes and feelings is how disconnected they are. These branches often thrive in "splendid isolation," as if the others did not exist. Cross-references by researchers in the different areas are, at best, sparse. (Fisher, 1990, p. 3)

We agree completely. The insights of the previous generations of body image scholars seem to exist in a not-so-splendid isolation from contemporary perspectives. Divergent theoretical positions and lines of research are seldom integrated. Moreover, much contemporary body image research has evolved from a "single problem" perspective—that is, in an effort to understand body image among individuals, especially women, with eating disorders and other weight-related concerns. Although this focus has produced many valuable advances in knowledge, it fails to capture the rich diversity of negative and positive body experiences that fall outside its lens. In creating this handbook, our intention is to lessen the isolation by bringing together a diverse group of experts to share their insights into body image with current and future body image scholars.

CONTEMPORARY PERSPECTIVES ON BODY IMAGE: ORGANIZATION AND CONTENTS OF THE HANDBOOK

Body image research has grown substantially over the past 50 years. Figure 1.1 graphs this dramatic expansion of the professional literature, showing the number of citations in psychological and medical databases for each of the past five decades. The sheer volume of research in the most recent decade is astounding. The variety of contexts in which body image is explored has broadened considerably. These impressive developments are expounded and elucidated by the contributors to this handbook. We have organized their chapters into eight substantive sections.

Conceptual Foundations

The first section of the book assembles an array of conceptual approaches for understanding human appearance and body image. Our contributors review important, wide-ranging perspectives, including sociocultural, neurocognitive, psychodynamic, cognitive-behavioral, information-processing, and feminist viewpoints. Authors thoughtfully articulate concepts, princi-

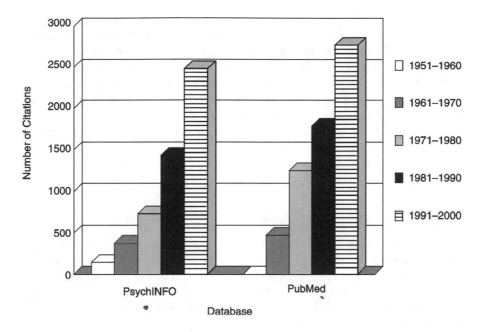

FIGURE 1.1. Citation rates for "body image" and "body satisfaction" in psychological and medical databases over the past 50 years.

ples, and propositions applicable to the empirical data and clinical observations presented throughout the book.

Developmental Perspectives and Influences

In the next section, contributors describe the development of body image across the lifespan, with special emphasis on understanding the unique body experiences of childhood, adolescence, and adulthood. These body image trajectories are further elucidated in chapters that carefully examine the influences of cultural media, family systems, and other interpersonal relationships, as well as the impact of sexual abuse. The developmental context is essential for understanding virtually all body image experiences, whether "normal" or impaired.

Body Image Assessment

The scientific study of body image requires thoughtful and precise measurement of its components and dimensions. In this section, the handbook reviews the extant literature on body image assessments across a spectrum of populations, including children, adolescents, and adults. Measurement techniques include those for assessing attitudes and perceptions as well as the use of objective and projective methodologies. Perhaps no other area of body image inquiry has seen such impressive and needed growth and refinement. These chapters offer comprehensive yet concise guidelines by which scientists and practitioners can understand both psychometric and practical issues in measuring body image. Accordingly, the authors provide foundations on which to build our future understanding of body image development and individual differences and disorders. The authors also identify assessments for documenting the efficacy of interventions designed to improve body image and its impact on the quality of life.

Individual and Cultural Differences

A comprehensive understanding of body image requires a deep appreciation of the cultural diversity and personal contexts of embodiment. This extensive section of the handbook examines a range of cultural and individual differences in body image related to gender, sexual orientation, and particular physical characteristics, including adiposity, muscularity, athleticism, as well as disfiguring congenital conditions.

Body Image Dysfunctions and Disorders

Many students of body image are interested in the myriad difficulties and disorders of body experience. In this section of the handbook, contributors comprehensively review the explosive growth of observations and evidence in the study of body image dysfunctions and disorders and consider the epidemiology of "negative body image" as well as its impact on social relations and sexual functioning. Contributors discuss difficulties that range from "common" body image discontentment to more severe disturbances, including eating disorders, body dysmorphic disorder, and somatic delusions.

Body Image Issues in Medical Contexts

One of the new frontiers of scholarship is the elucidation of the challenges to body image associated with physical diseases and disorders. An obvious but oft-neglected fact is that body image issues accompany changes in the appearance and functioning of the human body, and that these changes can dramatically affect quality of life. Such issues are routinely encountered in many medical specialties, including oncology, physical rehabilitation, obstetrics and gynecology, urology, endocrinology, dentistry, dermatology, as well as in the context of treating individuals with HIV and AIDS. The contributors to this unique section summarize the nascent state of scientific inquiry in these areas, outline specific directions for future research, and provide helpful guidance for clinical assessment and intervention.

Changing the Body: Medical, Surgical, and Other Interventions

This first of two sections on changes in body image focus on one central question: Does changing the body lead to a changed body image? Lessons from psychotherapy outcome research have taught us that it is more productive to frame our intervention efficacy questions more precisely: Which body change interventions are helpful, to what degree, for how long, in what areas of life, and for which specific individuals? These chapters in Part VII review the evidence regarding body image changes as a result of physical interventions, such as weight loss, fitness regimens, cosmetic surgery for "elective" appearance changes, reconstructive surgeries for congenital and acquired deformities, and psychopharmacological treatments.

Psychosocial Interventions for Changing Body Images

This second section on changes in body image offers an array of psychotherapeutic and psychoeducational interventions, including promising, albeit often overlooked, psychodynamic and experiential approaches. The well-documented and empirically validated cognitive-behavioral approaches to changes in body image are reviewed. Finally, two chapters tackle the topic of prevention—one delineates a psychoeducational approach, and the other, an ecological and activist approach.

Conclusions and Directions

The concluding chapter of this volume, "Future Challenges for Body Image Theory, Research, and Clinical Practice," provides an organized series of epigrammatic statements regarding our beliefs about the most important directions to pursue in expanding our understanding of body images.

INFORMATIVE READINGS

Cash, T. F. (1997). *The body image workbook: An 8-step program for learning to like your looks*. Oakland, CA: New Harbinger.—Cash's most recent version of his body image therapy program, applying contemporary body image concepts.

Cash, T. F., & Pruzinsky, T. (Eds.). (1990). *Body images: Development, deviance, and change*. New York: Guilford Press.—The editors' first compendium of body image theory, research, and clinical applications.

Fisher, S. (1970). *Body experience in fantasy and behavior*. New York: Appleton-Century-Crofts.—Presents theory and research pertinent to Fisher's psychodynamic perspective on body image.

Fisher, S. (1986). *Development and structure of the body image* (Vols. 1 & 2). Hillsdale, NJ: Erlbaum.—Comprehensive scholarly review of body image research and articulation of the author's own perspective and research.

Fisher, S. (1989). *Sexual images of the self: The psychology of erotic sensations and illusions.* Hillsdale, NJ: Erlbaum.—A thoughtful examination of body image influences on sexuality.

Fisher, S. (1990). The evolution of psychological concepts about the body. In T. F. Cash & T. Pruzinsky (Eds.), *Body images: Development, deviance, and change* (pp. 3–20). New York: Guilford Press.—The best historical review of the body image construct.

Fisher, S., & Cleveland, S. E. (1968). *Body image and personality* (2nd rev. ed.). New York: Dover.—Early review of body image research conducted primarily from a psychodynamic perspective.

Jackson, L. (1992). *Physical appearance and gender: Sociobiological and sociocultural perspectives.* Albany: SUNY Press.—Synthesizes theory and research on the social and psychological influences of physical appearance and body image.

Krueger, D. W. (1989). *Body self and psychological self: Developmental and clinical integration in disorders of the self.* New York: Brunner/Mazel.—A contemporary psychodynamically oriented perspective on body image development and treatment.

Krueger, D. W. (1990). Developmental and psychodynamic perspectives on body-image change. In T. F. Cash & T. Pruzinsky (Eds.), *Body images: Development, deviance, and change* (pp. 255–271). New York: Guilford Press.—A concise, clear, and compelling explanation of psychodynamic perspectives on body image development and treatment.

Schilder, P. (1935/1950). *The image and appearance of the human body.* New York: International Universities Press.—A reissued version of this classic and seminal text.

Shontz, F. C. (1969). *Perceptual and cognitive aspects of body experience.* New York: Macmillan.—A scientific exposition of concepts and research on body image perception and cognition.

Shontz, F. C. (1990). Body image and physical disability. In T. F. Cash & T. Pruzinsky (Eds.), *Body images: Development, deviance, and change* (pp. 149–169). New York: Guilford Press.—This chapter provides a very informative review of issues related to rehabilitation and body image, as well as a discussion of the terminological issues related to body image.

Thompson, J. K. (1990). *Body image disturbance: Assessment and treatment.* Elmsford, NY: Pergamon Press.—The author's first book, a concise overview of emerging perspectives and research on body image.

Thompson, J. K. (Ed.). (1996). *Body image, eating disorders, and obesity: An integrative guide for assessment and treatment.* Washington, DC: American Psychological Association. A detailed overview of critical assessment and treatment issues related to anorexia nervosa, bulimia nervosa, and obesity.

Thompson, J. K., Heinberg, L. J., Altabe, M., & Tantleff-Dunn, S. (1999). *Exacting beauty: Theory, assessment and treatment of body image disturbance.* Washington, DC: American Psychological Association.—A contemporary and comprehensive volume detailing theory and research on body image.

Thompson, J. K., & Smolak, L. (Eds.). (2001). *Body image, eating disorders, and obesity in youth: Assessment, prevention, and treatment.* Washington, DC: American Psychological Association.—Current perspectives and research on body image development in childhood and adolescents, particularly related to eating disorders and obesity among females.

2

Physical Attractiveness
A Sociocultural Perspective

LINDA A. JACKSON

All the beauty of the world 'tis but skin deep.
  —RALPH VENNING, *The Triumph of Assurance*

Beauty's only skin deep.

Judge not according to the appearance.
  —JOHN 7:24

Never judge a book by its cover.

Beauty is not judged objectively, but according to the beholder's estimation.
  —THEOCRITUS, *The Idyll*

Beauty is in the eye of the beholder.

THE SOCIOCULTURAL PERSPECTIVE
ON PHYSICAL ATTRACTIVENESS

The sociocultural perspective is an approach to understanding human behavior that focuses on how cultural values influence individual values and behavior. It encompasses a variety of theoretical approaches that share the premise that cultural values are important in understanding how individuals are perceived by others and how they perceive themselves. For example, if the culture values attractiveness in its members, then individuals will value attractiveness in themselves and others. If the culture admonishes against the importance of attractiveness, as the above cultural maxims suggest, then individuals will likewise consider it unimportant in judging themselves and others.

Three theoretical approaches within the sociocultural perspective have been used to conceptualize the role of physical attractiveness in everyday life; each is described briefly, followed by a review of the empirical evidence. The sociocultural perspective and research on body attractiveness is discussed, followed by a consideration of the practical and research implications for understanding body image.

Social Expectancy Theory

Social expectancy theory argues that cultural values influence perceptions of and behavior toward others, which in turn influence the behavior of others, which in turn influences the self-perceptions of others. This sequence of events, from the perceiver's perspective, is commonly known as the "self-fulfilling prophecy" or "interpersonal expectancy effects." For example, if the perceiver believes that the target (of perception) is lazy, then this expectation may lead to assigning fewer tasks to the target. The target, whose behavior has been constrained by the perceiver's expectations (i.e., the target is now performing fewer tasks), may, in time, internalize a self-view as "lazy." Thus the perceiver's expectations become the target's self-perceptions. This outcome, from the target's perspective, is commonly known as "the looking-glass self," which refers to those aspects of the self-concept that are primarily reflections of how others view the target.

Social expectancy theory offers the following hypotheses regarding the effects of physical attractiveness:

1. There is consensual agreement within cultures about who is attractive and who is not (i.e., beauty is not in the idiosyncratic eye of the beholder) but variability among cultures.
2. There are consensual expectations within cultures about attractive and unattractive others (i.e., a physical attractiveness stereotype) but variability among cultures.
3. People behave differently toward attractive and unattractive others (i.e., an expectancy–behavior link).
4. People's differential behavior toward attractive and unattractive others results in differences in how they respond.
5. These behavioral differences result in differences in the self-concepts (e.g., self-esteem, personal characteristics) of attractive and unattractive others.

Research on physical attractiveness has focused primarily on the first two hypotheses of social expectancy theory. Only a handful of studies has examined cultural differences, which constitute the core predictions of the sociocultural perspective. Moreover, although there is a plethora of research on how cultural institutions (e.g., mass media, diet and beauty industries) communicate the value of attractiveness, there is very little research on why attractiveness is valued, or why some faces and body characteristics are considered attractive and others are not. Even the sociocultural perspective is relatively silent on these issues.

Implicit Personality Theory

Implicit personality theory focuses on the knowledge structures that people use to make sense of their social world—that is, to understand and predict the behavior of others. Implicit theories are conceptualized as cognitive structures that consist of personal attributes (e.g., personality traits) and inferential relations that specify the degree to which attributes are related. For example, the attribute "intellectual" might be expected to covary more strongly with the attribute "studious" than with the attribute "nervous."

Implicit personality theory provides a framework for understanding the physical attractiveness stereotype. The category label *physically attractive* is presumed to be linked to a variety of attributes (e.g., social competence), the number and nature of which depend on the culture. Cultural information is transmitted through direct observations of attractive others and by exposure to cultural representations of attractiveness (e.g., via the media). The theory does not address why different cultures associate different attributes with attractiveness.

Status Generalization Theory

Status generalization theory evolved from sociological theories that addressed how external status characteristics influence social interaction and outcomes in informal, task-oriented groups. According to the theory, external status characteristics are used to generate expectation states regarding performance (i.e., "spread of relevance"), with or without prior association between these characteristics and performance (i.e., the "burden of proof" assumption), and with or without conscious awareness.

Status generalization theory views physical attractiveness as a "diffuse" status characteristic because it discriminates among individuals and establishes performance expectancies "without limit"—that is, without regard to the actual relevance of attractiveness to performance. From the status generalization perspective, physical attractiveness should be associated with a wide range of desirable attributes in both perceptions of others and self-perceptions.

Like social expectancy theory and implicit personality theory, status generalization theory predicts that people hold more positive expectations for attractive than unattractive others. All three theories predict that people behave more favorably toward attractive than unattractive others, and that more favorable treatment results in more favorable self-concepts for attractive people.

THE EMPIRICAL EVIDENCE

Recent meta-analytic reviews of the research on physical attractiveness provide some support for the predictions of sociocultural theories as well as revealing weaknesses in this perspective. In terms of the theories' hypotheses, conclusions can be summarized as follows:

First, contrary to the cultural maxim that "beauty is in the eye of the beholder" but consistent with the sociocultural perspective, there is considerable agreement within the U.S. culture about who is attractive and who is not. However, contrary to the sociocultural perspective, there is also considerable cross-cultural agreement, especially regarding facial attractiveness. Thus, either all cultures are communicating the same standards of attractiveness, or standards of attractiveness are determined by some mechanism other than culture such as fitness-related evolutionary mechanisms.

Second, contrary to the cultural maxim to "never judge a book by its cover" but consistent with the sociocultural perspective, attractive people are perceived as possessing a variety of desirable characteristics. Two meta-analytic reviews, spanning almost a decade, have concluded that attractive people are perceived as having greater occupational competence (adults) and academic competence (children), greater interpersonal competence, more social appeal, and better adjustment than their less attractive counterparts. Moreover, the physical attractiveness stereotype is applied equally to strangers and acquaintances, males and females, adults and children, and regardless of culture. Thus support for the sociocultural perspective is mixed. Although culture may be communicating favorable views of attractiveness, as suggested by this perspective, it is not clear why all cultures appear to be communicating identical views (i.e., associating similar attributes with attractiveness), or why the effects of attractiveness are uninfluenced by other category distinctions, such as gender, in any of the cultures studied thus far.

Third, not only do people judge others based on physical appearance, they also behave differently toward them. Attractive people are often treated more favorably than their less attractive counterparts, regardless of level of acquaintance, gender, age, or culture. Specifically, attractive children are treated as more competent, experience fewer negative and more positive interactions, and receive more attention and caregiving than less attractive children. Attractive adults receive more attention, positive interaction, help, and cooperation from others, and are less likely to experience negative interactions than unattractive adults. Again, implications for the sociocultural perspective are mixed. Although expectations do influence behavior, as predicted by this perspective, the universal effects of attractiveness on behavior suggest that universal mechanisms, rather than cultural transmission, are responsible.

Fourth, the traits and behavior of attractive people are "better" in ways consistent with their preferential treatment by others. Attractive children generally behave more positively and possess more positive characteristics than unattractive children. Attractive children are more popular, better adjusted, and evidence somewhat greater intelligence and competent performance than less attractive children, although the number of studies addressing these relationships is small. Attractive adults experience greater occupational success and popularity, and have more dating and sexual experience. They have higher social self-esteem, better social skills, better physical and mental health, and are somewhat more extraverted, self-confident, and intelligent than less attractive adults, regardless of gender. However, the effects of attractiveness are generally small, raising questions about whether the preferential treatment that attractive people experience is internalized (i.e., influences self-concept). Thus, *being* attractive or unattractive may differ from *experiencing* its advantages or disadvantages.

Missing from the research just summarized are studies that establish causal relationships between perceiver expectations, perceiver behavior, target behavior, and target characteristics. In short supply are studies of very young children (under age 6) and older adults, and studies using identical conceptual and operational variables to compare different cultures. Establishing causal links and cultural variability are critical to the sociocultural perspective. This perspective must also address the source of cultural values regarding attractiveness, and why there appears to be cross-cultural agreement in what constitutes physical attractiveness.

THE SOCIOCULTURAL PERSPECTIVE ON BODY ATTRACTIVENESS

The majority of research on physical attractiveness, summarized above, is actually research on facial attractiveness. There are at least three reasons for researchers' apparent neglect of studying "below the neck" body attractiveness. First, much of the early research on attractiveness focused on person perception—that is, on how attractive people are viewed by others. From this perspective, the face is more important than the body because the face is initially a more salient source of information and a more potent and differentiated source of information during social interaction. Second, because facial appearance is more stable than body appearance, both over the lifespan and within developmental stages, it was presumed to have more stable effects on both person perception and self-perception. Third, early research revealed that social ratings of overall attractiveness were largely determined by facial attractiveness. Thus, there appeared to be no compelling reason to include the body in establishing the effects of attractiveness.

In contrast to research on person perceptions, the research on self-perceptions of physical attractiveness has emphasized the body, as evident from the wealth of research discussed in this volume. From the sociocultural perspective, the culture defines what constitutes an attractive body, and self-perceptions of body attractiveness depend on these cultural definitions. The closer body self-perceptions come to the cultural ideal, the higher should be self-ratings of body attractiveness. Thus, body image should depend on cultural ideals and on how an individual perceives his or her own body in relation to these ideals.

Culture and Ideal Body Types

Consistent with the sociocultural perspective, research indicates that body ideals vary among cultures as well as within cultures across groups and time. Contemporary Western cultures idealize thinness for females and an average body type for males. The thin ideal for women replaced the more full-figured one of the 1950s, and may soon be replaced by a "fitness" ideal that began to emerge in the 1990s. Explanations for the thin ideal, elaborated elsewhere in this volume, include a desire to emulate the upper class, where thinness is equated with wealth and leisure; changing roles of women from maternal to more instrumental or masculine venues; a desire to appear youthful (where youthfulness is equated with small stature); and a perceived association between thinness and health, as promoted by the medical community. The potentially negative consequences of the thin ideal, also elaborated elsewhere in this volume, include negative body image, low self-esteem, and psychological and physical disorders of life-threatening proportions.

Variability in body ideals within Western cultures also supports the sociocultural perspective. In the United States, African American, Hispanic, and Native American women, despite having higher average body weights, are more satisfied with their bodies than are Caucasian women. Upper-social-class Caucasian women, particularly adolescents and young adults, are the most dissatisfied with their bodies.

Implications of Body Attractiveness

Research from the sociocultural perspective on the implications of body attractiveness has focused on the negative end of the attractiveness dimension and, to a lesser extent, on the effects of height on perceptions. Supporting this perspective is the negative stereotype of the obese and the negative self-perceptions among the obese, although the former is more firmly established than the latter. Also consistent with the sociocultural perspective is the variability within and among cultures in perceptions of the obese. The obese are perceived less unfavorably (if not favorably) in cultures where food is scarce, and in cultures and among groups within cultures where obesity is attributed to uncontrollable rather than controllable causes (e.g., genetic constitution rather than character weakness). Height stereotypes depend on gender and appear to have little influence on self-perceptions. Short men are perceived less favorably than tall or average height men in terms of social attractiveness and professional competence, but there is little evidence that they perceive themselves less favorably. Short females are perceived as less physically attractive, and tall females are perceived as more professionally competent. Again, there is no evidence that these perceptions by others influence self-perceptions.

Less attention has been given to the implications of overall body attractiveness as perceived by others than to the implications of self-perceived body attractiveness. Although it seems reasonable to assume that possessing the culturally defined ideal body leads to positive perceptions and behavior by others, just as possessing a pretty face does, these benefits have yet to be documented in the research, with one notable exception. Having an attractive body clearly increases dating and mating opportunities for both sexes, but especially for females. Moreover, body characteristics related to fertility and mothering for females, and to strength and dominance for males, increase self- and other-perceived physical and sexual attractiveness.

IMPLICATIONS OF THE SOCIOCULTURAL PERSPECTIVE FOR BODY IMAGE

The basic tenet of the sociocultural perspective is that cultural values influence individual values and behavior. Western cultures value physical attractiveness, and this value unequivocally influences how members of the culture think about and behave toward people who vary in attractiveness. Attractive people are the recipients of all manner of positive behaviors, and they appear to develop positive characteristics as a consequence, although causal links have yet to be established. But before concluding that plastic surgery is the answer to a better life for us all, consider the limitations of the sociocultural perspective and the research to date.

First, the sociocultural perspective is noticeably silent on the question of what constitutes an attractive face. Evolutionary perspectives, discussed by Nancy Etcoff in her 1999 volume, *Survival of the Prettiest: The Science of Beauty*, address this question directly. Findings from this perspective suggest that average faces are perceived as attractive, that facial characteristics associated with youth and good health are perceived as attractive, and that the preference for attractiveness is universal. The "good news" in these findings is that most of us are already attractive (i.e., average), and may enhance our attractiveness by engaging in eating and exercise behaviors that promote good health and a youthful appearance. Moreover, whether a trip to the plastic surgeon is still warranted depends on how much an increment in attractiveness is likely to net, compared to an increment in a more malleable characteristic, such as social skills. Indeed, research indicates that at least some of the benefits of being attractive are actually benefits of being socially skillful.

Second, for all the attention that body appearance has received in the research, we know very little about its importance in everyday life—beyond its role in finding a mate. The sociocultural perspective, which has focused on demonstrating cultural influences on ideal body types, has yet to address whether having a culturally ideal body causes others to behave differently toward us, or causes us to behave differently and to develop different characteristics. Moreover, because body characteristics are less distinctive, salient, and stable than facial characteristics, it may well be that they have less impact on person perception and social interaction than facial characteristics.

Third, the relationship between facial attractiveness and body attractiveness, whether socially perceived or self-perceived, requires additional research. Socially perceived attractiveness is only modestly related to self-perceived attractiveness, be it facial attractiveness or body image, suggesting that others' perceptions, or the "outsiders' view," is quite distinct from our own perceptions, or the "insiders' view."

Finally, to the extent that cultural messages about physical attractiveness are internalized and serve as personal ideals, they may adversely affect self-evaluations of (and satisfaction with) one's own physical appearance. The more discrepant one's self-evaluation is from the cultural ideal, the greater the dissatisfaction with appearance. As discussed elsewhere in the volume, body image dissatisfaction can have devastating effects on psychological and physical health.

INFORMATIVE READINGS

Eagly, A. H., Ashmore, R. D., Makhijani, M. G., & Longo, L. C. (1991). What is beautiful is good, but . . . : A meta-analytic review of research on the physical attractiveness stereotype. *Psychological Bulletin, 110,* 109–128.—A theoretical integration that identifies the relative strengths of components of the attractiveness stereotype and when the stereotype is most likely to influence person perception.

Etcoff, N. (1999). *Survival of the prettiest: The science of beauty.* New York: Anchor Books.—A comprehensive account of the bioevolutionary perspective on physical attractiveness that focuses on how physical characteristics are related to fitness from an evolutionary perspective.

Feingold, A. (1992). Good-looking people are not what we think. *Psychological Bulletin, 111,* 304–341.—A review and theoretical integration of research on the personal characteristics of attractive adults and children.

Halberstadt, J., & Rhodes, G. (2000). The attractiveness of nonaverage faces: Implications for an evolutionary explanation of the attractiveness of average faces. *Psychological Science, 11,* 285–289.—An experiment demonstrating a preference for prototypic exemplars, or typical members, across a variety of categories (e.g., dogs, wrist-watches), suggesting that the preference for average faces may reflect a more general tendency to like the familiar.

Jackson, L. A. (1992). *Physical appearance and gender: Sociobiological and sociocultural perspectives*. Albany: State University of New York.—Hypotheses derived from two theoretical perspectives are evaluated in light of physical appearance research from both self and other perspectives.

Jackson, L. A., Hunter, J. E., & Hodge, C. N. (1995). Physical attractiveness and intellectual competence: A meta-analytic review. *Social Psychology Quarterly, 58*, 108–122.—Examines whether attractive adults and children are actually more intellectually competent than less attractive, same-age others.

Langlois, J. H., Kalakanis, L., Rubenstein, A. J., Larson, A., Hallam, M., & Smoot, M. (2000). Maxims or myths of beauty?: A meta-analytic and theoretical review. *Psychological Bulletin, 126*, 390–423.—Contrasts research findings with common maxims about the importance of attractiveness in everyday life.

Langlois, J. H., & Roggman, L. A. (1990). Attractive faces are only average. *Psychological Science, 1*, 115–121.—Evidence that digitally combining many faces yields an "average" face that is perceived as attractive.

Wade, T. J. (2000). Evolutionary theory and self-perceptions: Sex differences in body esteem predictors of self-perceived physical and sexual attractiveness and self-esteem. *International Journal of Psychology, 35*, 36–45.—Body attributes related to fecundity and mothering for females, and to strength and dominance for males predicted self-ratings of attractiveness and esteem.

Webster, M., & Driskell, J. E. (1983). Beauty as status. *American Journal of Sociology, 89*, 140–165.—Provides evidence that attractiveness confers status in task-oriented groups.

Zebrowitz, L. A., Collins, M. A., & Dutta, R. (1998). The relationship between appearance and personality across the life span. *Personality and Social Psychology Bulletin, 24*, 736–749.—Evidence of modest stability in the relationship between attractiveness and personality.

The Brain and Body Awareness

MARCEL KINSBOURNE

The body image was described by Paul Schilder (1935, p. 11) as "the tridimensional image everyone has about himself": One can visualize one's body in front, side, and even back views, though not all three at the same time. Or one can feel one's body as an integrated percept, without separately experiencing the contributions of touch, position sense, and balance. A body part may fleetingly occupy the foreground of attention during pauses in action. Autonomic arousal in emotion is experienced as sensations attributed to the body. These are all instances in which the body is the object of attention. However, even when attending elsewhere than the body, one experiences one's body as an ill-defined somatosensory background, in which the body's parts are not registered individually. One can even lack a clear perception that a body part is absent. For example, even an amputee or someone who feels nothing below the level of a spinal transection feels that he or she is embodied and whole as a person.

IS BODY IMAGE LOCATED IN A SEPARATE NEURAL MODULE?

What neural activity is responsible for awareness of one's body? Is a specific part of the brain responsible for bringing the body into awareness? Is this module, which specifies what the body parts are, separate from the areas that represent where the largely unconscious postural adjustments occur that maintain the body in balance during action? Is it also separate from the cerebral locations of our assembled knowledge and beliefs about our bodies—the "body archive"? Or does the body image have no privileged localization?

Opposing the modular/localization view, the attentional perspective contends that when coordinated regions of the somatosensory maps (tactile, kinesthetic, and vestibular) distributed in the gray matter are simultaneously activated, they construct the body image. Coordinating the modalities into an articulated pattern might involve the right posterior parietal lobe. There is no need for a particular part of the brain to be specialized for representing the body image. We can selectively attend to sensations derived from different parts of the body at will. The brain has a readily available repository of information about itself, an "outside memory," like a handy reference library, in the body. The brain can sample this database as needed, rather than internalizing all the body information all the time, just in case some part of it becomes relevant. Comparable alternative accounts apply to our visual experience of the world. Do we construct an inner model of our surroundings, or do we use our surroundings as an "outside memory" to be drawn upon at will? The body and the environment are always present, and they contribute a background to the experience of the moment. Details of the body and the environment are picked up from the background, as needed.

The parts of the brain are highly differentiated in their functioning. Modules have been postulated across an enormous range of performance complexity. But to fit a brain module hastily to any activity of interest risks "kicking the problem upstairs"—that is, from behavior to brain. Perhaps the well-known somatosensory maps in the brain suffice to explain how we experience and identify the parts of our body. That is, perhaps no extra or additional module is needed to explain body experience. Neuropsychology can clarify this issue. Focal lesions can dissect a neural mechanism and expose its components. How does the experience of the body fall apart when the brain is damaged?

NEUROPSYCHOLOGY OF THE BODY IMAGE

If there is a localized body image neural module, lesions that disturb our experience of the body should be restricted to a particular part of the brain. Is there a place in the brain which, when totally destroyed, renders us altogether unaware of our bodies? When such a place is partially injured, do either negative or positive part-symptoms result, suggesting that the body image has been depleted or disorganized? Negative symptoms include unawareness and disuse of a body part. Positive symptoms include distorted and obtrusive awareness of that body part, including phantom awareness of an amputated limb.

Asomatagnosia refers to an overall body image impairment that may result in the inability to name one's body parts or indicate them when named, unawareness of body parts as one's own, and unawareness that one is para-

lyzed or numb. However, asomatagnosic patients are never completely unaware of their bodies. After left parietal damage, they typically have trouble
with simple body-related activities, such as naming the body parts, pointing
to them when named, and specifying their spatial interrelationships. Disso-
ciations are also found: Some patients can name the body parts but not find
them; others can find but not name them. Almost always, the problem
extends to the bodies of others as well as mannequins. In general, these patients are unable to link names with body locations: in some cases, the problem is semantic, in others, visuospatial.

If there were a modular body image, and it was partially damaged, partial asomatagnosias should result. All parts of the body image should be
vulnerable, and over time patients whose partial lesions collectively involve
the whole body should come to our attention. A candidate syndrome is unilateral neglect, in which patients with right posterior cerebral lesions may be
blatantly unaware of, ignore, disown, or fail to use their left-sided limbs.
However, there are no reports of patients with corresponding difficulties
with other body parts, such as chest, back, or top of the head. The static
modular model predicts diverse local asomatagnosias; the fact that they do
not exist counts against it. (I call this a "nonexistence proof.") The left unilateral neglect (mentioned above) is not a partial asomatagnosia but an
attentional bias (discussed below)—which directs us toward the alternative
model: the body image as a product of selective somatosensory attention.

Other examples of body distortion that do not appear to be based on
specific modules derive from the study of seizures, which may cause transi-
tory distortions of bodily sensations. Body parts may seem swollen, dis-
placed, or even disconnected. These positive manifestations are modality-
specific: For example, a limb may feel but not look grotesquely swollen.
Although this sensation occurs suddenly, it is not painful, as one would expect of a swollen limb. A limb may be experienced as positional in a physically impossible manner but feel neither awkward nor strained. The seizure
foci that engender these illusions of touch and position do not all arise from
the same brain area; rather, they are located within the primary cortical representation of the sensory modality within which the distortion is experienced. Thus evidence from seizures supports the view that body sensation
does not derive from a uniquely specialized brain area but instead reflects a
pattern of attention that encompasses the various somatic sensory modalities.

Interestingly, distortions in the body image do not assume every imag-
inable form. For example, patients do not report a scrambled body image,
such as might be anticipated were a dedicated module involved. No one has
reported feeling his or her body parts to be misarticulated, such as an arm
arising from the back, or the head confined in the bend of the elbow. Distortions are experienced when parts of the somatosensory cortex are abnor-
mally amplified, giving rise to anomalous sensations. These observations ar-

gue for a ~~theory of body image that does not depend on a specific,~~ localized ~~brain module.~~

BODY AWARENESS

How do people become aware of their previously unconscious, automatically controlled posture, if not by being sent to a specific neural "consciousness module"? The answer is clear: Attention amplifies the previously unconscious somatosensory signals. The contents of consciousness simply reflect the dominant pattern of brain activity. Preconscious somatosensory neural activity emerges into consciousness if any one of three conditions is met: (1) The stimulus provokes a sufficient amplitude of neural firing, and the firing lasts long enough; (2) the pattern of the evoked neural activity fits the existing context; and (3) the stimulus is biologically prepotent (for instance, it signals pain). Once again, there is no need for recourse to a specific body image module to explain body awareness; the concept of attentional redistribution provides a sufficient explanation.

Automatic motor performance is typically fluent. Its stages follow one another closely, and any one stage in the activity may last only a small fraction of a second, such as in postural rearrangements during action. These stages are unrelated to the awareness of body image; rather, they flow rapidly into one another, and no one of them persists long enough to become entrained in consciousness—except the ultimate one, when the action sequence has run its course. Postural rearrangements become conscious under difficult circumstances, as when we are hesitant, have injured one part or another, feel as if we are losing our balance, or deliberately arrest the action to monitor it. I propose that the same facilities that continuously rearrange the disposition of the body give rise to momentary awareness of the body when they are slowed down. Conversely, if we turn our attention to a body part that is engaged in fluent action, we risk arresting its activity. In the brain, attention works by amplifying and prolonging the relevant neural activity, which is then entrained in awareness. This prolongation slows down the succession of stages in the body's movement, causing it to falter. This is why attending to one's own skilled actions brings them into awareness *and* interrupts their fluency and flow.

PHANTOM LIMB

A brain-based theory of body image should account for phantom limb experiences. Most amputees continue to feel their amputated limbs, as though they were still attached, for years. The phantom limb obtrudes into their experience of their bodies and is more apt to attract attention than the real limbs. Moreover, the phantom is not a static or inert appendage. A person might even automatically "reach out" with his nonexistent arm, "extend" it to support himself as he stumbles and falls, or attempt to walk on the nonexistent leg. The phantom phenomenon demonstrates that the sense of owning a limb arises from the limb's representations in the brain, which can continue to be active even when the limb, now amputated, no longer provides feedback. What is this continuing neural activity? It is the "top-down" activation of motor representations that holds the limb in readiness to move. This readiness is a function of *intention*, the motor counterpart of attention. By its very nature, intention is conscious. Intention to move is normally matched against and rapidly cancelled by the feedback of the intended movement occurring. When there is no limb to move, there is no feedback and no cancellation. Because of the mismatch, the neural program for moving remains activated and the limb rises into consciousness.

The phantom limb phenomenon is not easily explained as a modification of a localized body image separate from the limb's sensorimotor control areas. Indeed, it arises from the continued functioning of such areas, under abnormal circumstances, inducing phantom limb as an aberration of attention.

UNILATERAL NEGLECT

The phenomenon of unilateral neglect highlights the role of attention in the experience of body part awareness and ownership. As noted, patients with unilateral neglect ignore, disuse, and disown the left side of their body, particularly the distal hand and forearm. This is as true of left-handed as of right-handed patients. Damage to the right hemisphere results in right neglect much less commonly, and the effect is far less striking and severe. Damage in the posterior right cerebral hemisphere skews somatosensory attention away from the left and toward the right side of the body. The patient cannot attend to the left-sided limb or intend to move it. Even if the limb is not paralyzed, it still does not respond automatically. Nor does it take part in the continual automatic rearrangements that control the ever-changing "body schema" (the term used to describe the constantly changing configurations of brain activity that underlie our perpetual postural adjustments). Precisely the reverse of the absent but experienced phantom limb, the neglected limb fails to attract attention or to move when the person attempts to move it intentionally. It no longer feels part of the person's body. When the experimenter forces the limb into the patient's attention, the patient dismisses it. (One patient used particularly picturesque and derogatory words: "Your limb, the nurse's, a monkey's, a snake, swollen and hideous," he responded, and hastily changed the subject.) Why does this happen?

The inability to attend to the left side of the body confronts the patient with an existential crisis: a flagrant conflict between what he feels and what he knows. He knows he has a left arm but does not feel that the limb he can see is his. His left hemisphere, adept at formulations that resolve conflict and permit ongoing activity to continue, constructs a cover story or confabulation. This narrative momentarily protects the individual from a "meltdown" of his sense of personal integrity, while he eagerly changes the topic and reverts to denying the disability.

If a limb does something that a patient did not intend, she may think it is being directed by an alien influence. In "alien hand" syndrome, the left hand acts independently. It even counteracts and thwarts what the right hand does and what the patient says she intended to do. Split-brain patients sometimes complain that their left-sided limbs are out of control.

The attentional basis of unilateral neglect is consistent with the attentional account of the body image. The body image is fashioned by coordinating the somatic senses with intention and action, at times supplemented by vision. When a person attends to a body part, it comes into focus and the rest of the body provides somatosensory background.

HOW DOES THE BODY IMAGE DEVELOP?

Awareness and experience of the body are the original anchors of our developing sense of self. The mind continues to mature until it can represent and reflect upon its own contents. Ultimately, the self becomes abstracted from the body and is intellectualized as the self-conscious mind. But the felt self and its body background continue to frame whatever is the current focus of attention.

Is body image innate, or is it constructed out of experience and learning? This fascinating question can be approached by examining the relatively rare experience of children who fail to develop one or more limbs (limb aplasia).

Some 15% of children with limb aplasia report phantoms, although they never had the opportunity to experience the absent limb in action. This suggests that body sensations are represented in the brain well before experiences have had a chance to elicit them. The presence of representations that correspond to the limbs before the limbs are experienced through action is classified as an instance of top-down influence. Initially these top-down representations serve no adaptive purpose. Prepared ahead of time, they are components of coordinated activities that will emerge later, such as reaching and grasping.

Children with limb aplasia usually have upper extremity phantoms. In infants there is an innate synergy between hand movement and mouth opening. If one component of the synergism is activated, then the remaining parts play out centrally in the brain, even if the limb that would normally implement the action in the periphery does not exist. It is clear, however, that the environment helps maintain these preprogrammed neural arrangements: Most children with aplasia do not experience phantoms, or at least do not report them when they are old enough to be able to do so. These children must have learned to modify their innate top-down expectation of the hand-to-mouth synergism. This modification again suggests a plastic and modifiable attentional process rather than a "hard-wired" structural component of a modular body image.

We can reconcile the apparent disparity between the view that the body image is innate and the view that it is learned by observing that the newborn child is equipped with a limited number of articulated movement patterns (synergisms). These synergisms become refined over time as the child matures. The mechanism of this refinement seems to be alterations in patterns of attention induced by activity. Experience differentiates additional movement patterns in a dazzling variety of combinations that modulate innate synergism in concert with further maturation of the nervous system. Attention is preparation for action. Concurrent with increasingly refined action, somatosensory attention becomes increasingly selective. Certain types of brain damage can render this attentional capability coarse and inaccurate, as if reverting to a developmentally earlier condition. Neuropsychological impairments of the body image reflect an attentional coarsening (except in the case of unilateral neglect, in which attention is biased).

THE ONTOGENY AND PREDOMINANCE OF SOMATIC SENSATION

This discussion has summarized evidence that body awareness depends on the ability to deploy somatosensory attention "online," not on an already stored repository of information about the body. Body awareness is a dynamic process; it is not a matter of retrieving information from a specialized area or module of the selectively attending brain. It follows that the sense of self as body is not something that is present from birth or that suddenly becomes available during maturation. Rather, it emerges gradually out of the increasing ability to attend selectively to various body parts. Infants may first experience themselves as individuals when they begin to move body parts against a background of undifferentiated body sensation. Looking at visible body parts may come later and appears to be less important in the appreciation of one's own body. Infants move body parts that they cannot see (such as facial features), and blind children have a sense of their bodies. Somatic sensation outranks vision in the phantom limb experience. The patient feels that he owns his phantom limb, even though he can plainly see that the limb does not exist. Similarly, the patient with unilateral neglect disowns her left arm, even though she can see that it is attached to her body—it does not feel like part of her body. The somatic sensations predominate over the visual sensations when the brain represents its body. It is by somatic attention that the body, and perhaps the self, enters awareness.

INFORMATIVE READINGS

Berlucchi, G., & Aglioti, S. (1997). The body in the brain: Neural bases of corporeal awareness. *Trends in Neurosciences, 20,* 560–564.—This article offers a neuroscience approach to body awareness.

Kinsbourne, M. (1994). Orientational bias model of unilateral neglect: Evidence from attentional gradients within hemispace. In I. H. Robertson & J. C. Marshall (Eds.), *Unilateral neglect, clinical and experimental studies* (pp. 63–86). New York: Erlbaum.— Explains the attentional basis of neglect.

Kinsbourne, M. (1995). Awareness of one's own body: An attentional theory of its nature. In J. L. Bermudez, A. Marcel, & N. Amir (Eds.), *The body and the self* (pp. 205–223). Cambridge, MA: MIT Press.—A more extensive treatment of the attentional theory of body awareness.

Melzack, R. (1992). Phantom limbs. *Scientific American, 266,* 90–96.—An accessible account of phantom limb.

Ramachandran, V. S., & Hirstein, W. (1998). The perception of phantom limbs. *Brain, 121,* 1603–1630.—Ingenious experiments that clarify phantom limb.

Schilder, P. (1935). *The image and appearance of the human body.* New York: International Universities Press.—The classic neuropsychological/psychodynamic treatment of body awareness.

Semenza, C. (2001). Disorders of body representation. In R. S. Berndt (Ed.), *Handbook of neuropsychology* (2nd ed., Vol. 3). Amsterdam: Elsevier.—An up-to-date treatise on the neuropsychology of body awareness.

Psychodynamic Perspectives on Body Image

DAVID W. KRUEGER

The body and its evolving mental representations form the foundation of a sense of self. While Freud recognized the ego as, first and foremost, a body ego, the more inclusive term "body self" refers to a combination of the psychic experience of body sensation, body functioning, and body image. Thus body image is the dynamically and developmentally evolving mental representation of the body self.

The body appears in the narratives of dreams, metaphors, and symptoms as a symbolic vision of inner landscapes, mysterious structures and configurations, and geographical terrain. An idea as well as a fact, the body is container and conduit of emotional experience, and the body image a Rorschach onto which fantasies, meaning, and significance are projected. The body self and image are ideas, like that of the ego; the body is a fact. The body self and its image are created by, and live within, the imagination, the map within the actual territory of the body. We experience life through the body and focus with it but not usually on it, for the body is usually in the background. People who are unattuned to their affective world may not have a way of understanding some of the affective states they experience; they may lack a representation of body self and psychological self that would allow them to integrate these emotions. Such individuals make their bodies the narrator of what words cannot say: of sensation for which there is no lexicon, of feelings they cannot tolerate in their conscious awareness, and of action language (i.e., speaking of action rather than feelings) rather than verbalization. When the body cannot be naturally integrated into psychological experience, it remains in the foreground, accentuated by asceticism and alienation (such as fasting or self-mutilation), or by becoming the instrument of action symptoms (such as the addictive use of activities or substances) or the subject of narcissistic investment and excessive rumination (such as body dysmorphic disorder), or brought into focus by pain, physical illness, age, or weight.

DEVELOPMENTAL ORIGINS OF THE BODY SELF AND IMAGE

The body self emerges through a developmental hierarchy of experience and intellectual mechanisms progressing from images to words to organizing patterns to superordinate abstractions and inferences that regulate the entire self-experience. The body image is the cumulative set of images, fantasies, and meanings about the body and its parts and functions; it is an integral component of self-image and the basis of self-representation. In the last two decades, neurophysiological research has produced salient data on the development of the body image and the differentiation of the mental self as a bridge between mind and body.

The close and careful attunement by the caretaker to all the sensory and motor contacts with the child forms the child's accurate and attuned body self as container and foundation for the evolving psychological self. The caregiver's sensory–motor interaction with the infant's body, providing physical and psychological soothing for all the sensations and secure holding, occurs before there are words or language. It is the accuracy and continuity of caregiver's empathic resonance with the child's body self that forms the foundation of the psychological self: the sense that we reside inside our bodies, that there is a unity of mind and body with evolving cohesion of body self and image, that the psychological self evolves with the use of symbols and language to communicate internal experiences. Dramatic developments in infant research, newer understandings of early development, and expanding awareness of neurobiological and intersubjective experience all inform this appreciation of the developmental building block of body image and body self.

The capacity to recognize and reflect on how our own mind is unique from others develops by ages 6–8. Developing this capacity to reflect on our own experience and behavior, as well as to conceive of others' feelings, intents, desires, knowledge, beliefs, and thinking, leads to an integration of the body self. This integration contributes significantly to affect and tension regulation, impulse control, self-monitoring, and the emergence of a sense of self-agency. The activation of this self-reflective function is dependent on the parents' mirroring of their child's mental states and independent thinking throughout the attachment process.

STAGES IN THE DEVELOPMENT OF THE BODY SELF

The development of a body self can be conceptualized as occurring in a series of three stages: the early psychic experience of the body; the early awareness of a body image that integrates inner and outer experience and forms body surface boundaries and internal state definition; and the integration of the body self as a container of the psychological self, which forms a cohesive sense of identity and continuity.

Stage 1. Early Psychic Experience of the Body

The earliest sense of self is experienced through sensations from within the body, especially via proprioception. These sensoriperceptive stimuli, particularly tactile sensations, enable infants to discriminate their bodies from the surroundings. Auditory and visual stimuli also play an important role as early development proceeds. The caretakers' hands outline and define the original boundary of the body's surface, and the caretakers' empathic resonance with the infant's internal experience provides a mirroring and reciprocity that not only reinforces and affirms but forms the infant's sense of boundary. The infant's internal state is also given form and definition by the accuracy of this empathic attunement.

   The impact of the absence of this empathic attunement by primary caretakers and its resulting experience of competence can be seen in adult patients who remain dependent on external referents, persistently searching for mirroring responses and tangible representations of the deficient internal affirmation. It is precisely when this development does not occur, or gets derailed, that psychosomatic symptoms or other forms of body stimulation or self-harm are created to bridge between mind and body, and to regulate affect and tension. In healthy development children locate themselves in their mother's eyes, movements, gestures, touches, words, expressions. Children who experience unhealthy development, in contrast, may not be able to find themselves in the vacant dissociative stare, the foggy mirror of preoccupation or disinterest, or the frightening window of anxiety. Such children may lose all sense of themselves as they strive to evoke response from an inattentive, nonresponsive, or rigid parent who offers neither hugs nor words.

Stage 2. Defining Body Surface Boundaries and Distinguishing the Body's Internal States

This stage of development begins at a few months and extends into the second year of life. It is characterized by the child's growing sense of reality that emerges as newly discovered body *boundaries* and *internal states* form an integrated sense of body self. Outer boundaries of the body become more specific and delimited, and inner and outer are differentiated.

Empathic parental mirroring and reciprocal interactions, with the child's experience as point of reference, shape both internal and body surface (skin) sensations into distinct and coherent functions of the child's evolving self and body image. The boundaries of the body provide a limiting membrane between what is "me" and what is "not me." The child's internal experience becomes unified, no longer a collection of parts, as criteria are learned for identifying the limits of the body self (where one's body ends and the rest of the world begins) and corresponding development and differentiation of psychic representation and functioning (psychological self) solidifying the cohesion of body self-development.

Stage 3. The Definition and Cohesion of the Body Self as a Foundation for Self-Awareness

Observational studies of infants describe a new level of organized self-awareness beginning at about 15–18 months, when the child discovers him- or herself in the mirror and begins to say "no." This inaugurates the process whereby the infant experiences his or her differentiation: "I am not an extension of you and your body or your desire; this is where you end and I begin—my body is mine and mine alone."

In normal development the experiences and images of the inner body and the body surface are organized and integrated into an experiential and conceptual whole. Consolidating a stable, cohesive mental representation of one's body is a key developmental task during this period, accompanied by a developing sense of distinctness and effectiveness. The body self-experience—body images and self-concept—cohere to form the sense of self overall, which is a prerequisite to an internalized sense of psychological self. This synthesis of body and psychological selves provides the experience of internal unity and continuity over time, space, and state.

Body image is inaccurately assumed to be something that one either has or does not have, as if it were a fixed representation that is either accurate or distorted. With the beginning of concrete operations at approximately 6 years of age, a definite sense of separation between self and object and a more distinct and accurate body image become possible as abstract ability crystallizes. The body image must develop accurately as the physical body matures, in relationship to its physical surroundings, and must be integrated with the development of the psychological self.

The body self seems to consist of a group of images that is dynamically and preconsciously centered on body experiences. A body image is a conceptual composite of all sensory modalities; the individual's sense of cohesion is also a conceptualization, because the entire body cannot be simultaneously retrieved from memory. In addition to the mental representations, later developmental influences include the reactions of others to one's appearance. Usually preconscious and uncritically internalized, a body image is not as static as the term *image* might imply. One's body self and body image are developmental processes that undergo gradual maturational change around a cohesive core, analogous to an intact psychological self. It is only when pathology is introduced in this process that change becomes abrupt, symptomatic, and prominent.

DEVELOPMENTAL DISRUPTIONS OF BODY SELF AND IMAGE

When developmentally disrupted individuals experiences regressed states such as narcissistic rage or depression, their body images and self-states oscillate. In such patients body image and emotional states appear to mirror one another; that is, during a time of emotional turmoil, their body image becomes more distorted, vague, or regressed. Over the course of successful therapy, the patient will undergo a process of body image maturation, involving increased cohesion and distinctness, which parallels developmental maturation.

Certain developmental disruptions in body self-formation, which manifest as psychopathology, may be linked to attempts to restore normal development. Early developmental arrests in the process of establishing a stable, integrated, cohesive body image seem to result from maladaptive interactions with primary caretakers. These pathological sequences cluster into three groups, with associated body self/image pathology and consistent symptomatic configurations. Although not mutually exclusive, the types of psychopathogenic interactions can be described in terms of the predominance of interactive patterns manifesting as (1) overintrusiveness and overstimulation, (2) empathic unavailability, and (3) inconsistency or selectivity of response.

Overintrusiveness and Overstimulation

Overly intrusive parents may attempt to remain psychologically merged with their children from infancy onward, impeding their pleasure of mastery and disrupting their individuation. Parents' behavior toward children is characteristically controlling, protective, and enmeshing, with predominant demands for conformity. When this pattern is extreme enough to produce developmental arrest, the body self and image are frequently experienced as indistinct, small, prepubescent, asexual, undifferentiated, and intermingled with a parental image. Anorexia nervosa illustrates this developmental disruption. People with anorexia experience their bodies as separate from themselves and easily invaded, so that they carefully guard their body integrity. They may attempt to establish their body self/image distinctness in rudimentary ways, such as exercising to feel physical sensation, refusing to eat, compulsive weightlifting to establish a firm body outline, or various sexual perversions, such as exhibitionism, that force recognition and response.

If development of a complete and distinct body self and image is arrested, a later compensatory attempt to supply this experience may employ intense sensory stimulation to provide perceptions of the body, such as the inordinate exercise often adopted by anorexic individuals, induction of physical pain, intense physical stimulation, such as cutting or bingeing, or extreme physical risk taking. At times of emotional stress, these individuals regress to body self-stimulation and body self-harm as an attempt to regulate affect, reduce tension, and reclaim control over their body. Stimulation and reintegration of the basic body self are the most primitive adaptive attempts at psychic reorganization.

Empathic Unavailability and Nonresponsiveness

The parent may be unable to resonate accurately and consistently with the infant's internal experiences or respond to the subtleties of emotional and physical experiences, movements, and affects. The child's experience does not become a point of self-reference. When body boundaries are not consistently or accurately defined by caress, touch, and secure holding, the infant cannot develop a reliable body boundary or sensory awareness. Later, the child's development and awareness of body self are incomplete, and the body image is distorted. These individuals' projective drawings reflect body images that are distorted, excessively large, without shape, and with blurred boundaries. These findings are most notable in individuals diagnosed as bulimic, borderline, or chronically depressed. Their body images often fluctuate with their mood and self-image, perhaps several times a day; the body image becomes several times larger when they are experiencing a depleted self-image.

Many behaviors regarded as impulsive or addictive are designed to evoke or establish boundaries that create rudimentary body experience and image. Active attempts to define the body surface involve stimulation of skin, the psychic envelope, to inscribe and outline a body boundary; wearing large, loose clothes to feel the brushing sensation, compulsive sexuality, weightlifting, and mutilation of the skin via cutting, burning, biting, wounding, or etching. Stimulation of internal body awareness may be achieved by bingeing, starving, vomiting, using laxatives or diuretics, and the sensations associated with extreme amounts of exercise.

Inconsistency or Selectivity of Response

Parental response to selective stimuli from the infant creates a selective reality. For example, the mother may ignore affective and kinesthetic stimuli, responding only to physical needs or physical pain. This response pattern

teaches the infant to perceive and organize experiences around pain and illness in order to obtain attention and affection. In this scenario effectiveness
is associated with the body self; affect regulation never gets desomatized.
The pattern of experiencing the body self and psychological self through
pain and discomfort becomes entrenched in the child's personality and characteristic modes of interaction, with a resulting predisposition toward psychosomatic expressions.

These three types of pathological sequences/interactions seem to result
in specific developmental arrests that impact the sense of self, at a basic
body self level, through the absence of a coherent, accurate, cohesive, organized body image. Individuals who undergo these developmental arrests
have a poor or absent sense of their body boundaries. Lacking internal evocative images of a body self/image or a cohesive, positive psychological self,
they rely on external feedback and referents, such as the reactions of others
to their appearance and actions or to mirrors. There is a distinct lack of object and image constancy, with the arrest in body self-development parallel-
ing the arrest in development of the psychological self.

The failure to achieve autonomy and separation stems from an early
nucleus of compromise when the nascent sense of self emerges from mirroring experiences with the mother in the first weeks and months of life. The
preverbal interactions in the first year of life have failed to acknowledge and
confirm a distinct and accurate body self. The more severely narcissistic individual may not have a consolidated body image or internal ideal to either
deny or achieve.

Disturbances in differentiating self and other affect the ability to consol-
idate a symbolic representation of one's self and body images, promoting a
particular kind of developmental arrest characterized by self-referential
thinking that is concrete, without the capacity for abstraction or representation of the body and its contents, including affect differentiation. Though
perhaps quite articulate and accomplished, these individuals may feel lost
when focusing internally, lacking a language for feelings.

Without a consistent, cohesive body self and psychological self representation, they may attempt to elicit a sense of self-representation and regulate affect via the felt experiences of their body. Their representation of self
must emerge from the body self-experience rather than through a symbolic
representation of the self.

These patients are not primarily denying body awareness and feelings,
for they never attained the desomatization and differentiation of affect and
bodily sensation; they have not as yet integrated mind and body enough to
split them defensively. When an emotional insult occurs, their organizing
function directs focus to the first and most basic organizer of ego experience
and structure: the body self.

INFORMATIVE READINGS

Krueger, D. (1989). *Body self and psychological self: Developmental and clinical integration in disorders of the self*. New York: Brunner/Mazel.—A description of the developmental origins of body self as the foundation of psychological self, the related psychopathologies, and clinical treatment.

Lichtenberg, J. (1989). *Motivation and psychoanalysis*. Hillsdale, NJ: Analytic Press.—From infant research, Lichtenberg describes fundamental building blocks of motivations and their development over time.

Mahler, M., Furer, M., & Pine, F. (1968). *On human symbiosis and the vicissitudes of individuation*. New York: International Universities Press.—The groundbreaking summary of direct infant observation regarding separation–individuation.

Main, M. (1995). Attachment: Overview, with implications for clinical work. In S. Goldberg, R. Mair, & J. Kerr (Eds.), *Attachment theory: Social, developmental, and clinical perspectives* (pp. 407–474). Hillsdale, NJ: Analytic Press.—This chapter and the book as a whole provide a theoretical and clinical overview of attachment theory.

McDougall, J. (1989). *Theatres of the body: A psychoanalytic approach to psychosomatic illness*. New York: Norton.—An eloquent treatise of mind–body interaction and psychosomatic illness as an attempted bridge in disrupted mind–body development.

Meissner, W. (1997a). The self and the body: I. The body self and the body image. *Psychoanalysis and Contemporary Thought, 20*, 419–448.—A very informative psychoanalytic perspective on body self and body image with clinical applications.

Meissner, W. (1997b). The self and the body: II. The embodied self—self versus non-self. *Psychoanalysis and Contemporary Thought, 21*, 85–111.—A very informative psychoanalytic perspective on body self and body image with clinical applications.

Meissner, W. (1998a). The self and the body: III. The body image in clinical perspective. *Psychoanalysis and Contemporary Thought, 21*, 113–146.—A very informative psychoanalytic perspective on body self and body image with clinical applications.

Meissner, W. (1998b). The self and the body: IV. The body on the couch. *Psychoanalysis and Contemporary Thought, 21*, 277–300.—A very informative psychoanalytic perspective on body self and body image with clinical applications.

Stern, D. (1985). *The interpersonal world of the infant*. New York: Basic Books.—An eminent child researcher describes unfolding development in the child from an intrapsychic point of view; attunement to the child's affect states creates accurate internal readings of self states and mental representations of the body.

Cognitive-Behavioral Perspectives on Body Image

THOMAS F. CASH

Most contemporary research on body image derives directly or implicitly from cognitive and/or behavioral paradigms in psychology. An integrative cognitive-behavioral viewpoint reflects no single theory but rather draws upon an enduring tradition of ideas and empirical evidence that emphasizes social learning processes and cognitive mediation of behaviors and emotions. This chapter summarizes key concepts, principles, and processes inherent in cognitive and behavioral conceptions of body image.

To articulate basic elements of a cognitive-behavioral model, it is first necessary to distinguish historical from proximal or concurrent factors that shape body image development. Historical factors refer to past events, attributes, and experiences that predispose or influence how people come to think, feel, and act in relation to their body. Salient among these factors are cultural socialization, interpersonal experiences, physical characteristics, and personality attributes. Through various types of social learning, historical factors instill fundamental body image schemas and attitudes, including dispositional body image evaluations and degrees of body image investment. *Body image evaluation* refers to satisfaction or dissatisfaction with one's body, including evaluative beliefs about it. *Body image investment* refers to the cognitive, behavioral, and emotional importance of the body for self-evaluation. In this model, proximal body image factors pertain to current life events and consist of precipitating and maintaining influences on body image experiences, including internal dialogues, body image emotions, and self-regulatory actions.

Figure 5.1 illustrates this distinction and the concepts and processes discussed in this chapter. However, this figure must be viewed with three important caveats in mind. First, it is a heuristic conceptual model, offered to

Historical, Developmental Influences

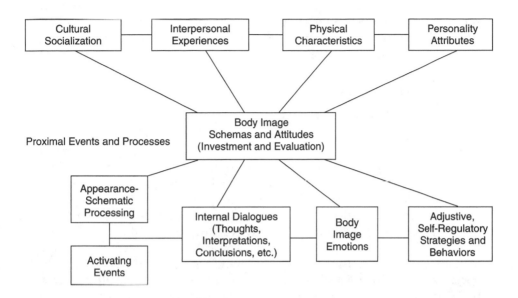

FIGURE 5.1. A cognitive-behavioral model of body image development and experiences.

help organize our thinking about body image and its multidimensionality. Second, the distinction between historical and proximal events is intended to differentiate prior cognitive social learning from more immediate body image experiences and reactions. However, just as today inevitably becomes yesterday, proximal body image events may be stored and contribute to one's cumulative body image history. Third, Figure 5.1 is intentionally presented without directional arrows because the causality is believed to be complex and reflect what social-cognitive theorist Albert Bandura and others term "triadic reciprocal causation." Within individuals there exists a reciprocally interactive causal loop connecting external (environmental) events, internal personal factors (cognitive, affective, and physical processes), and the individual's own behaviors. Therefore, while Figure 5.1 helpfully organizes the salient body image variables, it cannot possibly represent the complexity of interactions among them.

HISTORICAL AND DEVELOPMENTAL INFLUENCES

Historical factors largely pertain to socialization about the meaning of physical appearance and one's body-focused experiences during childhood and adolescence. However, people are not simply passive recipients of socialization. Formative body image experiences unfold as person–environment transactions and occur in the contexts of individuals' cognitive, social, emotional, and physical development. (See the book's detailed chapters on body image development in Part II.)

Cultural Socialization

As Jackson and other contributors to this volume affirm, cultural messages convey standards or expectations about appearance: which physical characteristics are and are not socially valued, and what it means to possess or lack these characteristics. Tiggemann concludes in her chapter that the media create and communicate these values in highly influential ways. Cultural messages not only articulate normative notions about attractiveness and unattractiveness but also express gender-based expectations that tie "femininity" and "masculinity" to certain physical attributes. Culture further prescribes the myriad body-altering means of attaining societal expectations (e.g., by dieting, exercising, using beauty and fashion products, etc.). As internalized by individuals, these cultural values foster the acquisition of basic body image attitudes, which predispose them to construe and react to life events in particular ways.

Interpersonal Experiences

Socialization about the meaning of one's body involves more than cultural and media-based messages. Expectations, opinions, and verbal and nonverbal communications are conveyed in interactions with family members, friends and other peers, and even strangers. Parental role modeling, comments, and criticism express the degree to which physical appearance is valued within the family, potentially establishing a standard against which a child compares him- or herself (see Kearney-Cooke's chapter on familial influences). Moreover, siblings can provide a social comparison standard for the appraisal of a child's looks. Siblings, especially brothers, are also frequent perpetrators of appearance-related teasing or criticism, and peer teasing regarding physical appearance is a common childhood and adolescent experience. In their chapter, Tantleff-Dunn and Gokee contend that interpersonal teasing and criticism predispose the recipient to body dissatisfaction. In this volume, Cash and Fleming further elucidate the reciprocal influences that flow between body image and social relations.

Physical Characteristics

Body image development is certainly affected by one's actual physical characteristics. As Jackson and a vast scientific literature attest, the attractiveness and social acceptability of a person's physical appearance impact how the person is perceived and treated by others. In 1990 Lerner and Jovanovic presented a "goodness-of-fit model" that proposed that how well one's appearance matches social standards of physical attractiveness may be pivotal in one's self-evaluations. In part, this process may be mediated by social feedback (e.g., overweight kids receive more social teasing and rejection). However, body image evaluations may also stem from self-appraisals in relation to internalized standards that the individual does not match. For example, as Schwartz and Brownell discuss in their chapter in Part IV, juvenile obesity often has an adverse and potentially lasting impact on body image.

Obvious but underappreciated is the ephemeral nature of the human body; from birth to death our bodies constantly change. Changes in physical competence and appearance are especially dramatic during youth. For example, pubertal maturation in adolescence, a period marked by rapid physical change, can affect body image development. (See chapters in this volume by Levine and Smolak and by Striegel-Moore and Franko.) Weight is not the sole physical factor affecting body image formation, however. As other contributors to this volume attest, countless characteristics can alter one's goodness-of-fit with personal and social expectations—deviations in stature and muscularity, conditions such as adolescent acne, and acquired disfigurements, to name a few. Adulthood may bring physical changes to the skin's elasticity or hair density, as Whitbourne and Skultety describe in their chapter. Simply stated, the body is a moving target. For better or worse, embodiment entails an ongoing process of adaptation to physical changes.

Personality Factors

Individual personality attributes also influence the formation of body image attitudes. Self-esteem may be the most pivotal of these factors. A positive self-concept may facilitate development of a positive evaluation of one's body and serve as a buffer against events that threaten one's body image. Conversely, poor self-esteem may heighten one's body image vulnerability. Perfectionism is another potentially influential personality trait that may lead the individual to invest self-worth in lofty or exacting physical ideals. Public self-consciousness—a disposition of attentional focus onto one's appearance and behaviors—increases self-monitoring and processing of appearance-related information. Furthermore, a need for social approval may increase one's investment in socially valued appearance standards. Similarly, as Cash and Fleming discuss in a chapter in Part V, an insecure attachment system, whereby individuals seek love and acceptance yet feel unworthy, may foster faulty body image attitudes. On the other hand, secure attachment may promote a more favorable body image. A final example of personality factors pertains to certain gender-based attitudes and values. My own research suggests that females who endorse traditional gender attitudes in their relationships with males (1) are more invested in their appearance, (2) have internalized cultural standards of beauty more fully, and (3) hold more maladaptive assumptions about their looks.

BODY IMAGE ATTITUDES AND SCHEMAS

Having examined the historical, developmental variables that predispose one to the acquisition of certain body image attitudes, let's consider how they operate in everyday life. As Figure 5.1 shows, these attitudes function as central organizing constructs in the interplay of cognitive, emotional, and behavioral processes in the context of environmental events. As mentioned previously, two basic attitudinal elements are body image investment and evaluation. *Investment* refers to the cognitive-behavioral importance persons place on their appearance. *Evaluation* refers to the positive-to-negative appraisals of and beliefs about one's appearance (e.g., body satisfaction-dissatisfaction). As Cash and Szymanski showed in 1995, body image evaluations stem from the degree of discrepancy or congruence between self-perceived physical characteristics and personally valued appearance ideals.

A higher-order attitudinal body image construct is that of self-schemas related to one's appearance. In 1977, Markus defined self-schemas as "cognitive generalizations about the self, derived from past experience, that organize and guide the processing of self-related information contained in an individual's social experience" (p. 64). A person who is schematic for a self-dimension (in our context, one's body and appearance) will process information pertinent to that dimension differently from someone who is not schematic. Moreover, as cognitive theorist Aaron Beck has articulated, implicit attitudes, assumptions, beliefs, and rules comprise schematic content and influence the substance of thought, emotion, and behavior. Body image schemas reflect one's core, affect-laden assumptions or beliefs about the importance and influence of one's appearance in life, including the centrality of appearance to one's sense of self. The Appearance Schemas Inventory, which I developed with Labarge, assesses this construct with such items as: "What I look like is an important part of who I am"; "My appearance is responsible for much of what's happened to me in my life"; and "I should do whatever I can to always look my best." I discuss these self-schemas further in my 1997 therapeutic program, *The Body Image Workbook*.

PROXIMAL EVENTS AND PROCESSES

Activating Events and Cognitive Processing

According to cognitive-behavioral perspectives, specific situational cues or contextual events activate schema-driven processing of information about, and self-evaluations of, one's physical appearance. Thus appearance schematic people place more importance on, pay more attention to, and preferentially process information relevant to appearance. (See Williamson and colleagues' enlightening chapter on body image and cognitive processing.) Precipitating events may entail, for example, body exposure, mirror exposure, social scrutiny, social feedback or comparisons, wearing certain clothing, weighing, exercising, mood states, or changes in appearance.

The resultant internal dialogues (which I have termed "private body talk") involve emotion-laden automatic thoughts, inferences, interpretations, and conclusions about one's looks. Among individuals with problematic body image attitudes and schemas, these inner dialogues are habitual, faulty, and dysphoric. Thought processes may reflect various errors or distortions, such as dichotomous thinking, emotional reasoning, biased social comparisons, arbitrary inferences, overgeneralizations, overpersonalization, magnification of perceived defects, and minimization of assets. (Again, see *The Body Image Workbook* for additional discussion of cognitive distortions.)

Adjustive, Self-Regulatory Processes

To manage or cope with distressing body image thoughts and emotions, whether anticipated or actual, individuals engage in a range of actions and reactions that may involve well-learned cognitive strategies or behaviors to accommodate or adjust to environmental events. Adjustive reactions include avoidant and body concealment behaviors, appearance correcting rituals, seeking social reassurance, and compensatory strategies. These maneuvers serve to maintain body image attitudes via negative reinforcement, as they enable the individual temporarily to escape, reduce, or regulate body image discomfort. Moreover, individuals engage in proactive self-regulatory behaviors to control evaluative body image and other self-reinforcing consequences.

Despite a vast and growing literature on coping processes, surprisingly little research has examined coping specifically in relation to body image. In an initial exploratory investigation, my students and I developed a 39-item self-report measure, the Body Image Coping Strategies Inventory. We asked 369 college women and men how they characteristically managed or coped with situations that challenged or threatened their body image experiences. Factor analysis identified three internally consistent coping subscales:

1. Avoidance—attempts to avoid the threat to one's thoughts and feelings about body image.
2. Appearance Fixing—attempts to change one's appearance by concealing, camouflaging, or "fixing" a physical characteristic perceived as disturbing.
3. Positive Rational Acceptance—actions or strategies that focus on positive self-care or rational self-talk and acceptance.

Dysfunctional body image schemas were significantly associated with the use of the first two types of coping but not with the use of rational coping. Furthermore, compared to rational coping, the other two coping patterns were more strongly associated with higher levels of body image discontentment and dysphoria across a range of situations for both sexes. One interpretation of our preliminary findings emphasizes the dynamic interplay (i.e., vicious cycle) of dysfunctional body image schemas and faulty coping strategies that merely reinforce negative self-evaluations and perpetuate body image distress.

People engage in a variety of purposeful actions to manage their appearance and produce reinforcing self-evaluations. One class of self-regulating body image behaviors that has seldom been studied is appearance self-management. Appearance self-management is negatively motivated only in cases where concealment or correction of "offending" physical characteristics and avoidance of self-conscious thoughts and emotions are the goals. For many individuals, everyday grooming behaviors provide favorable and reinforcing affective, cognitive, and interpersonal consequences. Appearance self-management (with clothing, cosmetics, hairstyling, jewelry, body art, etc.), whereby people experience pleasure and pride in their physical appearance, is ubiquitous across cultures. Human appearance is not entirely biogenetically assigned; it is also continually created by the individual.

CONCLUSIONS AND DIRECTIONS

Applications to Prevention and Treatment

Cognitive-behavioral perspectives have demonstrated great utility in our scientifically productive understanding of body image. Most chapters in this book delineate ideas and evidence emanating from this paradigm. This fact attests not only to the validity of its principles and concepts but also to the scientific value system inherent in a cognitive-behavioral viewpoint. Several chapters discuss the utility of its application to prevent and ameliorate human suffering. Winzelberg and colleagues describe how cognitive-behavioral perspectives can be used in psychoeducational programs to prevent body image problems. Levine and Smolak critically examine the use of these principles in ecological and activism approaches in preventing body image difficulties. Cash and Strachan offer an overview of cognitive-behavioral body image therapy and review evidence of its efficacy in various formats.

Cognitive-Behavioral Perspectives and Positive Psychology

The study of body image has always been a pathology-focused endeavor—from historical attempts to understand the aberrant experiences of patients with brain injury or phantom limbs to the more recent boom in the investigation of eating disorders. Researchers, myself included, typically describe findings in terms that refer to negative body image rather than in equally accurate terms reflecting body acceptance or satisfaction. Of course, this "glass half empty" bias is not unique to body image research. As Martin Seligman and other proponents of the current positive psychology movement argue, this bias permeates psychology and other behavioral sciences.

Cognitive-behavioral perspectives are not intrinsically oriented toward pathology. This framework can be applied just as readily to understand the development and experience of a positive relationship between individuals and their bodies. My hope is that we will do so, thereby enhancing our knowledge of the trajectories whereby people create fulfilling experiences of embodiment. Currently, Emily Fleming and I are conducting a large-scale study to identify the historical-developmental and personality characteristics of young women who have a "positive body image."

INFORMATIVE READINGS

Bandura, A. (1977). *Social learning theory.* Englewood Cliffs, NJ: Prentice Hall.—Discusses the informative foundations of Bandura's cognitive social learning perspective.

Bandura, A. (1986). *Social foundations of thought and action: A social cognitive theory.* Englewood Cliffs, NJ: Prentice Hall.—Explicates contemporary principles and processes in the author's theory.

Cash, T. F. (1997). *The body image workbook: An 8–step program for learning to like your looks.* Oakland, CA: New Harbinger.—The author's most recent version of his body image improvement program, which delineates and applies elements of a cognitive-behavioral model.

Cash, T. F. (2002). Women's body images. In G. Wingood & R. DiClemente (Eds.), *Handbook of women's sexual and reproductive health* (pp. 175–194). New York: Plenum Press.—Summarizes ideas and research evidence relevant to the current cognitive-behavioral model.

Cash, T. F., & Labarge, A. S. (1996). Development of the Appearance Schemas Inventory: A new cognitive body-image assessment. *CognitiveTherapy and Research, 20,* 37–50.—Describes the development and validation of an assessment of dysfunctional body image schemas (available at *www.body-images.com*).

Cash, T. F., & Szymanski, M. L. (1995). The development and validation of the Body-Image Ideals Questionnaire. *Journal of Personality Assessment, 64,* 466–477.—Discusses and assesses evaluative body image in relation to self-ideal discrepancies (available at *www.body-images.com*).

Dobson, K. S. (Ed.). (2001). *Handbook of cognitive-behavioral therapies* (2nd ed.). New York: Guilford Press.—A comprehensive volume that describes the historical, theoretical, and empirical foundations of a cognitive-behavioral paradigm, as well as its clinically rich applications.

Follette, W. C., & Hayes, S. C. (2000). Contemporary behavior therapy. In C. R. Snyder & R. E. Ingram (Eds.), *Handbook of psychological change* (pp. 381–408). New York: Wiley.—Discusses the foundations and advances in behavioral perspectives in a compelling and future-looking volume on psychological change and psychotherapy.

Lerner, R. M., & Jovanovic, J. (1990). The role of body image in psychosocial development across the life span: A developmental contextual perspective. In T. F. Cash & T. Pruzinsky (Eds.), *Body images: Development, deviance, and change* (pp. 110–127). New York: Guilford Press.—Discusses an interesting "goodness-of-fit" model of the developmental roles of bodily attributes and body images in cultural contexts.

Markus, H. (1977). Self-schemata and processing information about the self. *Journal of Personality and Social Psychology, 35*, 63–78.—Offers an excellent foundation for understanding the nature and operation of self-schemas.

Seligman, M. E. P., & Csikszentmihalyi, M. (Eds.) (2000). Positive psychology [Special issue]. *American Psychologist, 55*(1).—A thought-provoking series of articles on positive psychology, pertinent to points made in the present chapter.

Thompson, J. K., Heinberg, L. J., Altabe, M., & Tantleff-Dunn, S. (1999). *Exacting beauty: Theory, assessment, and treatment of body image disturbance.* Washington, DC: American Psychological Association.—Extensively covers underpinnings, evidence, and applications of cognitive-behavioral perspectives on body image.

6

An Information-Processing Perspective on Body Image

DONALD A. WILLIAMSON
TIFFANY M. STEWART
MARNEY A. WHITE
EMILY YORK-CROWE

Over the past decade, several authors have described a cognitive information-processing model for body image in relation to eating disorders. Figure 6.1 illustrates a model that integrates our perspectives with those of Thompson and Vitousek. In this model, body image (as it is usually assessed) is one type of cognitive bias that stems from a self-schema that includes memory stores related to body size/shape and eating that are easily activated and readily accessible for retrieval from memory. This self-schema is presumed to draw the person's attention to body and food-related stimuli and to bias interpretations of self-relevant events in favor of fatness interpretations. This model postulates that disturbed body images are one type of cognitive bias that is most similar to selective interpretational biases: Individuals come to a conclusion based upon the "evidence," but the conclusion is one that is not shared by most people. The model assumes that cognitive biases occur without conscious awareness and that the person experiences the cognition as "real."

As shown in Figure 6.1, the model hypothesizes that certain types of stimuli are more likely to determine cognitive bias in "susceptible people": (1) body- or food-related information, (2) ambiguous stimuli, and (3) tasks that require self-reflection. Most body size estimation tasks, questionnaires, and naturally occurring situations that trigger "body image reactions" have

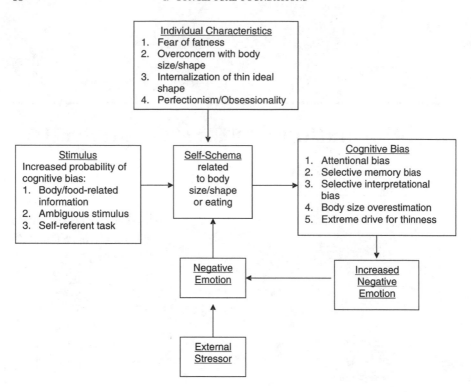

FIGURE 6.1. Cognitive model of body image as it applies to eating disorders.

these stimulus characteristics. Stimuli with these characteristics are hypothesized to activate the self-schema related to body size/shape and eating. People who are most susceptible to cognitive biases related to body image are hypothesized to have the following characteristics: (1) fear of fatness, (2) overconcern with body size/shape, (3) internalization of a thin ideal size/shape, and (4) perfectionism/obsessionality. The types of cognitive biases that are hypothesized to result from these conditions are (1) attentional bias, (2) selective memory bias, (3) selective interpretational biases, (4) body size overestimation, and (5) extreme drive for thinness. The model hypothesizes that negative emotion interacts with the self-schema to increase the probability of certain cognitive biases and particular aspects of disturbed body image. In addition, the model postulates that the activation of cognitive bias also activates negative emotion. Thus it is possible for cognitive biases to activate negative emotion and the self-schema for body size/shape or eating, which in turn activates cognitive bias. This feedback loop may be experienced as an obsession.

HYPOTHESES DERIVED FROM THE MODEL

• *In normal-weight or underweight people who are very concerned about body/size shape, a variety of cognitive biases, including body image disturbances, are present.* This hypothesis has been supported by many studies conducted over the past 10 years. Furthermore, these cognitive biases are often of comparable severity to those in people diagnosed with eating disorders. Therefore, cognitive biases are not exclusive to eating disorders but also affect individuals of normal weight who are preoccupied with body size. Research in our laboratory has found that cognitive biases in nonclinical people may be more easily modified than in those with clinical eating disorders.

• *Some cognitive biases are labile (in people overly concerned with body size/shape), and other cognitive biases are relatively stable across a variety of situations and emotional states.* Recent studies support the hypothesis that the lability of cognitive biases is most frequently observed in people who are very concerned (obsessed) with body size/shape. These studies have found that when cognitive biases are labile, reactions occur in response to stimuli that activate the body schema and stimuli that elicit negative emotions. The implications of these findings are discussed later.

• *Cognitive biases and body image disturbances are more likely to be observed in response to tasks or stimuli that are self-referent than in other-referent tasks.* Information-processing theories of body image hypothesize that people who are obsessed with body size/shape are most likely to misinterpret body-related information in regard to self. Most studies have instructed participants to think about the experimental stimuli in terms of relevance to self as opposed to others. We were unable to identify studies that directly compared self- versus other-related encoding strategies. Thus it is our observation that this hypothesis has not been directly tested.

• *Cognitive biases and body image disturbances are more likely to be observed in response to ambiguous stimuli/situations.* Body image assessment typically involves "projecting" one's visual self image upon an ambiguous representation of that image, such as a small silhouette or a measure of width that reflects the size of a body area (e.g., thigh or abdomen). Research shows that women with eating disorders and/or high levels of preoccupation with body size have a cognitive bias for body-related interpretations of ambiguous stimuli. However, no studies were identified that compared responses to ambiguous versus nonambiguous stimuli. It is our conclusion that this hypothesis has not been directly tested.

• *Cognitive biases and body image disturbances in people who are overly concerned with body size/shape are a specific response to stimuli that are body- or eating-related.* Tests of this "content specificity" hypothesis have compared control stimuli that were unrelated to body size/shape, such as concerns about health, with stimuli that have content specifically related to body size/shape or eating. In general, the results of these studies have supported this hypothesis.

IMPLICATIONS FOR FUTURE RESEARCH

Body Image and Emotion

As noted in the previous section, some aspects of body image, as well as some cognitive biases related to body shape information, are not stable over time and across situations. For example, induction of negative mood states influences current body size estimation but does not influence other cognitive processes, such as attention and memory bias for body-related stimuli. Therefore, estimation of body size appears to be labile, whereas attention to, encoding, and retrieval of body-related information appear to be more stable cognitive variables.

Cognitive theories pertaining to information networks, or schemas, offer some explanation for the lability of cognitive phenomena. A cognitive schema can be thought of as a mental structure pertaining to particular information that serves as a mental shortcut. A schema is representational and therefore subject to perceptual and informational biases. Research has shown that the more frequently a schema is activated, the more likely it will come to be associated with external events or internal cues, such as hunger or negative emotion. Further, higher frequency of activation should result in a dense, highly integrated network of memories that is easily activated and very accessible for retrieval. When more associative cues are connected to a schema, it is more likely that the schema will be activated by a wide variety of external stimuli (e.g., tight clothing) and internal cues related to fullness.

According to cognitive theory, schemas are interconnected. It may be useful to think of them as overlapping webs connecting bits of information to form an overall concept. Therefore, relevance of body-related information to environmental events or situations may influence the frequency of activation. For example, the body self-schema is more likely to be activated when an individual is trying on clothes than when the individual is taking a timed math test. This theory offers an explanation for the finding that body image is labile across mood states. Because negative body images are likely to induce negative mood states such as anxiety and depression, the activation of a negative mood can activate the body self-schema, resulting in the exacerbation of body image disturbances. As illustrated in Figure 6.1, this feedback loop can result in constant distress about body-related information. Thompson and Heinberg refer to this phenomenon as the "hurricane effect."

According to the information-processing perspective, the more frequently negative body information is activated, the stronger the associative network will become. Less well understood is why some aspects of body image, such as estimation of body size, are reactive to the activation of body self-schema and/or negative emotions, while other aspects of body image, such as the selection of ideal body size, are relatively stable. Williamson, in 1996, suggested that the selection of ideal body size may be a "standard" or "anchor" that serves as a point of comparison for current body size estimates. This type of cognitive variable may be less vulnerable to emotional influences. This hypothesis has not been tested, however.

Sociocultural Differences in Body Image

The relationship between frequency of activation of the body self-schema and the occurrence of body image disturbances provides explanation for gender, developmental, sexual orientation, and cultural differences in body image. The emotional significance of body-related information varies across ages, cultures, and genders. Some people value thinness more than others. Individuals who greatly value thinness are more likely to access the body self-schema, resulting in a dense, highly integrated network of memories that is easily activated and more vulnerable to the formation of cognitive biases. Recent research has found that beauty ideals among African American women are more flexible than those held by Caucasian women, and that African American women have more positive body images in comparison to Caucasian women with similar body size. (See this volume's chapter by Celio, Zabinski, and Wilfley.) Other research has reported that homosexual men are more concerned with thinness as a positive characteristic of physical appearance, and more dissatisfied with their bodies, than are heterosexual men; the finding was attributed to a heightened emphasis on thinness in male homosexual cultures. (See Rothblum's chapter in this volume.)

IMPLICATIONS FOR TREATMENT

Early Intervention

Research in the past 10 years has identified a wide variety of risk factors for eating disorders. These include early onset of puberty, dietary restraint, perfectionism, low self-esteem, exposure to media influences promoting thinness, and activities that promote a thin ideal (e.g., gymnastics, dance, modeling). Extreme concern (obsession) with body size/shape has been identified as one of the strongest risk factors for the development of eating disorders in children and adolescents. A recent study from our laboratory found that the relationship between concern with body size and cognitive biases related to body size/shape exists in children as young as 8 years old. As noted, extreme concern with body size/shape has been found to be associated with a wide variety of body image disturbances and cognitive biases.

These findings from the risk factor literature, in the context of findings from the cognitive bias literature, lead to the following conclusion: The earliest signs of an eating disorder may be the development of a dense, highly integrated body self-schema stemming from frequent activation (often described as preoccupation, rumination, or obsession) of body-related information relevant to the self. The implications of this observation are twofold: First, children who are preoccupied with body size/shape may be the best targets for prevention of an eating disorder. Second, the content of eating disorder programs should emphasize (1) counteracting the cultural pressures that promote dieting and a thin body ideal (e.g., recognition of fad diets, resisting peer pressure to diet); (2) challenging assumptions about appearance and cognitive distortions related to body; (3) promoting healthy interpersonal relationships; (4) teaching healthy coping strategies to effectively handle stress and negative social aspects of body image; and (5) enhancing self-esteem separate from body esteem. Furthermore, instruction about healthy weight regulation via a balanced diet/nutrition and exercise should be promoted as a positive alternative to dieting and the use of extreme methods for weight regulation. A recent study by Varnado-Sullivan and colleagues found that preadolescent girls who were highly concerned with body size/shape benefited most from this type of intervention. For further observations about prevention, consult this volume's chapters by Levine and Smolak and by Winzelberg and his colleagues.

Treatment of Body Image in Clinical Eating Disorders

Several researchers, particularly Cash and Rosen, have developed outpatient cognitive-behavioral treatment programs for body image disturbances and body dissatisfaction. As Cash and Strachan indicate elsewhere in this volume, these programs have been validated using obese patients and women of average weight who are dissatisfied with their bodies. Hospital-based treatment programs for eating disorders often include some type of body image treatment as one aspect of a comprehensive therapeutic approach.

Cognitive biases and body image disturbances are very treatment-resistant. Recently, our research group developed a "Body Positive" treatment program that targeted cognitive biases and body image disturbances in women who had been "successfully" treated for an eating disorder but had persistent body image concerns that made them vulnerable for relapse. The Body Positive program included relaxation and rebreathing training, self-monitoring of body image experiences, cognitive-behavioral treatment for body image concerns, mirror exposure to distressing body areas, prevention of body checking rituals, and relapse prevention. This program included in vivo exposure to the body and exposure to feared situations in sessions and in homework assignments. Preliminary results indicated improvement of body image, which suggests that body image therapy can be effectively utilized to treat persistent weight/shape concerns in people who have partially recovered from an eating disorder but remain at risk.

Body Image and Emotion: Implications for Body Image Therapy

The relationship between cognition and emotion with regard to body image is an unexplored area in the treatment literature. As noted earlier, emotions may be linked to specific representations (body self-schema) that serve as "triggers" for negative body image experiences. It has been suggested that cognitive-behavioral techniques should be directed towards aiding individuals in the management of unwanted affective states as well as helping them to access other, more positive affective states. To accomplish these goals, there is a need to develop methods that explore and access the implicit meanings of emotions that may not be completely obvious to the clinician or the patient.

From this perspective, there are several implications for body image treatment. Initially, treatment may emphasize management of existing affective states and body image reactions to provide some sense of control over these "automatic" reactions. However, in order to modify the body self-schema, it may also be necessary to activate affective states deliberately (via exposure to "threatening" body stimuli) to identify the connection between certain thoughts and feelings. Once this connection has been established, the therapist can directly challenge thoughts, expectations, and other cognitions that are now more easily accessed and therefore experienced with a higher level of awareness. Traditional cognitive-behavioral approaches for body image have focused more on management of emotions and body image reactions than on altering the body self-schema. We believe that this type of treatment must be conducted in individual therapy sessions, where the duration and specific characteristics of the body image "triggers" or exposure stimuli can be carefully controlled.

In conclusion, when using this approach for body image treatment, individuals are encouraged to develop alternative perspectives that might aid in challenging maladaptive schemas. The goal of treatment—of targeting the relationship between emotion and body image—is to break the cycle of perceived threat and reaction to body image, including reactive behaviors that confirm the perceived threat. In order to accomplish this outcome, the memory store must be activated to elicit emotion. Once the emotion is present, treatment focuses on preventing behavioral responses and reducing the intensity of the emotional reaction, thereby breaking the cycle of rumination about body size, eating, and extreme negative emotions. Emotion is an important part of the body image experience. Although it is necessary to elicit emotion in therapy, it should be done in a very controlled manner so that the individual learns the connection between certain thoughts and memories and intense body image and emotional reactions. Individuals can be trained to cope with emotion associated with difficult body image experiences using relaxation and other anxiety management techniques. Ultimately, this therapy should address the separation of the emotional and cognitive domains of the body image experience in order to disrupt the feedback loop that is depicted in Figure 6.1.

INFORMATIVE READINGS

Cash, T. F. (1997). *The body image workbook: An 8–step program for learning to like your looks.* Oakland, CA: New Harbinger.—A cognitive-behavioral self-help program for the improvement of body image concerns.

Rosen, J. C. (1997). Cognitive-behavioral body image therapy. In D. M. Garner & P. E. Garfinkel (Eds.), *Handbook of treatment for eating disorders* (2nd ed., pp. 188–201). New York: Guilford Press.—A chapter that reviews cognitive-behavioral treatment for body image.

Thompson, J. K., Heinberg, L. J., Altabe, M., & Tantleff-Dunn, S. (1999). *Exacting beauty: Theory, assessment, and treatment of body image disturbances* (pp. 271–310). Washington, DC: American Psychological Association.—A book that provides extensive coverage of cognitive-behavioral perspectives; see especially the chapter, "Cognitive-Processing Models" (pp. 271–310).

Varnado-Sullivan, P., Zucker, N., Williamson, D. A.., Reas, D., & Thaw, J. (2001). Development and implementation of the Body Logic Program for adolescents: A two-stage prevention program for eating disorders. *Cognitive and Behavioral Practice, 8,* 248–259.—A study investigating the effectiveness of a prevention program for eating disorders in adolescents.

Vitousek, K. B., & Hollon, S. D. (1990). The investigation of schematic content and processing in eating disorders. *Cognitive Therapy and Research, 14,* 191–214.—An early position paper on the possible relevance of cognitive research for eating disorders.

Williamson, D. A. (1996). Body image disturbance in eating disorders: A form of cognitive bias? *Eating Disorders, 4*(1), 47–58.—A research review of cognitive biases associated with body dysphoria and eating disorders.

Williamson, D. A., Muller, S. L., Reas, D. L., & Thaw, J. M. (1999). Cognitive bias in eating disorders: Implications for theory and treatment. *Behavior Modification, 23*(4), 556–577.—A review of the evidence pertaining to cognitive-behavioral theories of eating disorders and the implications of this research for the treatment.

Williamson, D. A., Perrin, L., Blouin, D. C., & Barbin, J. M. (2000). Cognitive bias in eating disorders: Interpretation of ambiguous body-related information. *Eating and Weight Disorders, 5,* 143–151.—A study investigating the relationship of eating disorders and selective interpretation biases.

Feminist Perspectives and Objectified Body Consciousness

NITA MARY MCKINLEY

Feminist social critique has historically pointed out how the body has served as a locus of control in women's lives. Current feminist theory contends that women's normative body dissatisfaction is not a function of individual pathology but a systematic social phenomenon. In this chapter, I review this feminist theory, outline the use of this theory to develop a measure of women's body experience, report empirical evidence supporting this theory, and make suggestions for future research and prevention of negative body experience.

FEMINIST PERSPECTIVES: THE SOCIAL CONSTRUCTION OF THE BODY

Feminist theorists have found the social construction perspective useful in understanding women's body experience and its relationship to gendered power relations. This perspective focuses on how societies create meaning. For example, Western societies construct a duality between mind and body, and women are associated with the body and men with the mind. This allocation presumably occurs because of women's reproductive function, a "truth" that ignores the fact that many men are also reproductive and not all women are. Western societies also define men's bodies as the standard against which women's bodies are judged, and women's bodies are constructed as deviant in comparison. This meaning can be observed by examining cultural values and practices. For example, the body the media portray as attractive is slim and muscular, a body type more common in men than in women. The mature female body with fat on the hips and thighs is considered unattractive. In a subtler example of the deviance of the female body, we define normal female biological functions, such as menstruation and menopause, as medical events.

The perceived deviance of the female body and the association of women with the body create the context for women's body experience. This context encourages the construction of women and girls as objects to be watched and evaluated in terms of how their bodies fit cultural standards. This construction begins early when girls are praised for their appearance and learn that they are judged by how they appear to others. (One can understand the power of this norm by trying to congratulate new parents of a baby girl without mentioning her appearance.) Girls learn to watch their own bodies from this outside perspective to avoid negative judgment. This construction of women as objects to be watched and evaluated both shapes women's consciousness and makes them dependent on others for approval.

The social construction perspective particularly fits a feminist understanding of women's lives because it stresses the social context of women's discontent, rather than individual pathology. The social context, in which women are defined as objects to be watched and unattainable body standards are constructed as "normal," makes the normative negative body experience of women understandable.

PSYCHOLOGY AND OBJECTIFIED BODY CONSCIOUSNESS

Feminist theory on how women and girls come to view their bodies as objects to be watched has had an important impact on psychological research on body image. For example, I have used this theory to study the internalization of social constructions of women's bodies and have developed a measure of what I call *objectified body consciousness* (OBC), which includes body surveillance, internalization of cultural body standards, and appearance control beliefs (McKinley, 1998, 1999; McKinley & Hyde, 1996).

Body surveillance is watching oneself as though one were an observer. Watching one's appearance is presumably associated with self-love and individual achievement for women. However, research shows that when people pay attention to how others perceive them, they try to meet relevant standards, feel bad if standards are not met, and are susceptible to influence by others. Thus body surveillance is about control, not self-love. Fredrickson and Roberts argue that habitual self-monitoring of the body shapes women's psychological experience, increasing shame and anxiety while reducing peak motivational states and awareness of internal bodily states.

The second facet of OBC is the *internalization of cultural body standards*. A woman who internalizes these standards experiences them as coming from her own desires, which makes the standards difficult to challenge and conceals the external pressures to conform, such as the discrimination against women who do not "measure up." Furthermore, this internalization predisposes women to connect achievement of these standards with their sense of self-worth. Because the standards are narrow and difficult to achieve, women experience a sense of empowerment as they approximate them but more often shame when they do not.

The final component of OBC, *appearance control beliefs*, is the assurance that, given enough effort, cultural body standards can be achieved. To establish the legitimacy of judging women in terms of their bodies, body standards must be believed to be attainable. Regardless of the extent to which women actually control their appearance, control beliefs may provide benefits to women in the form of relief from the stress of working to attain sometimes impossible standards and a sense of competence in controlling their bodies.

Empirical Evidence for OBC

The ability of the OBC theory to predict women's body experience has been shown through survey data with predominantly European American undergraduates. Three eight-item OBC Scales measure body surveillance, body shame, and appearance control beliefs. Their internal consistency, test–retest reliability, and the factorial structure have been established.

A woman who is high in body surveillance believes that how she looks is more important than how she feels. For young women, higher body surveillance is related to lower body satisfaction, more eating problems, and lower levels of some measures of psychological well-being, such as autonomy and self-acceptance. Body surveillance is a consistent predictor of negative experience for young women.

To the extent that a woman has internalized cultural body standards, she presumably experiences shame if she does not achieve them; therefore, body shame is used to measure degree of internalization. However, greater body shame is related to more personal endorsement of cultural body standards, and body shame is more strongly related to body satisfaction than is endorsement of standards. Across samples, body shame is consistently and pervasively related to higher body surveillance, lower body satisfaction, lower psychological well-being, and more eating problems in young women. Body shame is typically the strongest of the three OBC scales in predicting women's body experience and psychological well-being.

A woman with high appearance control beliefs endorses the idea that she can control her appearance if she tries hard enough. The results for appearance control beliefs are less consistent than those for body surveillance and body shame. These beliefs are associated with an increased frequency in restricted eating and in eating problems in young women. However, appearance control beliefs are usually unrelated to surveillance or body shame and are related to *greater* body satisfaction for some samples. Although the relationships are weaker than those for surveillance or body shame, control beliefs are also related to *higher* levels on some measures of psychological well-being. Given the context of a requirement for body control in women, such beliefs may serve to help women feel good about themselves while simultaneously encouraging problematic eating practices. Because these are correlational rather than causal data, it also may be that women who feel good about themselves, or whose bodies meet certain standards, believe they control their appearance.

One limitation of my studies and others like them is their correlational design, which does not allow us to determine whether body surveillance causes negative body experience, or if those who feel bad about their bodies engage in more surveillance. Fredrickson and her colleagues conducted an experimental study to test whether surveillance was causally related to body shame, restricted eating, and math performance. They randomly assigned undergraduate women to try on either a swimsuit or a sweater; trying on a swimsuit presumably evoked self-consciousness in terms of appearance, which is closely related to body surveillance. Compared to the sweater group, the swimsuit group had increased body shame, ate less, and also had decreased performance on a math test. This latter finding is especially important because the relationship of body practices to cognitive functioning is an understudied but consequential component of women's body experience.

Age Differences in OBC

Although the social construction of women's bodies as objects to be watched is likely to affect women of all ages, developmental differences between young and middle-aged women suggest the likelihood of variations in their body experience. A number of factors may account for differences in body experience of young and middle-aged women. There are differences in life tasks; young women may be initiating heterosexual relationships and middle-aged women may be maintaining long-term relationships. Those who conform more closely to cultural body standards, as young women do, have greater visibility. Moreover, there are cohort differences in body standards, with decreasing body size standards for younger generations.

As expected, middle-aged women have lower levels of body surveillance and body shame compared to undergraduate women, but no difference in control beliefs. Body shame has very similar relationships to other variables in middle-aged women, but body surveillance is unrelated to body satisfaction, and higher control beliefs are related to greater body satisfaction. The relationships between OBC and measures of autonomy and self-acceptance are similar for young and middle-aged women, but the relationship with surveillance is stronger for younger women. Thus OBC is also meaningful for middle-aged women but somewhat better describes young women's experience.

Gender Differences in OBC

That women are not as satisfied with their bodies as are men is well established; OBC provides a theoretical understanding of why this difference might occur. As stated earlier, men are viewed as connected with the mind, whereas women are connected with the body. Furthermore, because boys are not routinely evaluated in terms of their appearance, they do not internalize an observer's view of their bodies, as girls do. Therefore, men should show lower levels of OBC than women and weaker relationships between OBC and body satisfaction.

Although the OBC scales were developed using a theory of women's experience and were validated on samples of women, they are internally consistent and factorially sound for college men as well. Relationships between body surveillance, body shame, control beliefs, and body satisfaction are similar for women and men. However, relationships between surveillance, body shame, and body satisfaction are stronger for women. Men have lower levels of body surveillance and body shame but similar levels of control beliefs. Moreover, when levels of OBC are statistically controlled, gender differences in body satisfaction are eliminated. In the study by Fredrickson and her colleagues described earlier, men were also asked to try on a bathing suit or a sweater. The researchers did not find relationships between this experimentally manipulated body surveillance and body shame, eating behavior, or math performance, as they did for women. These findings suggest that OBC is useful for understanding some of the body experience differences between women and men, and that OBC does not predict men's body experience as well as that of women in experimental situations.

FUTURE RESEARCH DIRECTIONS

The research on how women objectify themselves, while promising, needs to be expanded in scope. We know very little about women who do not fit the profile of the modal U.S. college student. Thus, we know little about women of color, lesbians, bisexual women, women of nonprivileged classes, women with disabilities, adolescents, and older women. We need to include more groups of women not only in our participant database but also in our theorizing. For example, how might dominant social constructions of women's bodies interact with other constructions, such as those of race and class?

Social constructions are not monolithic; at any given time, multiple meanings may coexist. We need more research, both qualitative and quantitative, to understand how diverse women think about their bodies and how women resist narrow definitions of themselves as bodies. Studying resistance helps to clarify how dominant constructions work as well as how they can be effectively counteracted. However, we also need to remember the power differentials that exist between institutionally supported social constructions and individual resistance. Changing how she thinks or acts will not change very real patterns of discrimination a woman faces based on her appearance. Bordo also warns that romanticizing resistance can distract us from examining the normalizing power of dominant constructions.

Although it is important to document women's objectification of their own bodies and the psychological consequences of this body consciousness, we also need to acknowledge that this focus creates a context in which body dissatisfaction and OBC continue to be understood as *psychological problems of individual women*. This frame leads to an assumption that the solution is one of simply helping women change how they think about their bodies. Thinking about themselves differently may sometimes be useful to certain women, but this strategy ignores the very real social pressures women experience not only to display certain types of bodies but even to think about their bodies in certain ways. We need to expand our theorizing and research to include the social context itself: how particular types of social situations might encourage women and men to objectify other women, and how this objectification of women is learned. Without this broad research agenda, we risk changing labels—from "women like their bodies less than men" to "women objectify their bodies more than men"—without addressing the greater social issues.

PREVENTING BODY IMAGE DISTURBANCE

Fredrickson and Roberts make a convincing case that body surveillance can account for many of the mental health risks associated with being female, including depression, sexual dysfunction, and eating problems. An understanding of how OBC shapes women's experience allows us to account for the tenacity of women's body discontent.

We need to think of women's body problems as a social justice issue for women. Working to achieve cultural body standards deprives women of time, energy, and economic resources. We also know that standards for women's bodies reflect biases of race and ethnicity, class, age, sexual orientation, and ability. Given these biases, the definition of women in terms of the body helps maintain status differences among women.

Feminism focuses on changing social systems rather than the individual. The social construction perspective underlines the belief that the source of women's negative body experience lies in the social context rather than in individual pathology. Individual women may feel better about themselves by learning a cultural analysis of women's body issues and strategies for resistance. However, changing the context itself through political activism and the creation of body-positive communities may also be important for changing women's body experience.

INFORMATIVE READINGS

Bartky, S. L. (1988). Foucault, femininity, and the modernization of patriarchal power. In I. Diamond & L. Quinby (Eds.), *Feminism and Foucault: Reflections on resistance* (pp. 61–86). Boston: Northeastern University Press.—A Foucauldian analysis of women's body experience and how surveillance is translated into social control.

Bordo, S. R. (1993). *Unbearable weight: Feminism, Western culture, and the body.* Berkeley: University of California Press.—A collection of essays on the cultural meanings attached to gendered bodies.

Fredrickson, B. L., & Roberts, T. (1997). Objectification theory: Toward understanding women's lived experiences and mental health risks. *Psychology of Women Quarterly, 21,* 173–206.—A theoretical analysis of the pervasive relationship of objectified body consciousness to women's psychological well-being.

Fredrickson, B. L., Roberts, T., Noll, S. M., Quinn, D. M., & Twenge, J. M. (1998). That swimsuit becomes you: Sex differences in self-objectification, restrained eating, and math performance. *Journal of Personality and Social Psychology, 75,* 269–284.—An experimental study showing a causal relationship between surveillance, eating behavior, and cognitive performance.

McKinley, N. M. (1998). Gender differences in body esteem: The mediating effect of objectified body consciousness and weight discrepancy. *Sex Roles, 39,* 113–123.—Reports reliabilities of OBC scales for men and gender differences analyses.

McKinley, N. M. (1999). Women and objectified body consciousness: Mothers' and daughters' body experience in cultural, developmental, and familial context. *Developmental Psychology, 35,* 760–769.—Reports age differences on OBC scales as well as the relationship between daughters' OBC and their parents' approval of their appearance.

McKinley, N. M., & Hyde, J. S. (1996). The objectified body consciousness scale: Development and validation. *Psychology of Women Quarterly, 20,* 181–215.—Psychometric analyses of the OBC scales for young and middle-aged women.

Rodin, J., Silberstein, L., & Striegel-Moore, R. (1985). Women and weight: A normative discontent. In T. Sonderegger (Ed.), *Psychology and gender: Nebraska symposium on motivation* (pp. 267–307). Lincoln, NE: University of Nebraska Press.—Describes the reasons weight has become a ubiquitous problem for women and argues that shame is an important component of women's body experience.

Spitzack, C. (1990). *Confessing excess: Women and the politics of body reduction.* Albany: State University of New York Press.—A Foucauldian discourse analysis of weight loss literature and interviews with women that concludes that women must "confess excess" in order to gain acceptance.

Thompson, J. K., Heinberg, L. J., Altabe, M., & Tantleff-Dunn, S. (1999). *Exacting beauty: Theory, assessment, and treatment of body image disturbance*. Washington, DC: American Psychological Association.—Chapter 7 reviews feminist themes in research about body issues, research findings, and feminist approaches to assessment.

Wolf, N. (1991). *The beauty myth: How images of beauty are used against women*. New York: Anchor Press.—A popular account of the political context of women's body experience.

II

Developmental Perspectives and Influences

Body Image Development in Children

LINDA SMOLAK

There are many reasons to be interested in the development of body image during childhood. We might assume, for example, that a positive body image is related to global self-esteem. Furthermore, it is evident that by early adolescence, negative body image predicts the development of depression and eating disorders. Presumably, adolescent negative body image is rooted in childhood body image.

Unfortunately, the empirical support for these assumptions is quite limited. There is certainly research concerning body image development during childhood. However, it is rarely of the type that allows us to examine causal relationships, either in the etiology or the outcomes of negative body image. In other words, there is very little prospective, longitudinal research. With this caveat in mind, this chapter focuses on the development of body image as it occurs in children age 11 and under. In the United States, these children are generally in elementary school. The emphasis here is on the sequence of development within gender and ethnic group as well as on potential biological and sociocultural influences.

THE DEVELOPMENT OF BODY IMAGE

Researchers have looked at both overall body image and specific measures of weight and shape concerns among children. The measures of overall body image, often referred to as "body esteem" or "appearance esteem," tend to include items concerning facial features, hair, and general appearance. A child could be dissatisfied with weight or shape and obtain a relatively high score on these measures. Other measures tend to focus more specifically on weight and shape; these may examine overall body shape, specific body areas, or how worried a child is about being or getting fat. These measures are often referred to as "body dissatisfaction" or "weight and shape concerns" assessments, though they, too, are sometimes termed "body esteem" scales. It is noteworthy that such measures are more likely to ask about being overweight than about being too thin.

These two types of measures tend to show different developmental patterns. Global measures of body esteem show few changes until, perhaps, late elementary school. Furthermore, girls and boys typically show comparable levels of overall body esteem throughout much of childhood. Body esteem appears to be substantially correlated with global self-esteem.

However, when body esteem is measured in terms of satisfaction with weight and shape, a very different picture emerges. Most currently available research uses these measures. Many studies indicate that a significant minority of white American, Australian, and British children is dissatisfied with body shape or weight. Studies routinely find that about 40% of elementary school girls and 25% of elementary school boys are dissatisfied with their size and want to be thinner. Even girls who are underweight by statistical standards are sometimes concerned about being too fat.

Children as young as 6 express body dissatisfaction and weight concerns. In general, though not unanimously, research finds that girls in late elementary school (fourth grade and beyond) express more concern about being overweight and a stronger desire to be thinner than do younger girls. Indeed, by the end of elementary school, it is not uncommon to find that half or more of the girls are unhappy about their weight and shape—a comparable finding to the levels of body dissatisfaction observed among adolescent and adult females, which may indicate that at least some components of disturbed eating may be internalized at fairly young ages. Indeed, body satisfaction in late elementary school may predict body esteem as well as eating problems in early adolescence.

Most studies of body image among girls have examined Caucasian samples. The sparse data available concerning African American girls, however, generally suggest that despite higher BMIs (body mass index) and more advanced pubertal development, they suffer body dissatisfaction less than or equal to that of Caucasian girls. Interestingly, some studies find that more black than white girls are unhappy with their bodies because they are too small. These girls, who are a minority within any sample of girls, want to be *larger* than their current size. Overall, black girls generally indicate a larger ideal body size than do white girls. Thus, the data suggest that, as in the adult literature, black girls may be somewhat protected from developing certain eating problems because they espouse a less severe ideal body type. However, though the data are extremely limited, there appear to be no differences in body dissatisfaction between Hispanic and white girls, thus underscoring the potential diversity of body image experiences across ethnic groups.

Among boys, body satisfaction may also decrease throughout the elementary school years, though not all studies find this trend. Several issues must be considered in interpreting this finding. First, following puberty, boys may experience a plateau or even an increase in body esteem, whereas girls continue to experience decreases, suggesting that growth may be viewed more positively by boys. This possibility raises a second issue. Some of the body dissatisfaction seen among boys may reflect feeling too small rather than too big. Several, but not all, studies have indicated that elementary school boys want to be bigger, a desire that may be more pronounced during childhood than adolescence. Many researchers fail to differentiate direction of dissatisfaction. Furthermore, those studies that have asked about being bigger have not effectively differentiated larger size in terms of fat, muscle, or just normal physical development. Finally, it is more difficult to draw definitive conclusions about the development of body esteem in boys because there is less research on boys than girls.

Data concerning body image in males of ethnic minorities are very limited; one study reported comparable levels of body satisfaction among black, Hispanic, and white fourth-grade boys. Research consistently indicates that boys are more satisfied with their weight and shape. Among black and white children, boys seem more satisfied with their body shape and less concerned about their weight; white girls were more concerned about their weight than were black girls.

CONTRIBUTORS TO BODY IMAGE PROBLEMS

Any model of the development of body image problems needs to explain at least two factors. First, there are developmental trends in body dissatisfaction, body esteem, and weight concerns. At least among white girls, there are fairly steady decreases in body satisfaction accompanied by an increase in weight concerns throughout the elementary school years and immediately following puberty. Second, these trends vary by gender and ethnic group and are important because they presage those of eating disorders. Sociocultural models of eating problems have given more attention to these developmental and demographic patterns than have the biological models.

Biological Contributors

BMI

It is unlikely that there are any direct biological contributors to body image problems. However, given that body weight and shape have a strong genetic basis *and* that heavier body weights and shapes are seen as socially undesirable (especially for females), BMI may well be an indirect biological contributor to negative body image—one that operates through social psychological mechanisms.

By age 6, and probably earlier, children are aware of the societal bias against fat people and will frequently express this bias themselves. This prejudice may increase with age. Not surprisingly, young children who are heavy begin to internalize this message. Even in early elementary school, overweight children report more body dissatisfaction and wish they were thinner. Although overweight children appear to be unhappy with their bodies, this does not necessarily reduce their overall self-esteem, at least until early adolescence.

The correlation between BMI and body esteem is probably created by a third variable: societal attitudes toward fat people. Poor body esteem is not part of a pattern of poor mental health; overweight and obese people are not inherently more prone to psychopathology or poor mental health. Furthermore, the relationship between BMI and body esteem varies by gender and probably by ethnicity, even in childhood, further suggesting that societal attitudes may moderate this relationship.

The issue of social reactions to increasing BMI may be particularly important during puberty. In early adolescence, current pubertal status is related to body image. Recent data suggest that an increasing percentage of elementary school girls, especially black girls, are experiencing breast development. If this breast development is accompanied by a weight spurt, then some of the body image issues related to puberty may be increasingly common among elementary school girls. This is an issue for future research.

Temperament

Some prominent theorists have suggested that there are personality predispositions for severe body image disturbances and eating disorders. Since such work primarily deals with pathological states, it falls beyond the scope of this chapter. However, if we assume a continuum of eating problems, beginning with body dissatisfaction and weight concerns and culminating in eating disorders, then it becomes reasonable to at least acknowledge the potential contribution of these personality characteristics to body image problems.

There is little research on these relationships among elementary school-children. Several studies have examined the relationship between depression and body dissatisfaction in childhood, but the results are too inconsistent to draw any conclusions. The well-established findings that gender differences in depression do not emerge until adolescence while those in body image are evident in elementary school will need explanation if depression and body image disturbance are to be linked by genetics. It is possible that the gender differences in body image contribute to the later gender difference in depression.

High levels of social anxiety and social comparison tendencies show concurrent relationships to poorer body esteem during childhood. This relationship has only been evaluated in girls. The importance of considering the development of body image separately for boys and girls is underscored by longitudinal data suggesting that negative emotionality during childhood may be related to adolescent girls', but not boys', drive for thinness.

Sociocultural Influences

Gender, ethnicity, cross-cultural, historical, and age differences in levels of body esteem all suggest that culture and society play a major role in the construction and hence the development of body image. Likely sociocultural influences include parents, peers, and media.

Parents

Parents can influence body image development by selecting and commenting on children's clothing and appearance, or by requiring the child to look certain ways and to eat or avoid certain foods. Although parents of young children are generally pleased with their child's appearance, many parents do comment on their children's weight. They might also actively encourage their children to slim down. This is true for both mothers and fathers, for boys and girls, and in black and white families (although some researchers have suggested that African American mothers may place less emphasis on body shape). Surprisingly, some studies of white families have found that daughters are not more likely than sons to be encouraged to control their weight.

In addition to direct comments, parental modeling of weight concerns may contribute to body esteem problems in children. Parents might remark on the appearance of their own bodies or might engage in calorie-restrictive dieting or exercise solely for the purpose of weight loss. Such behavior could teach children to focus on and be unhappy with their body shape.

Parent comments about children's weight appear to be related to children's body satisfaction. Data concerning parental modeling are more ambiguous. Despite the fact that parents do not clearly encourage weight control in their prepubertal daughters more than their sons, daughters may be more affected by parental weight-related behavior than sons. Girls may be particularly affected by their mothers' behavior, and direct comments appear to be more powerful than parental modeling.

Peers

Although peers may be less influential during the elementary school than adolescent years, they are still relevant to children's development. Social comparison appears as a factor by very early elementary school. This is probably one reason why even young children are aware of whether they are overweight and why they feel bad about it. Peer influences probably also contribute to children's awareness of the negative stereotypes associated with body fat. Thus it is reasonable to expect that peer messages concerning body shape might affect children's body esteem. Peer messages may take a variety of forms: comments from peers about weight and shape, discussions about body shape, and modeling of weight concerns and weight control techniques.

Concurrent data are quite consistent in supporting a relationship between peer messages and body dissatisfaction. Again, this may be truer of girls than boys. In fact, girls may be more exposed to, aware of, and sensitive to weight-related messages from peers. Sensitivity to the messages may be more important than objectively measured amount of exposure.

Not surprisingly, teasing is positively correlated with body dissatisfaction in elementary school. Apparently some girls take such teasing more to heart, and these girls appear to have higher levels of weight concerns. Furthermore, peer modeling and teasing may be more strongly related to body dissatisfaction than is perceived parental concern about girls' weight, even in elementary school. In addition, teasing can be considered to be part of the cultural objectification of the female body, which feminists argue contributes to the development of eating disorders. More specifically, treating girls as sexual objects in a way that is threatening, dehumanizing, and demeaning might focus girls on their bodies, encourage comparisons to the cultural ideal and to other girls, and ultimately result in body dissatisfaction and low body esteem. In elementary schoolchildren, such objectification might take the form of peer teasing that resembles later sexual harassment. For example, boys might prevent girls from walking in the halls, flip up their skirts, comment on their appearance, and call them ugly. Research suggests that frequency of sexual harassment is negatively associated with body esteem for elementary school girls but not for boys. Furthermore, girls are more likely to report being scared by these experiences. Those girls who report being scared have lower levels of body esteem as do girls who report being uncertain as to how a victim of such an experience would feel. Objectification theory may explain how some girls (e.g., those who are more frightened or silenced by harassment) might become more negatively focused on their bodies. Clearly, peer influences in childhood deserve much more research attention, particularly given their potential role in prevention programs.

Media and Toys

Even among adolescents and adults, drawing a conclusion about the influence of media images on body esteem is a complex and confusing issue. It is even more complicated in children, partially because research is severely limited.

Like adults, children see skewed gender roles on television, including presentations of the "ideal," and even the typical, woman as slender. By late elementary school, girls may start reading the "teen" magazines that routinely present a particular appearance ideal as well as address appearance concerns. Up to half of late elementary school girls may read these magazines at least occasionally, with as many as 25% reading them twice a week. Obtaining beauty and weight information from magazines has been related to body image in late elementary and early adolescent girls. Girls do compare themselves to fashion models and feel bad about the comparison. Girls who make such comparisons may have higher levels of weight concerns.

Consider Barbie, a doll owned by about 90% of girls ages 3–11: Fewer than 1 in 100,000 women are likely to have proportions similar to Barbie's. It is not only Barbie's appearance that may increase young girls' weight and shape consciousness. The primary way to "play" with Barbie is to change her clothes, which focuses girls even more selectively on the importance of appearance and "looking good" in clothes. Research has not clearly examined the link between Barbie and body image issues. As with other sociocultural influences, the relationship is likely to be moderated, and perhaps mediated, by each girl's beliefs about thinness and success as well as her exposure to other sources that emphasize thinness.

A similar statement might be made about the action figures played with by boys. These male figures have become unrealistically muscular during the past two decades and may be presenting boys with an unattainable and potentially damaging body ideal. Limited evidence suggests, however, that internalization of media images is less related to body image in boys than in girls.

CONCLUSIONS

The conclusion to be drawn from the currently available literature on the development of body image during childhood is that more girls than boys are concerned about being or becoming fat. Girls appear to receive stronger and more consistent messages about the importance of having the "right" body than do boys, particularly from peers and media. The effects of such messages may be particularly pronounced among those girls who more readily compare their own appearance to that of others.

Even these modest conclusions can only be considered tentative, however. Most studies have employed cross-sectional designs and thus have looked at age group differences rather than age-related changes. Many studies have included only girls among their participants, and the vast majority of research has been done with all white samples. Thus even the simplest demographic questions are unresolved.

When the focus shifts to etiology and outcome, the situation is even murkier. Again, most of the etiological research, which is already very limited, involves cross-sectional concurrent data rather than prospective longitudinal designs. It is impossible to adequately assess causal relationships with the available data.

Any future research needs to acknowledge the possibility, perhaps even probability, of gender and ethnic group differences not only in levels of body dissatisfaction but, more importantly, in the process of body image development. There is evidence to suggest that sociocultural factors, including peer and media messages, help to shape body image development. If this is true, then groups that experience different levels, types, and interactions of sociocultural influences are likely to develop body image differently. Furthermore, while most of the body image research focuses on weight and shape concerns, other body-related factors, such as athletic competence, may mediate the relationship between etiological factors and body image. So, for example, the higher levels of athletic self-esteem found among boys may help to explain why they are less invested in appearance than are girls. Describing and understanding these links are primary challenges for future research.

INFORMATIVE READINGS

Cohane, G., & Pope, H. (2001). Body image in boys: A review of the literature. *International Journal of Eating Disorders, 29,* 373–379.—Most studies reviewed in this article deal with adolescents; however, important methodological issues concerning assessment of body image among boys are also raised.

Field, A., Camargo, C., Taylor, C., Berkey, C., Frazier, L., Gilman, M., & Colditz, G. (1999). Overweight, weight concerns, and bulimic behaviors among girls and boys. *Journal of the American Academy of Child and Adolescent Psychiatry, 38,* 754–760.—One of the few large-scale studies investigating body image in both boys and girls.

Martin, G., Wertheim, E., Prior, M., Smart, D., Sanson, A., & Oberklaid, F. (2000). A longitudinal study of the role of childhood temperament in the later development of eating concerns. *International Journal of Eating Disorders, 27,* 150–162.—One of the few longitudinal studies of possible childhood etiological factors of adolescent eating problems.

Ricciardelli, L., & McCabe, M. (2001). Children's body image concerns and eating disturbance: A review of the literature. *Clinical Psychology Review, 21,* 325–344.—This is a thorough review of the etiology and outcomes of body image concerns reported by children.

Smolak, L. (1999). Elementary school curricula for the primary prevention of eating problems. In N. Piran, M. P. Levine, & C. Steiner-Adair (Eds.), *Preventing eating disorders: A handbook of interventions and special challenges* (pp. 85–104). Philadelphia: Brunner/ Mazel.—This chapter considers the importance of, and approaches to, the prevention of body image and eating problems among elementary schoolchildren.

Smolak, L., & Levine, M. P. (2001). Body image in children. In J. K. Thompson & L. Smolak (Eds.), *Body image, eating disorders, and obesity in youth: Assessment, prevention, and treatment* (pp. 41–66). Washington, DC: American Psychological Association.—This chapter reviews research on the etiology and outcomes of childhood body image, including a brief presentation of longitudinal data linking elementary school body image to later body image and eating disorders.

Thompson, J. K., & Smolak, L. (2001). *Body image, eating disorders, and obesity in youth: Assessment, prevention, and treatment.* Washington, DC: American Psychological Association.—This book contains review chapters covering a variety of issues related to body image in children, including body image development, ethnic group differences in body image and eating problems, the relationship of sexual abuse to body image, measurement issues, and prevention. Its focus on children and adolescents is unique.

Body Image Development in Adolescence

MICHAEL P. LEVINE
LINDA SMOLAK

Body image is a very important aspect of psychological and interpersonal development in adolescence, particularly for girls. This chapter summarizes the research findings on body image in girls and boys ages 12–17.

No large-scale epidemiological studies have assessed the multidimensional aspects of body image in adolescent girls and boys. However, we do know that approximately 40–70% of adolescent girls are dissatisfied with two or more aspects of their body. Discontentment typically focuses on sites of substantial adipose tissue in the middle or lower body, such as hips, buttocks, stomach, and thighs. In various developed countries, between 50% and 80% of adolescent girls would like to be thinner, and the point prevalence of self-reported dieting varies from 20% to 60%. Thus the widespread nature of weight and shape dissatisfaction in adolescent girls (and adult women) can be fairly characterized as a "normative discontentment." There is little research on the meaning and correlates of positive body image.

Boys and young men also wish to avoid being (or appearing) fat, flabby, or out of shape. However, among boys who are dissatisfied with their weight and shape, at least an equal number, and perhaps considerably more, seek to *gain* weight and to develop bigger upper arms, chests, and shoulders.

DEVELOPMENTAL FACTORS

Age Trends

Pubertal development in girls is accompanied by an average weight gain of 50 pounds. This includes 20–30 pounds of fat, much of it deposited in the hips, thighs, buttocks, and waist. This normal biological process moves most girls away from the dominant white ideal body shape. In contrast, as boys mature physically, their bodies have a greater chance of developing toward the broad-shouldered, tall, and muscular ideal. Longitudinal studies reveal that, for girls, satisfaction with body parts and overall appearance declines significantly over the years 12–15, before leveling off or even increasing slightly in middle and later adolescence. This increase in dissatisfaction appears to be less pronounced and less linked to increasing body mass for African American girls, whereas the increase persists for white girls and is accompanied by an increasing drive for thinness (even after BMI [body mass index] is statistically controlled). The very limited data available for boys suggest either no correlation of body satisfaction with age or a slight dip in early adolescence, followed by a modest increase over middle and late adolescence.

Early Adolescent Transition

Early adolescence is an important period for the development of body image, especially for girls. For girls and boys a number of normative developmental challenges influence, and are influenced by, body image, including pubertal development, emerging sexuality, incipient identity formation, gender role intensification, and exploring realistic possibilities for success in various realms.

In general, this transition is more stressful for girls than boys because girls confront more of these demands (e.g., pubertal weight gains, dating, the move to middle school) simultaneously or in rapid sequence. Additionally, girls as a group experience more limited options for success in careers and in sports, more threatening sexual harassment and abuse, and other reminders of lower status. All these experiences increase insecurity, limit confidence, and increase a girl's tendency to define herself in terms of the social and economic value of her body.

Girls' development through the stages of puberty in early adolescence is associated with increased body mass, a more negative body image, and higher levels of drive for thinness and dieting. Pubertal timing, however, does not consistently correlate with body dissatisfaction, nor has it been shown to consistently predict negative body image in middle or late adolescence. With respect to the impact of synchronous stressors, girls who begin middle school, begin puberty early, and begin dating during the same year report more body dissatisfaction at the time. Furthermore, this disadvantage increases over the middle school period (ages 11–14). A significant minority of girls enters the pubertal transition with weight and shape concerns, an investment in thinness as an important part of beauty and health, and a history of experimenting with dieting. Developmental psychologists have shown that the pubertal transition accentuates previously existing vulnerabilities and problems.

There is far less research on the development of body image in adolescent boys, and this research is inconsistent as to the impact of pubertal timing. Overall it appears that the timing of puberty does not have a strong or lasting effect on boys' body image. More research is needed on body image as a function of actual and perceived pubertal development, gender, and ethnicity. Interestingly, Siegel and colleagues have found that white girls who perceived themselves as early developers felt less positive about their bodies, whereas there was no relationship between white boys' perceived timing and their body image. On the other hand, black girls and black boys who perceived themselves as late developers had a more negative body image.

SOCIAL MARKERS

Gender

There are striking gender differences in body image, even when levels of depression and negative self-esteem are controlled statistically. For example, adolescent girls have a more differentiated body image. They think about and evaluate their bodies in terms of more parts, and they have stronger negative feelings about more individual parts (e.g., hips, face).

Feingold and Mazzella conducted a meta-analysis of gender differences in self-rated physical attractiveness and in global satisfaction with body or appearance. From the 1970s into the mid-1990s there was a significant increase in the tendency of females (relative to males) to have lower ratings, more variable ratings, and an especially poor body image. These disparities were greater in adolescents than in adults, even though adolescent females were rated by observers as being more objectively attractive than adolescent males.

Gender and Ethnicity

In developed countries no ethnic minority group is immune to developing negative body image and disordered eating. Some studies of adolescent girls find no differences across ethnic groups in body dissatisfaction; others find that differences are explained by variability in BMI across ethnic groups or socioeconomic categories. A significant minority of black and Hispanic adolescent girls wants to be thinner, in part because these girls are prone to high rates of obesity while coping with a dominant white culture that idealizes thinness as one form of feminine achievement. Some studies indicate that Asian and Hispanic girls do not differ from white girls in their average dissatisfaction, perhaps because "thin" and "small" are also valued aspects of "femininity" in Hispanic and Asian cultures.

That said, a substantial literature indicates that, compared to white and

Asian American females, and to some extent, Hispanic females, black adolescent females have a higher body mass and are more likely to (1) associate positive characteristics with large, more buxom women; (2) define beauty in terms of "working with what you've got" instead of a narrow range of slender body types; and (3) want to gain weight in order to have more substantial hips, thighs, and buttocks. Although some of these differences reflect positive features of black adolescents' body acceptance, others may contribute to high levels of binge-eating, obesity, diabetes, and high blood pressure among young and middle-aged black women.

The data on ethnicity and body image in adolescent males are quite limited and in need of clarification. For example, several studies suggest that African American boys are more satisfied with their bodies than other ethnic groups. African American boys also tend to have a larger ideal shape, so that when they are dissatisfied, it is because they want to gain rather than lose weight. However, a recent large scale study of male adolescents by Neumark-Sztainer and colleagues found that, compared to white males, all the minority groups (including African American, Asian American, and Hispanic) reported more disordered weight management behavior, such as self-induced vomiting.

BODY IMAGE, ACTUAL BODY MASS, AND PERCEIVED OVERWEIGHT

Many postpubertal females are dissatisfied with their body shape and weight, despite being of "normal" weight or even underweight. The *beliefs* that weight and shape are important and that one is overweight have a strong connection to body dissatisfaction, dieting, and low self-esteem in adolescent girls, regardless of the degree of their actual overweight. For both boys and girls, and across Asian American, Hispanic, black, and white adolescent groups, there is a small but meaningful inverse correlation between an index of body mass and body image. In girls, BMIs prospectively correlated with body dissatisfaction and being teased about one's weight.

BODY IMAGE, HEALTH, AND WELL-BEING

Self-Esteem and Depression

In industrialized cultures, body image, including perception of overall physical appearance, is probably the most important component of an adolescent's global self-esteem. This connection may be stronger during adolescence than in other age periods. In general, negative body image is correlated with various facets of neuroticism, such as low self-esteem, depression, anxiety, fear of negative evaluation, and obsessive–compulsive tendencies.

Moreover, across adolescence, the correlation of body image, self-esteem, and negative affect is significantly greater for girls than boys. This correlation may explain why despondency following interpersonal rejection or failure at school is more likely to find expression in negative body image among females than males. More important, the well-documented tendency for females to be more depressed than males, beginning around age 14, is clearly attributable to the tendency of adolescent females to feel less positively about their changing body's shape and competence. Having a negative body image (independent of BMI) increases the risk of both subsequent depression and sustained depression in adolescent girls.

Dieting and Disordered Eating

In adolescent girls, dissatisfaction with weight, shape, and individual body parts is a moderately strong correlate and predictor of the perceived need to be thinner and the actions of dieting and purging. This finding is true for a variety of ethnic groups. In contrast, even among overweight male adolescents who know they are overweight, a surprisingly small percentage is significantly motivated to lose weight. In combination with other variables (e.g., fear of fat, a commitment to dieting, negative relationship with parents), negative body image in girls is a prospective predictor of subclinical but chronic eating problems across adolescence and into young adulthood. Negative body image, fueled by teasing and adolescent self-consciousness, also motivates some girls and boys to avoid physical activity and to fast, binge-eat, or eat too often. In developed cultures negative body image is an essential link between eating disorders and the growing problems of adolescent and adult obesity.

CULTURAL AND INTERPERSONAL INFLUENCES

Internalization of Dominant Cultural Ideals

In the United States and other patriarchal, industrialized cultures, the attributes that characterize the ideal of feminine beauty are: white, young, tall, firm but not too muscular, and somehow both slender and full-breasted. For adolescent and young adult females, a discrepancy between the mental image of their body and the representation of this ideal is correlated with body dissatisfaction, a tendency to overestimate their body size, depressive affect, and bulimic behavior. Stice found that both internalization of the slender beauty ideal and perceived pressure to be thin (emanating from family, friends, dating partners, and media) predicted significant short-term increases in body dissatisfaction in girls ages 14–17. These factors were also concurrently associated with body dissatisfaction, which in turn predicted increases in dieting and negative affect.

The icon of masculine beauty is harder to define. This suggests that body type and looks in general are less important for self-definition of males, and it certainly means that there is less pressure on males to attain a particular type of physique. Despite this gender difference, short stature and fat are certainly less acceptable characteristics. Some research suggests an increasing preference for a moderate to great degree of well-defined muscularity. The nature and general psychological impact of this cultural change has not been well established. Our own preliminary research indicates that, in general, internalization of a muscular ideal is less correlated with negative body image in young adolescent boys than is internalization of a slender ideal for young girls.

Mass Media

In cultures as diverse as the Ukraine and Fiji, the institution of a market-driven mass media is associated with internalization of the slender beauty ideal and resultant increases in body dissatisfaction among girls. In developed countries mass media such as fashion–entertainment magazines and situation comedies are particularly appealing to adolescent girls ages 11–15. These girls are engaged in a rational struggle to understand the significance of pubertal weight and shape changes in a culture full of confusing messages about female sexuality and female desires, including hunger. For example, how is a girl to accept and value her body when the culture glorifies thinness while offering contradictory encouragement to impulsively consume a wide variety of fattening or otherwise unhealthy foods and beverages?

In early adolescence, girls who consider magazine articles and advertisements to be an important source of information for defining and obtaining the perfect body are more likely to be dissatisfied with their body. Many adolescent girls compare themselves to the slender, glamorous women in magazines and on TV. This "upward" social comparison makes them feel worse about their own weight and shape, especially if they already have a negative body image. Thus, for white adolescent girls, there is a cyclical and destructive process of focusing attention on cultural standards, making social comparisons, and experiencing body dissatisfaction. It is unknown whether these findings apply to different ethnic groups and to boys.

Athletics and Dance

In general, participating in sports and dance improves self-esteem. However, for adolescent girls there is no difference in body satisfaction and disordered eating between athletes and nonathletes. Some sports and forms of dance do encourage preoccupation with a slender shape and weight management in order to gain a competitive edge. Female dancers and female athletes at the highest, elite levels of competition are at significant risk for negative body image and disordered eating. Conversely, adolescent females competing in sports that do not emphasize leanness and who are not at the elite level have more positive body images.

Males involved in sports emphasizing bulk, power, and muscular definition may also be susceptible to negative body image arising from a disparity between self-perceived size (and rate of development) and the steroid-based, hypermuscular ideal featured so prominently in wrestling, action movies, and body-building. This discrepancy sets the stage for the use of worthless or unhealthy "fat-burning" products, as well as for binge-eating, compulsive exercising, abuse of food supplements and steroids, and the emergence of body dysmorphic disorder.

Family Factors

Some studies find that parents' attitudes and behaviors in regard to their own body image are correlated with body image in their adolescent children. Nevertheless, the evidence is too inconsistent to support parental modeling as a key source of social influence on body image. Direct comments about body, weight, and eating are more potent sources of parental influence. Most parents think their children are physically attractive, but as girls proceed through puberty and become adolescents, they receive less praise for their appearance and more criticism.

Across cultures, teasing and other negative verbal comments by family members have both short- and long-term negative effects on body image. Brothers are particularly likely to be perpetrators, and the face, head, and weight of females are the most likely targets. Although larger, heavier girls are more likely to be teased, teasing is a strong predictor of body dissatisfaction independent of BMI. There is a cumulative effect in that teasing has a more negative impact on those who are already anxious and self-conscious about their bodies.

A significant minority of girls is subject to sexual abuse within the family. In early adolescence girls are particularly vulnerable to sexual abuse and sexual harassment from family and peers. The consequences of sexual abuse—anxiety, shame, and loss of control over one's body—clearly contribute to negative body image, weight concerns, and disordered eating. (See chapter by Fallon and Ackard in this volume.)

Peers

Appearance and attractiveness are especially important topics for girls as they make the transition from childhood to adolescence. A significant percentage of adolescent girls talk with friends at least occasionally about weight, shape, and dieting. Although direct encouragement by girls to diet and direct, public comments about others' girls bodies are rare, exchanging information about weight control is common, as is "fat talk," in which girls voice their anxieties about being or becoming "fat." These exchanges provide an intimate, powerful context for learning and consolidating body disparagement. In this regard, there is evidence that girls who are best friends and who are part of friendship groups have similar levels of body image concerns, drive for thinness, and dietary restraint. Male and female peers also tease each other, and boys are more likely than girls to make critical, harassing comments to girls and boys about weight and shape. There is a strong, concurrent, and predictive relationship between this type of negative verbal commentary and body dissatisfaction.

Multiple Sources of Objectification

Females in developed countries receive a clear message from multiple sources that the female body, much more so than the male body, is to be looked at, evaluated, possessed by men, and, in general, treated as an object. White adolescent girls ages 12–14 who reported receiving more messages from peers, family, and mass media about weight and shape have very high levels of body dissatisfaction and disordered eating.

FUTURE RESEARCH DIRECTIONS

Given that body image is profoundly influenced by cultural ideals and social experiences, it should be possible to prevent or minimize negative body image. Research suggests that prevention programs for girls ages 12–17 can have a positive *short-term* effect on knowledge of cultural determinants, on body image, on healthy attitudes (e.g., a reduced drive for thinness), and on eating behaviors. However, achievement of long-term behavioral changes and full prevention effects remains an elusive goal. The limited research on the prevention and treatment of negative body image in adolescents is reviewed in later chapters.

A vast literature on the development of weight and shape concerns and disordered eating in adolescents is currently available. For adolescents more so than for children, body image is a multidimensional construct embedded in the larger, integrative construct of identity. Consequently, there is a clear need for psychologists and other mental health professionals to expand the scope of their research on this construct. We need more data and better integration of existing studies in regard to the impact on body image of phenomena such as acne, breast development for girls, male sexual development, physical ability in athletics and recreation, tattoos and body piercings, and diseases such as asthma and type 1 diabetes.

INFORMATIVE READINGS

Feingold, A., & Mazzella, R. (1998). Gender differences in body image are increasing. *Psychological Science, 9,* 190–195.—Statistical and theoretical review of the literature (excluding differences in perceived vs. ideal size) on female versus male differences in appearance esteem and self-rated attractiveness.

Graber, J. A., Petersen, A. C., & Brooks-Gunn, J. (1996). Pubertal processes: Methods, measures, and models. In J. A. Graber, J. Brooks-Gunn, & A. C. Petersen (Eds.), *Transitions through adolescence: Interpersonal domains and context* (pp. 23–53). Mahwah, NJ: Erlbaum.—Concise introduction to the study of puberty in girls and boys, including its impact on body image.

Neumark-Sztainer, D., Story, M., Falkner, N. H., Beuhring, T., & Resnick, M. D. (1999). Sociodemographic and personal characteristics of adolescents engaged in weight loss and weight/muscle gain behaviors: Who is doing what? *Preventive Medicine, 28,* 40–50.—Survey of dieting, exercising, unhealthy weight management, weightlifting, and steroid use among over 9,000 adolescent boys and girls from various ethnic backgrounds.

Pope, Jr., H. G., Phillips, K. A., & Olivardia, R. (2000). *The Adonis complex: The secret crisis of male body obsession.* New York: Free Press.—Blends research, clinical observations, and cultural commentary into a theory about ways in which changes in Western ideals of masculine beauty are creating significant body image problems in males.

Siegel, J. M., Yancey, A. K., Aneshensel, C. S., & Schuler, R. (1999). Body image, perceived pubertal timing, and adolescent mental health. *Journal of Adolescent Health, 25,* 155–165.—This large-scale, methodologically sophisticated study elucidates the relationship between body image and depression in girls, as well as the nature of positive body image among African American girls and boys.

Smolak, L., & Levine, M. P. (1996). Adolescent transitions and the development of eating problems. In L. Smolak, M. P. Levine, & R. Striegel-Moore (Eds.), *The developmental psychopathology of eating disorders: Implications for research, prevention, and treatment* (pp. 207–233). Mahwah, NJ: Erlbaum.—Uses a review of research on girls' body image and disordered eating to construct vulnerability–stressor models of risk at the early and late adolescent transitions.

Thompson, J. K., Heinberg, L. J., Altabe, M., & Tantleff-Dunn, S. (1999). *Exacting beauty: Theory, assessment, and treatment of body image disturbance.* Washington, DC: American Psychological Association.—Analyzes the cultural, social, and individual factors that influence body image and offers a model for directing further treatment and further research.

Thompson, J. K., & Smolak, L. (Eds.). (2001). *Body image, eating disorders, and obesity in youth: Assessment, prevention, and treatment.* Washington, DC: American Psychological Association.—Reviews many topics pertaining to body image and disordered eating in children and adolescents, including risk factors, gender, ethnicity, and prevention.

10

Body Image Development
Adulthood and Aging

SUSAN KRAUSS WHITBOURNE
KARYN M. SKULTETY

The concept of body image holds important promise for understanding fundamental issues of aging and identity. Yet, body image has not received much attention in the gerontological literature. While much research has been done to elucidate the self as an abstract concept, little scholarly or empirical research exists on how individuals respond to the physical changes constantly occurring throughout adulthood. This chapter explores how identity process theory can help us better understand how adults conceptualize the self as both a mental and physical entity.

COMPONENTS OF BODY IMAGE IN ADULTHOOD

Although most people regard themselves as having completed physical development by their teenage years, the fact is that the body continuously changes up until death. Evaluating how people react to changes in body shape, appearance, and functioning is central to fully understanding psychological adaptation throughout adulthood.

Three components of body image requiring evaluation in adulthood are appearance, competence, and physical health. Physical appearance provides many important external cues to the self and others, including information regarding age and attractiveness. The internal feelings of body competence are based, in part, on the physical sensations associated with aging, including feelings of agility, endurance, and power. The experience of physical health or disease has profound implications for quality of life (e.g., experiencing pain or weakness) and dramatically influences an individual's thoughts and feelings about the end of life.

NORMAL AGE-RELATED BODILY CHANGES

Changes in appearance due to aging, such as wrinkling and sagging of the skin, loss of height, and redistribution of body fat from the extremities to the torso, are universal. Physical competence is affected by loss of muscle strength and aerobic capacity at a rate of 1% per year. Bones become weaker and more brittle, and joints can become painful and stiff. Additionally, the respiratory system becomes less efficient, and bladder expandability decreases. There are alterations in hormonal function (especially evident in women), sleep patterns, and decreased ability to tolerate extreme temperature fluctuations. Mental functions, including working memory, attention, and decision making, are affected by changes in the brain. (However, Alzheimer's disease is relatively uncommon; 5–7% of the over-65.) Some diseases appear to be overestimated, such as gastrointestinal disorders, which are more related to dietary practices than intrinsic age-related changes. Nonetheless, many health-related changes do occur in conjunction with the aging process.

PREVENTION AND COMPENSATION

In virtually all areas of the body, compensation and especially prevention play important roles in minimizing the effects of aging. For example, losses in aerobic capacity and muscular strength can be cut in half by participating in regular aerobic exercise. Memory losses can be compensated by mnemonic strategies, and changes in information processing that would affect decision making, problem solving, and intelligence are generally more than offset by increased experience. The quality of "wisdom" may emerge in late life, as individuals gain greater understanding of how to resolve practical and interpersonal problems that affect the psychological well-being of themselves and others.

　　Through the actions they take, individuals can either slow down or accelerate the aging process. In the case of physical appearance, for instance, individuals can alter the rate at which they experience photoaging, the damaging effect of ultraviolet rays on the skin. It is well known that adults who use preventive measures (including sunscreen) show a slower rate of facial wrinkling than those who do not. Therefore, one of the most significant outward signs of aging can be mitigated through actions taken by the individual. Similarly, there is a wide range of preventive actions adults can take, starting in young adulthood and continuing throughout life, to minimize changes within the body. The most successful of these is aerobic exercise. A convincing array of findings testifies to the benefits of active participation in an aerobic exercise program. In addition to its effects on the body, involvement in exercise can promote positive self-esteem, as shown in research by Shaw and collaborators. A sense of self-efficacy may develop as the result of exercise participation, further enhancing the older individual's self-perception of physical attractiveness, as shown by McCauley and associates.

The effects of exercise, among other preventive measures, also benefit physical health and reduce the likelihood of chronic disease. Thus, preventive measures can be employed to control, to some degree, the rate at which both aging and disease progress, and to maintain a positive (i.e., healthy and competent) internal body image.

IDENTITY PROCESS THEORY

What determines whether individuals engage in preventive and compensatory activities that offset the effects of aging and maintain a positive body image? Identity process theory proposes that those adults who maintain a consistent sense of the self over time, while making behavioral and psychological adjustments to the aging process, are most likely to take advantage of methods of prevention and compensation for age-related changes in physical functioning. Identity process theory proposes that the adult's sense of identity is composed of feelings about physical, psychological, and social functioning.

Two mechanisms are involved in the way that the individual's identity interacts with the aging process. In the process of identity assimilation, the individual attempts to maintain a consistent view of the self when interpreting an age-related experience, such as detecting wrinkles in the face. The importance of the experience is minimized, and the individual does not give it a great deal of thought. Certainly the experience does not cause a shift in identity. In the process of identity accommodation, the experience overwhelms the individual and causes a reexamination or redefinition of the sense of self. Wrinkles may set off alarms that one's face, if not body, is getting "old." In the ideal state, the individual's sense of self remains relatively stable, even while incorporating information about the aging process into that sense of self. This is the process of identity balance, which is theorized to be positively related to a favorable view of the self, or high self-esteem.

According to identity process theory, there are risks attached to over-reliance on either identity assimilation or accommodation. Individuals who use identity assimilation exclusively are likely to deny or ignore signs of aging to which they *should* pay attention. Because they define themselves as "young," they do not see the relevance of using preventive or compensatory measures. On the other hand, they might become very involved in exercise programs designed to maintain their youthful appearance, though without reflecting on their reasons for participating in such programs. However, as long as they take advantage of behavioral strategies to maintain their physical health and functioning, they might avoid the negative outcomes that would otherwise occur.

Individuals who rely exclusively on identity accommodation are more likely to suffer negative consequences of the aging process. These individuals prematurely define themselves as "old" and "over the hill." They will be unlikely to regard exercise or other forms of prevention and compensation as holding hope for having beneficial effects. Another possibility is that they adopt the identity of "old person" and become preoccupied with their aging and health problems. Rather than take advantage of exercise or other preventive measures, they are likely to worry excessively and perhaps overmedicate themselves. Identity assimilation may therefore be a more favorable approach to the aging process, at least in terms of preserving feelings of well-being and a positive body image.

Research by Whitbourne and Collins on identity processes in adulthood has confirmed that there is a positive relationship between identity balance and self-esteem across the adult years. However, identity assimilation also relates positively to self-esteem, particularly with regard to appearance, and particularly for women, as we have found subsequently. For women, not thinking about the meaning of age-related bodily changes seems to be a favorable way of preserving self-esteem. This is not to say necessarily that denial is the optimal strategy, but that acknowledging changes, without giving great thought to their psychological meaning, seems to preserve self-esteem. This process may be particularly important as a way of insulating older adult women from the bias and stereotypes they face regarding society's views of the attractiveness and desirability of aging females (see below). In addition, by maintaining their identities, women may be more likely to continue to engage in activities that make them feel more satisfied with their bodies.

Wilcox found a positive relationship between age and body satisfaction in women who engaged in exercise, and a negative relationship in those who did not. By continuing to engage in exercise, these women are not allowing age-related physical changes to limit their activities. In this way, they maintain their existing identities and are able to feel satisfied with their bodies. In contrast, those women who do not engage in exercise may be accommodating or even overly accommodating age-related changes, such that they come to believe that their bodies are less competent and attractive—

which, in turn, leads them to experience less bodily satisfaction and, presumably, lower self-esteem. Unfortunately, throughout adulthood women are more likely than men to engage in identity accommodation, thus placing women at greater risk for the doubts and questions about their identities that can lower their self-esteem. However, in later adulthood, and particularly with regard to the aging body, women seem to be better able to use identity assimilation to maintain a stable identity and thereby boost their feelings of self-worth. Franzoi and Koehler found that although men have more positive body images than women in both older and younger age groups, the gender difference becomes less pronounced for those over the age of 65. Thus identity assimilation may be aiding older women to incorporate age-related changes into their existing identities, rather than becoming discouraged and feeling negatively about themselves.

Although men may be less likely to suffer from the negative effects of aging on body image with regard to outward appearance, they may be more vulnerable to the effects of aging on bodily competence and health. Because they are less likely to use identity accommodation than are women, they may be unable to make the changes that are necessary to adapt their body image to the effects of aging on their strength, mobility, and endurance. Although using identity assimilation may prevent men from becoming depressed, it will also increase their chances of experiencing age-related deleterious changes in the functioning and health of their bodies. Should they then experience a sudden loss of functioning or disease onset, for example, through a stroke or heart attack, they may be required to use identity accommodation to adapt and, in response, feel hopeless and despondent by the change in their identities. Eventually, if they are able to regain a sense of balance, they should be able to move forward and incorporate changes in their bodily functioning into their identity and simultaneously embark on a sensible program of exercise and dietary control.

One area, in particular, in which older adult men may be particularly vulnerable is that of sexual functioning. Men who experience sexuality as an important part of their physical identity and who are unaware of the normal effects of aging on sexual function may place themselves at risk for developing secondary impotence, which is a condition of erectile dysfunction resulting from psychogenic rather than physical causes. Because they are not used to accommodating, they are unable to use this process of adjusting when they encounter an occasional episode of erectile dysfunction. The episode leads them to conclude the worst—that they have lost their sexual potency. In this case, it is likely that identity assimilation, in which the older man dismisses or minimizes the significance of such an episode, would be a preferable response. Of course, if there is a physical and treatable problem underlying the dysfunction, it is advantageous for the man to accommodate or react in a balanced manner by seeking medical attention.

SOCIAL CONTEXT AND THE AGING BODY IMAGE

Society's definitions of desirable female and male attributes play a large role in influencing the way in which aging individuals interpret changes in physical functioning. For women, social attitudes of aging women as unattractive cause them to regard the outward appearance of their aging bodies in a negative manner. Allaz and colleagues found that many older women continue to engage in dieting, despite being at a normal weight. This finding reflects the continued pressure felt by women to lose weight. For men, physical strength is valued as a male attribute, and therefore loss of muscle strength and agility has the potential to cause older men to feel that they are weak and useless. For both sexes, social attitudes toward death and dying create an environment in which it becomes difficult to acknowledge the changes associated with the aging process that bring the individual closer to death. In addition, media portrayals of older adults as suffering from the mental incompetence of Alzheimer's disease further prey on the fears of older adults that they will lose their dignity and independence. Self-acceptance and a positive body image are thus difficult to achieve for both women and men but for somewhat different reasons.

Do older adult women and men, in fact, have negative body images? As discussed above, the process of identity balance protects older individuals from the negative self-evaluations that would otherwise accompany the aging of the physical self. As reported in the 1999 volume of *Health, United States*, the majority of older adults do *not* express negative self-evaluations of their health, well-being, or ability to carry out the tasks of daily life. It would seem, then, that the identity processes are working well. On the other hand, it is possible that older adults have become immune to the evidence presented by their own bodies that they are "losing" (as socially defined) their attractiveness, strength, and health. There is evidence that middle-aged individuals are more sensitive to fears of aging than are the older adults who are actually experiencing the effects of the aging process.

In addition to the possibility that aging brings with it a more relaxed and accepting view of physical changes is the idea that the current cohort of older adults never was as concerned about their bodily functioning and appearance as is the current cohort of middle-aged individuals. The so-called "baby boomers" are reaching middle adulthood at a time in history when youth and beauty are revered more than ever. Furthermore, this generation has dominated the social and cultural landscape since their coming of age in the 1960s. Having defined the social standards in which youth is the pinnacle, it may be particularly difficult for this generation to accept the fact that changes happen within their bodies due to forces outside their control. On the other hand, current cohorts of middle-aged individuals, at least those with higher levels of education, have embraced the values of exercise and dietary control. Therefore, they may be less likely to experience the challenges to identity presented by changes observed among historically less fit older cohorts.

THE FUTURE OF AGING AND BODY IMAGE RESEARCH

Clearly, more systematic investigation of the body image in middle-aged and older adults is needed. Research in the area of physical identity provides some insight into the inner experience of older adults, as they experience the changes in the functioning and efficiency of their body's systems. Moreover, it is clear that the aging experience, at least in contemporary society, is different for women and men. Whether or not future generations of older persons will "age better," the issue of the effects of aging on body image remains one of great fascination for those who study the aging process. Ultimately, aging presents the greatest challenge to the individual's sense of the integrity of the physical self.

INFORMATIVE READINGS

Allaz, A. F., Bernstein, M., Rouget, P., Archinard, M., & Morabia, A. (1998). Body weight preoccupation in middle-age and ageing women: A general population survey. *International Journal of Eating Disorders, 23,* 287–294.—Examines dieting behavior in women across age groups.

Cash, T. F., & Henry, P. E. (1995). Women's body images: The results of a national survey in the U.S.A. *Sex Roles, 33,* 19–28.—Examines women's body satisfaction across age groups and looks at differences among African American and Caucasian groups.

Franzoi, S. L., & Koehler, V. (1998). Age and gender differences in body attitudes: A comparison of young and elderly adults. *International Journal of Aging and Human Development, 47,* 1–10.—Compares men and women of different age groups in degree of body esteem, exercise behavior, and body satisfaction.

McAuley, E., Blissmer, B., Katula, J., Duncan, T. E., & Mihalko, S. L. (2000). Physical activity, self-esteem, and self-efficacy relationships in older adults: A randomized controlled trial. *Annals of Behavioral Medicine, 22,* 131–139.—One of the few controlled studies examining the relationships among exercise, self-efficacy, and perceptions of physical attractiveness.

McKinley, N. M. (1999). Women and objectified body consciousness: Mothers' and daughters' body experience in cultural, developmental, and familial context. *Developmental Psychology, 35,* 760–769.—Examines age-related differences in women in how they have incorporated society's emphasis on appearance in themselves and how it relates to self-esteem.

National Center for Health Statistics. (1999). *Health, United States 1999.* Hyattsville MD: National Center for Health Statistics.—Annual publication presenting survey data on how older adults feel about their physical abilities.

Pliner, P., Chaiken, S., & Flett, G. L. (1990). Gender differences in concern with body weight and physical appearance over the life span. *Personality and Social Psychology*

Bulletin, 16, 263–273.—First study including older adults in examining gender differences in body image, eating, and self-esteem.

Shaw, J. M., Ebbeck, V., & Snow, C. M. (2000). Body composition and physical self-concept in older women. *Journal of Women and Aging, 12,* 59–75.—Examines the effects of changes in body mass (as the result of involvement in weight-bearing exercise) on self-esteem among women.

Thompson, S. C., Thomas, C., Rickabaugh, C. A., Tantamjarik, P., Otsuki, T., Pan, D., Garcia, B. F., & Sinar, E. (1998). Primary and secondary control over age-related changes in physical appearance. *Journal of Personality, 66,* 583–605.—Examines coping strategies that involve control processes in men and women in response to appearance and physical changes.

Tiggemann, M., & Lynch, J. E. (2001). Body image across the life span in adult women: The role of self-objectification. *Developmental Psychology, 37,* 243–253.—Presents model on body satisfaction and body monitoring in women to explain stability of body satisfaction despite changes in body mass index.

Whitbourne, S. K., & Collins, K. C. (1998). Identity and physical changes in later adulthood: Theoretical and clinical implications. *Psychotherapy, 35,* 519–530.—Presents identity theory and the relationship between self-esteem and identity processes in various realms of physical functioning and appearance.

Wilcox, S. (1997). Age and gender in relation to body attitudes: Is there a double standard of aging? *Psychology of Women Quarterly, 21,* 549–565.—Examines gender differences in body attitudes during aging and the role exercise plays in these attitudes.

Media Influences on Body Image Development

MARIKA TIGGEMANN

The mass media pervade the everyday lives of people living in Western societies. Most adults read newspapers daily, and magazines have huge circulations. Media surveys indicate that fashion magazines, in particular, are read by the majority of women and girls (estimates up to 83%). Virtually every home has a television set, switched on for an average of 7 hours per day, with individuals each watching 3 or 4 hours. Over a year, children and adolescents spend more time watching television than in any activity other than sleeping. Such high consumption is likely to affect the consumers in some way. This chapter describes the influences of various media on body image development and difficulties.

AVENUES OF INFLUENCE

Media Content

There is no doubt that current societal standards for female beauty inordinately emphasize the desirability of thinness—and thinness at a level that is impossible for most women to achieve by healthy means. In their pervasiveness, the mass media are powerful conveyors of this sociocultural ideal. A casual flick through any fashion magazine reveals a preponderance of young, tall, long-legged, and extremely thin women. Formal content analyses of visual media document this trend toward thinness in all of women's magazines, film, and television (including children's television). It has been argued that this media presentation of thin images as the ideal is a major contributor to current high levels of body dissatisfaction and eating disorders in women.

For men, there is evidence that the cultural norm for the ideal body has become increasingly muscular during the 1990s, with some male ideals exceeding the upper limit of muscularity attainable without the use of anabolic steroids. Young, lean, and muscled male bodies are becoming more common in fashion magazines and advertising. Thus men and boys are also increasingly subject to media images that prescribe an ideal body shape: in their case, mesomorphic, broad shouldered, well-developed upper body, flat stomach, and narrow hips.

Influence Processes

The media's omnipresent idealized depiction of thin female figures may influence women's body image in a number of ways. Similar processes potentially operate in mediating the influence of muscular ideals in men. In increasing scope of influence, these processes include social comparison, internalization of the thin ideal, and investment in appearance for self-evaluation. When women compare their body with an image presented in the media, they almost invariably find themselves wanting. Repeated exposure to such images may lead women to internalize the thin ideal such that it becomes accepted by them as the reference point against which to judge themselves. Furthermore, thin ideals are not offered in a void but rather as part of complex cultural scripts that link thinness and attractiveness to happiness, desirability, and status. Acceptance of this cultural schema—that appearance and thinness are absolutely vital for success and happiness—means that self-worth becomes equated with a woman or girl's self-perceived attractiveness. Thus appearance becomes a core basis of self-evaluation, with self-worth contingent on meeting the societal ideals. This schema is likely to exert particular salience in adolescence, when the major developmental task is the establishment of identity and when puberty moves girls away from, rather than toward, the thin ideal.

These three processes have perceptual, affective, cognitive, and behavioral consequences for body image. There may be perceptual distortion whereby women view themselves as fat when they are not. In the affective realm, the failure to meet important but unrealistic size and weight goals leads to body dissatisfaction and negative mood. In the cognitive domain, investment in appearance as the central criterion of self-evaluation results in selective attention to appearance messages. In terms of behavior, women typically pursue the thin ideal through dieting or other weight loss measures. Indeed, studies confirm that social comparison, internalization of the thin ideal, and investment in appearance are related to body dissatisfaction and disturbed eating in adult and adolescent women and girls as young as 8.

Not only do media influence behavior indirectly, they also offer explicit instruction on how to attain the beauty ideal. Leading women's magazines contain a large number of diet and exercise articles. In accord with the muscular male ideal, advertisements and articles in men's magazines focus more on changing body shape than losing weight. These all promote the belief that people can, and indeed should, control their body shape and weight. The methods (and accompanying beliefs) are also taught implicitly through modeling and vicarious reinforcement. An analysis of prime-time situation comedies found that 12% of female characters dieted, with many making negative comments about themselves.

EMPIRICAL EVIDENCE OF MEDIA EFFECTS ON BODY IMAGE

A number of different evidentiary sources—women's own accounts, correlational studies of media exposure, and experimental studies of the immediate impact of idealized images—converges to provide strong evidence for a link between the images presented in the media and women's negative body experience.

Perceived Media Pressure

Certainly women themselves say that their body image is adversely affected by idealized images portrayed in the media. For example, in Garner's large 1997 survey of 4,000 readers of the magazine *Psychology Today*, nearly half the women (and one-third of the men) reported that very thin or muscular magazine models make them feel insecure and want to lose weight. In open-ended interviews with young women, the media and fashion models are spontaneously nominated as the most potent source of the pressure to be thin; disclosures are usually accompanied by considerable anger, frustration, and hurt. Women with diagnosed eating disorders also often point to the models in fashion magazines as a trigger for their disorder.

A large prospective study of more than 12,000 children, ages 9–14 years, demonstrated that media involvement actually preceded the development of weight concerns. Alison Field and her colleagues found that both girls and boys who reported making considerable effort to look like their same-sex figures in the media were more likely than their peers to have become very concerned about their weight over a 1-year period. For girls, these efforts were also predictive of beginning to purge at least monthly, and for boys, of starting to think frequently about wanting bigger muscles.

Media Exposure and Body Image

A number of studies has examined the relationship between women's body image and independently assessed indicators of media exposure, such as frequency of magazine reading or hours spent watching television. Both composite and specific measures of media use are correlated with a variety of body image indices, including body dissatisfaction, perceptions of overweight, and eating disorder symptomatology. More sophisticated statistical modeling by Stice and his colleagues found a direct link between media exposure and eating disorder symptoms, as well as an indirect pathway between internalization of the thin-ideal standard and the experience of body dissatisfaction.

However, other studies have found no relationship or inconsistent relationships. In one study, magazine reading but not television exposure was related to eating disorder symptomatology, with the opposite pattern for body dissatisfaction. Studies of adolescent girls find that time spent watching specific programs, particularly music videos, rather than total television-watching time, is related to weight and appearance concerns. Music videos may be a potent source of modeling; content analyses reveal high levels of eroticism and sex role stereotyping, with women usually depicted as thin, beautiful, and often scantily clad.

As a whole, the research supports a link between media exposure and body image. However, effect sizes are small and dependent on the specific measures. Although these results are generally taken to support the position that exposure to a large dose of idealized images leads to negative body experience, the converse causal assumption is equally plausible: That is, those women and girls who are most dissatisfied or invested in appearance seek out particular media content. This assumption is particularly likely in regard to the consumption of those types of media such as fashion magazines (and perhaps music videos) that offer explicit depictions of beauty and instruction on appearance enhancement, but less likely for television programs such as situation comedies and movies where thin ideal messages are implicit.

Experimental Studies

In an attempt to determine the direction of causation, several experiments have manipulated exposure to idealized images of thinness and assessed the immediate impact. Although an earlier comprehensive review by Levine and Smolak concluded that there was little support for the proposition that viewing photographs of thin models makes girls and women immediately feel worse about their bodies, a sizeable amount of research demonstrating negative impact has accumulated.

Brief exposure to print media images of thin female models from fashion magazines has been shown to produce a number of immediate negative effects, including greater concern about weight, body dissatisfaction, self-consciousness, negative mood, and decreased perception of self-attractiveness. Some studies have found effects only for some groups of women— those who are heavier, more concerned with self-presentation, and have high levels of trait–body dissatisfaction. In one study similar effects were found for men exposed to photographs of stereotypically attractive male fashion models, although the response was less than that of the female participants.

Given the ubiquity of television, it is surprising that there have been fewer studies of exposure to televised images. Among studies that compared the effects of appearance-related commercials (containing women who epitomize societal ideals of thinness and beauty) with non-appearance-related commercials, four out of five experiments reported negative consequences for at least some participants: specifically, greater anger, anxiety, depressed mood, and appearance dissatisfaction; more self-to-model comparisons; and self-perception of increased body size. Similar negative effects on body image have been found for appearance messages presented in auditory (radio-like) format.

Although not all women are equally affected, there is now sufficient evidence to conclude that brief exposure to idealized media images (less than one night's television viewing or a single issue of a fashion magazine) does have short-term deleterious effects on mood and body satisfaction. It seems likely that naturally occurring episodes of brief media exposure serve continually to maintain and reinforce levels of insecurity and concern about shape and weight.

INDIVIDUAL DIFFERENCES

The pervasiveness of the media ensures that nearly all girls and women are exposed to a substantial dose of idealized images of thinness and beauty, yet not all develop extreme preoccupation with their weight and only a minority develops clinically diagnosable eating disorders. Similarly, the experimental studies show that not all women are equally vulnerable to adverse effects when exposed to media images. These studies have identified a number of individual characteristics that determine or moderate responsiveness to media images: weight (heavier women are more negatively affected by media images), disordered-eating symptomatology, trait–body dissatisfaction, self-consciousness, a tendency toward social comparison, and high dispositional levels of internalization regarding thinness ideals.

Some body image researchers have suggested that this list of characteristics can be subsumed under the concept of "appearance schematicity." *Appearance schemas* refer to cognitive structures concerning appearance that organize and determine the processing of self-relevant information. People for whom appearance is crucial and integral to the self-concept ("appearance schematics") selectively attend to the appearance-related aspects of any presented material. In particular, their more complex and highly developed appearance schemas are readily activated by idealized media images. This hypothesis was confirmed in two experiments, which found that appearance schematic women suffered greater negative consequences of media exposure than did their aschematic peers. In sum, the research indicates that it is those women already most heavily invested in their appearance who are the most vulnerable to the effects of idealized media images. This suggests a downward spiral in which negative body image is exacerbated by further exposure to idealized media images. Conversely, those women with low investment in their appearance are relatively immune to media effects.

UNANSWERED RESEARCH QUESTIONS

At a practical level, there is an urgent need for systematic research in several areas. Media impact on the body image of men and boys awaits investigation; the lean but muscular male ideal increasingly portrayed in advertising and other media may be as harmful for men as thin ideals are for women. In another arena, most of the experimental research has been conducted with college students. Similar research with adolescents and children should focus on identifying the variables that mediate and moderate the potentially adverse effects of exposure to idealized images of thinness for young people.

At a theoretical level, identifying the causal direction of media effects remains a challenge. The experimental studies show that brief exposure to idealized thin media images of thinness does have short-term deleterious consequences. Here the causal direction is clear: *from* media *to* body image (moderated by various individual characteristics). Unfortunately, however, this research finding does not address the development of body image, which necessarily takes place over time. Naturally occurring media exposure cannot be manipulated experimentally. What is required to clarify the media's role is *prospective research* that traces the development of both variables (body image and media exposure) over time, as well as their relationship to the mediating processes of internalization and investment in appearance. Most likely, the media play multiple and differing roles at different times in the development process. Ideally, to capture important developmental transitions, such investigations should begin in early childhood and proceed through late adolescence.

CLINICAL IMPLICATIONS FOR TREATMENT AND PREVENTION

The evidence shows that media images contribute to negative body image. The most obvious preventive strategy would be to reduce exposure to idealized images of thinness by encouraging the media to present a wider and more realistic range of female body shapes as acceptable and even beautiful.

Surveys indicate that women and girls, as well as more formal advocacy groups, are calling for this change. However, economic pressures make it unlikely that such input will be heeded in the short-term. Women and girls can also reduce their own exposure to potentially damaging images, for example, by not buying or reading fashion magazines.

An alternative strategy is to equip young people with media literacy skills that make them resistant to media images. These skills need to go beyond the ability to recognize airbrushing and other image distortion techniques. Young people need to be able to think critically, to deconstruct the images and messages presented to them—specifically, those glorifying slenderness and harmful practices such as dieting. To be successful as a preventive measure, such media literacy needs to begin in childhood, before beauty ideals are internalized and appearance becomes crucial for self-evaluation.

Further, the moderators identified by the experimental work (e.g., appearance schematicity) offer targets for intervention in the treatment of women with negative body image. Cognitive-behavioral techniques challenging underlying assumptions that appearance is central to identity can be used to reduce investment in appearance, self-monitoring, and comparison with others' bodies. These approaches do not attack the media directly but do serve to make people less vulnerable to negative effects of media images.

Research shows that the media are a potent force in the development of body image. In principle, then, it should be equally possible to use the media to promote a positive body image. Large-scale media-based interventions promoting healthy body image have the potential to reach farther and have greater impact than other methods.

INFORMATIVE READINGS

Berel, S., & Irving, L. M. (1998). Media and disturbed eating: An analysis of media influence and implications for prevention. *Journal of Primary Prevention, 18,* 415–430.—A review of media effects, including a feminist perspective.

Field, A. E., Camargo, C. A., Taylor, C. B., Berkey, C. S., Roberts, S. B., & Colditz, G. A. (2001). Peer, parent, and media influences on the development of weight concerns and frequent dieting among preadolescent and adolescent girls and boys. *Pediatrics, 107,* 54–60.—One of several reports on a large prospective cohort study.

Garner, D. M. (1997, January/February). The 1997 Body Image Survey results. *Psychology Today,* 30–44, 75–80, 84.—A survey of 4,000 people showing widespread body dissatisfaction.

Grogan, S. (1999). *Body image.* London: Routledge.—Contains a review of media effects on body image, including original research (Chapter 5).

Hargreaves, D., & Tiggemann, M. (2002). The effect of television commercials on mood and body dissatisfaction: The role of appearance-schema activation. *Journal of Social and Clinical Psychology, 21,* 328–349.—An experimental study of the effects of televised images from a schema perspective.

Harrison, K., & Cantor, J. (1997). The relationship between media consumption and eating disorders. *Journal of Communication, 47,* 40–67.—A correlational study of magazine and television exposure and disordered eating in women and men.

Leit, R. A., Pope, Jr., H. G., & Gray, J. J. (2001). Cultural expectations of muscularity in men: The evolution of *Playgirl* centerfolds. *International Journal of Eating Disorders, 29,* 90–93.—A study of the male models in *Playgirl* magazine, from 1973 to 1997, confirming increasingly muscular ideals of the male body.

Levine, M. P., & Smolak, L. (1996). Media as a context for the development of disordered eating. In L. Smolak, M. P. Levine, & R. Striegel-Moore (Eds.), *The developmental psychopathology of eating disorders: Implications for research, prevention, and treatment* (pp. 235–257). Mahwah, NJ: Erlbaum.—A comprehensive review from a developmental perspective.

Stice, E., Schupak-Neuberg, E., Shaw, H. E., & Stein, R. I. (1994). Relation of media exposure to eating disorder symptomatology: An examination of mediating mechanisms. *Journal of Abnormal Psychology, 103,* 836–840.—Structural equation modeling of direct and indirect effects of media exposure on body dissatisfaction and eating disorder symptomatology.

Thompson, J. K., Heinberg, L. J., Altabe, M., & Tantleff-Dunn, S. (1999). *Exacting beauty: Theory, assessment, and treatment of body image disturbance.* Washington, DC: American Psychological Association.—Contains a comprehensive review of the media as a sociocultural influence on body image (Chapter 3).

Tiggemann, M., Gardiner, M., & Slater, A. (2000). "I would rather be size 10 than have straight A's": A focus group study of adolescent girls' wish to be thinner. *Journal of Adolescence, 23,* 645–659.—A qualitative study highlighting the importance of perceived pressure from the media.

12

Familial Influences on Body Image Development

ANN KEARNEY-COOKE

The translation of the physical body into the mental representation of the body and then into attitudes and behaviors toward the body is a complex and emotionally charged developmental process. Despite considerable research on body image formation, we are left with unanswered questions. What happens in human development that leads to a mental picture of the body that is quite different from the actual physical appearance of the body? Why are some individuals so intensely dissatisfied with their body that they structure their life around changing it, while others with a similar body type express dissatisfaction, wish they would lose 20 pounds, but let it go and get on with their day? Why do some individuals experience shifts in the image of their body while others tend to have a more stable body image? I believe that these types of discrepant perspectives are based on a mental image of the body that was formed by intrapsychic and/or interpersonal experiences strong enough to override the individual's perception of reality.

Figure 12.1 offers a proposed model of the factors that contribute to the development of a negative body schema and its effects on perceptions, cognitions, affect, and behavior. The predominance of unrealistic standards of beauty in the culture, in conjunction with processes such as internalization, identification, and projection, lead to the development of a negative body schema. Once a negative body schema is formed, it affects feelings, thoughts, behaviors and perceptions of the body. A negative body schema serves a powerful function in maintaining body image disturbances because it determines what we notice, attend to, and remember of our experiences.

Researchers agree that body image is multidetermined; in this chapter I

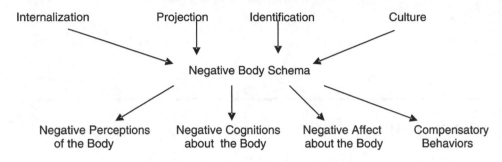

FIGURE 12.1. Model for the development of body image disturbance.

address one sector of these determinants: familial influences on body image development, as mediated by the processes of internalization and identification.

INTERNALIZATION

Internalization is defined as a progressive process whereby interactions between the person and outer world are replaced by inner representations of the self and body. The following quote from a 43-year-old woman effectively captures the process of internalization:

> "Being around critical people leaves its scars. Both my parents were very critical of their children. They tended to focus on everything negative about us. As a result, when I am critiquing myself, I focus on what's wrong. Instead of saying to myself, 'I have a nice figure,' I say, 'I have a big butt.' It's very hard to break this habit. It's as if the critical words are being *burnt* into your heart and mind. These words can be with you the rest of your life. It's like being *branded* for life."

Social learning theory proposes that parents are important agents of socialization who influence their children's body image through modeling, feedback, and instruction. Fisher, Fisher, and Stark proposed that body image involves parents' preconceived images of what sex they would like the baby to be and how they want the baby to look. When the baby is born, the parents will welcome the baby into the world if enough similarities exist between their ideal image and the baby's actual appearance. The baby's emotional needs can then be met in a loving environment, which leads to feelings of personal worth; these feelings, in turn, are the basis of a secure body image. The physical requirements desired by parents seem to be a resemblance to other members of the family and absence of deformity.

The expectations that parents have about their unborn children continue as their children age through parental attitudes, comments, and behaviors. Classic perspectives by MacGregor and colleagues and by Kolb have stressed the parents' role in affecting the child's attitude toward his or her body and the subsequent effect on self-image caused by the parents' praising or degrading of particular attributes. In 1990, Spitzack observed that while both parents influence their children's physical appearance and eating, "mothers criticize and fathers compliment" (p. 83). However, several recent studies have failed to confirm such a difference.

In 1953, MacGregor and her colleagues interviewed the mothers of daughters who had facial deformities. The daughters expressed exceptionally negative feelings about their entire bodies, even though their deformities were strictly facial. The authors suggested that these mothers placed great value on beauty and the importance of appearance. It has been argued that children will see their defects as their parents see them. Even without any "defects," children will internalize messages about their bodies from their parents. In 1986, Levinson, Powell, and Steelman examined the relationship between parents' evaluations of their children's weight (normal, overweight, or underweight) and the adolescent's perception of his or her weight. They found that parental assessment of adolescents' weight was a more powerful predictor of adolescents' self-perceptions of weight than either demographic characteristics or their physician's determination.

Striegel-Moore and Kearney-Cooke found that, as their children age, parents have increasingly negative perceptions of and attitudes toward their children's physical appearance. Respondents with the youngest children evaluated their child's physical appearance, eating, and exercise habits most positively and reported the highest level of praise and lowest level of criticism. Consistently, grade school-age children were rated less favorably than their younger peers but more favorably than adolescents. This pattern of parental views may contribute to the progression of negative body schema seen in girls, as they internalize the increasing criticisms of their parents.

The way parents respond to a child through touch also plays an important role in body image development. The infant has practically no knowledge of his or her body and must distinguish it from other objects in the environment through kinesthetic, visceral, and motor sensations. Adequate somatic–sensory stimulation, such as rocking, massaging, and water play, are crucial for the development of body image in infants. Spitz's work on the high mortality rate of institutionalized infants deprived of maternal care demonstrated dramatically the importance of the nurturing environment. It has been suggested that psychic life develops on the stage of somatic reactions, or to put it more precisely, in interplay with them.

In summary, the affirming or nonaffirming reactions of parents toward their children, whether by words, nonverbal communications, or touch, contribute to the development of the child's body image. Children internalize the way they are touched, talked about, and accepted or rejected by family members throughout their developing years.

IDENTIFICATION

The process of identification has been described by many theorists. Freud described it as one in which children adopt their same-sex parent's characteristics and incorporate his or her values. It is a process of becoming like someone in one or several aspects of thought and behavior. Typically, a child's parents are the objects available with whom he or she can identify.

The following quote from a 26-year-old woman captures the essence of identification:

> "My mother has always been critical of her body and even more critical of mine. She is always talking about how fat she is. She talked about how, when growing up, her best friend was gorgeous but she was plain—she got stuck with the guys that her friend didn't want. She told me how she couldn't go to her first few job interviews after college because she was too fat. Even though people tell me I am attractive, I feel unattractive and fat. I always wanted to be one of those girls who stood out, was really pretty, but I feel invisible most of the time when I am with people."

Schilder maintained that the interaction between mother and child affects the child's body image specifically because the child incorporates and identifies with the parent's body image as part of his or her own body image. A daughter is more likely to identify with her mother than her father. The strong mother–daughter connection is likely to be a result of the mother's involvement in childbearing and her greater availability. In 1985, Chernin suggested that girls strive to retain connectedness with their mother and generally tend to adopt their mother's lifestyle and values as they grow older. Girls will identify with many aspects of their mother's attitudes and behaviors, including those that the mother has toward her own body. In short, when mothers criticize their own bodies, daughters identify with this process and criticize their own bodies as well.

Today's young women are the first generation to be raised by mothers who typically reject their own bodies and are often concerned about the size of their daughter's bodies from the moment of birth. This phenomenon was illustrated in a 1984 *Glamour* magazine survey of body image. Mothers who were critical of their own bodies were also more critical of their daughter's body. Daughters who reported that their mothers were critical of their body showed a poorer body image, a greater use of severe dieting techniques, and a higher incidence of bulimia. Further research in this area has suggested strong associations between mothers' behaviors and attitudes toward their bodies and their daughters' behaviors and attitudes toward their own bodies. In 1986, Levinson and colleagues found mothers' encouragement of daughters' dieting to be associated with increased dieting behavior and disordered eating. In 1988, Smetana found that mothers were seen by their spouses and children as being in charge of family norms concerning physical appearance. In 1991, Pike and Rodin found that mothers of bulimic girls reported more disordered eating, had themselves begun dieting at an earlier age, and had been concerned with dieting for a significantly longer period of time than mothers of girls without eating disorders. Further, mothers of the eating-disordered girls rated their daughters as less attractive than the girls rated themselves, and felt that their daughters should lose more weight than did the mothers of girls who were not eating-disordered.

The value of being connected and having a relational capacity is central to women's development. This value includes the father–daughter relationship. As daughters enter adolescence, they may turn to their father for attention and in search of his support for her maturing body. The father's reaction to his daughter and her maturing body plays an important role in shaping her feelings about her body and the reality of becoming a woman. The quality of the emotional engagement between father and daughter may become a template for future relationships with men. The father's views on the "ideal" body for women, his attitudes toward women's bodies, his reactions to his daughter's changing body, and his comments about her maturity have an impact her body schema and are likely to influence her body image development in either positive or negative ways.

The following section offers suggestions found useful for parents.

WHAT PARENTS CAN DO TO PROMOTE CHILDREN'S POSITIVE BODY IMAGE

• *Provide adequate sensory stimulation* for young children, such as rocking, massaging, and water play. Express love in a physical way, provide body-to-body contact, movement, and quiet according to the baby's needs. When parents provide consistent, soothing bodily contact, they teach their children that the body is a source of pleasure and comfort.

• *Encourage children to explore their own physical strengths.* Feelings of body competency occur as a function of having ample opportunities to master one's body. Let children experiment with different types of movement experiences, such as dance, soccer, or martial arts. Give them opportunities to experience their bodies as a positive, effective part of themselves. Levels of strength, responsiveness, health, coordination, and stamina are part of experiencing one's physical effectiveness. A person with a high level of body effectiveness is likely to experience him- or herself as strong, healthy, coordinated, and energetic.

- *Teach children to pay attention to sensations occurring within their body.* Body awareness is crucial for the establishment of identity and mental health. Encourage children to monitor their internal signals indicating hunger, satiation, fatigue, and so on. Emphasize the importance of responding appropriately to physical signals, such as eating when they are hungry, resting when tired.
- *Do not allow teasing about appearance in the house.* Individuals with high levels of body dissatisfaction often report a history of being teased as a child. Teach children what to do if they are teased at school. Take an active the community, helping teachers, coaches, and other community leaders understand the detrimental effects of teasing, and working to minimize this negative experience.
- *Teach children how to criticize the media constructively*, how to deconstruct the messages that advertisements, television shows, music videos, and even character roles in books tell us about how we should feel, act, or look.
- *Encourage children to define their own body image* by choices they make each day rather than how others respond to their appearance. Encourage them to write down the positive body behaviors they engage in each day and to think about ways they can engage in positive body behaviors the next day, such as exercise, healthy eating, or sports.
- *Educate teenagers about bodily changes* they can expect during puberty. One effective means of educating children is for parents to share their stories about how they felt when their body was changing during puberty. Sharing strategies to help children handle this period and develop perspective is equally useful. Remind them that judgments based solely on appearance happen less often after middle school and high school.
- *Model a healthy self-perception.* Parents can help their children indirectly by determining a realistic weight and shape for themselves (based on genetic background, bone structure, and age) and following a healthy eating regimen, exercising, and resting each day. They can also teach others how to talk about and treat their body. This kind of consistent modeling increases the chance that children will feel good about their body through the identification process.

FUTURE RESEARCH

Recent research suggests that the mother can have a positive influence on her daughter's self-image, body image, and eating attitudes, even if the mother does not feel positively about herself in these areas. Maternal identification seems to be a complex process that requires further research. Is it the mother's positive feelings about her own body that affect her daughter's body image? Or is it simply a healthy mother–daughter relationship, with its increased closeness, sharing, and expression of feelings, that buffers a daughter against body dissatisfaction and eating disorders? Future research is needed to better understand the complexity of the identification process and how it may change as a girl moves through adolescence into adulthood. Moreover, much remains to be studied in understanding boys' body image development.

There is a dearth of empirical literature exploring the role of the father in body image development. Traditionally, the father represented a view of the external world; his expectations and reactions to his child were seen as playing a major role in shaping the child's perceptions of society's expectations. As an increasing number of women work outside the home and fathers become more involved in child rearing, we should study the role of the father's own feelings bout his body and his attitudes toward his children's bodies. If men are increasingly dissatisfied with their bodies, we must ask how their children are affected.

Future research should also focus on the role of siblings in body image development. Against the backdrop of siblings, each child in the family assesses and compares his or her own physical attributes. How does being the most athletic, least athletic, most attractive, least attractive sibling affect the body image of a child? A 1996 study by Rieves and Cash suggests that such sibling comparisons may indeed affect one's body image development. Development and maintenance of children's body image is dependent on how others respond to their body. For example, Rieves and Cash observed that brothers may frequently be a prime source of appearance teasing in families. How does the way siblings talk about and treat each others' bodies influence individual body image development?

There is much anecdotal clinical evidence and some scientific data to suggest the importance of internalization and identification processes in the development of a body schema. However, further longitudinal research is needed to understand these pathways. Such research should examine risk factors as well as protective factors, so that strategies can be identified to promote healthy body image in young individuals. As other contributors to this volume have argued, prospective primary prevention studies will allow us to examine the factors in body image development of children; in addition, the central roles of parents and siblings must be considered for any comprehensive theory of positive body image development.

INFORMATIVE READINGS

Chernin, K. (1985). *The hungry self: Women, eating, and identity.* New York: Time Books.—Provides a feminist analysis of the connection between identity, body image, and eating disorders.

Fisher, G., Fisher, J., & Stark, R. (1980). The body image. In *Aesthetic plastic surgery* (pp. 1–32). Boston: Little Brown.—Describes the role of parents in the development of body image.

Fisher, S. (1986). *Development and structure of the body image* (Vol. 1). Hillsdale, NJ: Erlbaum.—Review and analysis of the body image literature from 1969 to 1986.

Fisher, S. (1986). *Development and structure of the body image* (Vol. 2). Hillsdale, NJ: Erlbaum.—Description of the testing and evaluation of major theoretical concepts related to body image.

Freud, S. (1935). *A general introduction to psychoanalysis*. New York: Washington Square Press.—Provides an overview of the basic concepts of the theory of psychoanalysis.

Hahn-Smith, A. M., & Smith, J. E. (2001). The positive influence of maternal identification on body image, eating attitudes, and self-esteem of Hispanic and Anglo girls. *International Journal of Eating Disorders, 29,* 429–440.—Studied the role of maternal identification in the development of girls' body image, eating attitudes, and self-esteem.

Kearney-Cooke, A. (1989). Reclaiming the body: Using guided imagery in the treatment of body image disturbance among bulimic women. In E. Baker & L. Hornyak (Eds.), *Experiential therapies for eating disorders* (pp. 11–34). New York: Guilford Press.—Describes factors that affect body image development and how guided imagery can be used to treat body image issues of clients struggling with eating disorders.

Kearney-Cooke, A., & Striegel-Moore, R. H. (1997). The etiology and treatment of body image disturbance among eating disordered clients. In D. M. Garner & P. E. Garfinkel (Eds.), *Handbook of treatment for eating disorders* (2nd ed., pp. 295–305). New York: Guilford Press.—Describes the role of internalization and projection in the etiology of body image disturbance among eating-disordered clients.

Kolb, L. (1959). Disturbances of body image. In S. Arieti (Ed.), *American handbook of psychiatry*. New York: Basic Books—Describes the role of parents in body image development of the child, especially a child with physical disfigurement.

Levinson, R., Powell, B., & Steelman, L. C. (1986). Social location, significant others and body image among adolescents. *Social Psychology Quarterly, 49,* 330–337.—Provides a description of research on the relationship between parents' evaluation of their children's weight and adolescents' perception of his or her weight.

MacGregor, F. C., Abel, T. M., Bryt, A., Laver, E., & Weissman, S. (1953). *Facial deformities and plastic surgery*. Springfield, IL: Thomas.—Describes research that found that daughters with facial deformities see their defects as their mother did.

Pike, K. M., & Rodin, J. (1991). Mothers, daughters, and disordered eating. *Journal of Abnormal Psychology, 100,* 198–204.—Studied the relationship between mothers' attitudes and behaviors that relate to disordered eating among their adolescent daughters.

Rieves, L., & Cash, T. F. (1996). Social developmental factors and women's body image attitudes. *Journal of Social Behavior and Personality, 11,* 63–78.—Studied appearance teasing, maternal modeling, and sibling social comparisons as factors influencing females' body image development.

Schilder, P. (1950). *The image and appearance of the human body*. New York: International Universities Press.—Describes the role of identification in the development of body image.

Schwartz, D. J., Phares, V., Tantleff-Dunn, S., & Thompson, J. K. (1999). Body image, psychological functioning, and parental feedback regarding physical appearance. *International Journal of Eating Disorders, 25,* 339–343.—Examined the possible effects of mothers' and fathers' negative appearance-related feedback on both daughters' and sons' body image.

Smetana, J. G. (1988). Concepts of self and social convention: Adolescents and parents reasoning about hypothetical and actual family conflicts. In M. R. Gunnar & W. A. Collins (Eds.), *Development during the transition to adolescence.* Hillsdale, NJ: Erlbaum.— Reports on research in which parents and their adolescent children were interviewed that found that mothers were seen by their spouses and by their children as being in charge of enforcing family norms concerning family appearance.

Spitz, R. A. (1951). The psychogenic diseases in infancy. *Psychoanalytic Study of the Child, 6,* 255–275.—Describes high mortality rates of institutionalized infants deprived of maternal care, which demonstrates the importance of tactile nurturance early in life.

Spitzack, C. (1990). *Confessing excess.* Albany State University of New York.—Provides a description of parental influence on children's physical appearance and eating habits.

Striegel-Moore, R. H., & Kearney-Cooke, A. (1994). Exploring parents' attitudes and behaviors about their children's physical appearance. *International Journal of Eating Disorders, 15,* 377–385.—Provides descriptive information regarding parents' evaluations of children's physical appearance, eating habits, exercise behaviors, and their efforts to influence their children's physical appearance.

Thompson, J. K., Heinberg, L. J., Altabe, M., & Tantleff-Dunn, S. (1999). *Exacting beauty: Theory, assessment, and treatment of body image disturbance.* Washington, DC: American Psychological Association.—Chapters 5 and 6 review research pertinent to familial influences on body image development.

13

Interpersonal Influences on Body Image Development

STACEY TANTLEFF-DUNN
JESSICA L. GOKEE

Our interpersonal relationships, the way we see ourselves in comparison to others, and the feedback we receive all contribute to our self-concept, including how we feel about our physical appearance. This premise is underscored when we consider what *really* makes us anxious about our appearance. More often than not, we are nervous about how others will evaluate the way we look. A passing comment can either elevate or dampen our mood and self-confidence: Hearing "You look great!," we feel uplifted, our confidence renewed; hearing, "You look tired today," we may feel *more* fatigued as well as self-conscious. A growing body of literature suggests that others' opinions have a profound impact on how we view and feel about our bodies. For example, Rosen and his colleagues conducted a comprehensive study on body image influences; of the 19 critical experience categories identified, more than half were tied to interpersonal factors such as feedback on appearance and peer or familial competition.

This chapter reviews the interpersonal processes that shape body image and examines evidence that explicit and implicit messages regarding appearance have an important effect on an individual's body image. The unique influences of peers, romantic partners, and strangers are described, implications for assessment and treatment offered, and directions for future research explored. (Kearney-Cooke discusses familial influences in the preceding chapter in this volume.)

INTERPERSONAL PROCESSES THAT SHAPE BODY IMAGE

Three primary interpersonal processes that play significant roles in the development of body image are reflected appraisals, feedback on physical appearance, and social comparison. The *reflected appraisal* process refers to the notion that others' opinions of us (or our perceptions of how others view us) have significant influence on how we see ourselves. In the area of physical attractiveness, research findings suggest that, for both children and adults, *perceptions* of others' evaluations have a significant impact on self-evaluations; indeed, others' actual appraisals have significantly less impact than individuals' often inaccurate perceptions of them.

Receiving *feedback on physical appearance* is often the means by which people develop perceptions of how others view them. This feedback may come from parents, siblings, peers, romantic partners, coaches, employers, or even complete strangers. Feedback may range from outright teasing or criticism to ambiguous comments or subtle body language. Regardless of the source or variety, any negative feedback about appearance can be damaging. The negative consequences associated with disparaging feedback have been well documented. Researchers have found that being teased is one of the most commonly reported precipitants of body dissatisfaction. A history of frequent teasing has been linked to higher levels of body dissatisfaction, eating disturbance, depression, and lower self-esteem in both adolescent and college females across numerous studies conducted in several countries. In a 3-year longitudinal investigation, Cattarin and Thompson found that being teased predicted increases in body dissatisfaction. In another line of research, people with physical deformities and body dysmorphic disorder have reported that being teased precipitated their body image symptoms.

Social comparison is yet another process through which self-appraisals of physical attractiveness are formed. Social comparison theory suggests that, within the realm of body image, the propensity to compare one's physical appearance to others moderates the extent to which the pervasive representation of the thin, attractive ideal results in body image disturbance. Research has shown that individuals who compare themselves to others whom they view as physically attractive rate their own attractiveness lower than individuals who compare themselves to others viewed as unattractive. Correlational studies have consistently found that higher levels of comparison are related to greater body dissatisfaction. In theory, targets of comparison should be important variables in determining how people feel about themselves. However, experimental manipulations of the social comparison process have led some researchers to suggest that it is the general tendency to compare oneself with others that plays a critical role in body image dissatisfaction, not to whom those comparisons are made. In a recent study by

Cattarin and colleagues, participants who were encouraged to compare themselves to thin models in commercials became more dissatisfied with their bodies than participants who were distracted or shown non-appearance-related commercials. (For further discussion of media influences, see Tiggemann's chapter in this volume.) Additional research has identified the frequency of appearance comparison as a predictor of body image and eating disturbances, thereby explaining more unique variance than do maturational status, teasing history, or awareness and internalization of sociocultural pressures for thinness and attractiveness.

INTERPERSONAL RELATIONSHIPS

Body image development is a lifelong process inevitably influenced by the significant others who play the most central roles at different times in our lives. Thus young children may be most influenced by parents, whereas adolescents' body images may be more affected by interactions with peers. Adults' body images are likely to be influenced by romantic partners, who are often important sources of feedback and support. With these interpersonal processes in mind, the specific influences of peers, romantic partners, and strangers is discussed.

Peers

The influence of peer groups can be paramount, particularly throughout adolescence. The most obvious, direct manner in which peers may influence body image is through feedback on physical appearance. Teasing, in particular, is an experience common to most children and foreign to few adults. According to a study by Rieves and Cash on social development factors that contribute to women's body image, peers and friends are among the most frequent and "worst" perpetrators of teasing, second only to brothers. Being teased by peers is associated with greater concerns about physical appearance and more dieting behaviors.

Research findings suggest that the link between receiving appearance-related feedback from peers and the development of disturbance may not be direct. Rather, perceptions regarding peer acceptance may serve to elevate concerns about appearance. Studies have found that girls more often than boys believe that thinness increases likeability, and the extent to which this belief is held predicts weight and body image concerns. Girls in middle school report engaging in more body- and weight-related interactions than boys, and these interactions can become associated with weight and shape concerns later in development. In a recent study by Vincent and McCabe, surprisingly boys reported receiving more negative commentary from peers about weight and shape than girls did. However, in studies of adults, females typically report receiving more feedback on physical appearance than males. Ricciardelli and colleagues found that, regardless of quantity, boys viewed feedback from female friends as having a positive impact on body image, whereas they viewed feedback from male friends as more important in influencing body change methods, such as eating and exercise patterns.

In addition to appearance-related feedback, peers' modeling behaviors may influence body image and eating behaviors. Studies have shown that girls are more likely than boys to report peer modeling of weight loss behaviors. Paxton and colleagues' research on peer influences revealed that adolescent girls within friendship cliques are similar in the degree to which they are concerned about body image and engage in dieting behaviors. Studies of college-age women have also found similar levels of disordered eating among friends. Such findings lead to questions as to whether members within peer groups influence one another, or whether choice of peer groups reflects preexisting body image attitudes and eating behaviors. C. S. Crandall's study on the social contagion of binge eating found that, upon joining a sorority, its members' eating behaviors were uncorrelated, but after living together for a time, a member's binge eating could be predicted by the bingeing behavior of her friends.

Romantic Partners

Romantic partners spend a great deal of time together, share experiences, and allow themselves to be vulnerable in a way they rarely do with other people. Thus it seems likely that perceptions of how romantic partners feel about one another's looks and their feedback on each other's appearance will have a substantial impact on how they feel about themselves, their bodies, and their relationship. In fact, research in this area suggests that greater body dissatisfaction is associated with lower relationship satisfaction. Consistent with findings that suggest men place more emphasis on physical attractiveness than women, men's relationship satisfaction is significantly related to satisfaction with their partner's shape.

Research has also shown that both men's and women's perceptions of the opposite sex's body ideals are inaccurate. Women think their romantic partners prefer thinner figures than their partners actually prefer, and men and women both overestimate the breast/chest size preferred by the opposite sex. In a study designed to examine such perceptions, Tantleff-Dunn and Thompson investigated discrepancies between self-ratings and romantic partner ratings in relation to body image disturbance. We found that, for females, the discrepancy between self-rating and their *perception* of their partner's ideal explained the majority of variance in body dissatisfaction, eating disturbance, and general psychological functioning. In contrast, the discrepancy between males' self-ratings and their female partners' *actual* ratings of the ideal male figure predicted males' body image. We speculated that females may provide their partners with more direct feedback that subsequently highlights this discrepancy.

Rieves and Cash developed the Physical Appearance in Intimate Relationships Scale (PAIRS) to measure one's perceptions of the partner's attitudes and behaviors vis-à-vis one's own appearance. More negative PAIRS scores were associated with greater body dissatisfaction and less relationship and sexual satisfaction for both sexes. The specific relationship between body image and dynamics within romantic relationships has yet to be empirically evaluated, but relevant qualitative data and anecdotal evidence suggest that body image distress may parallel characteristics of eating disorders in couples. As Thompson and his colleagues hypothesized in *Exacting Beauty*, individuals may knowingly or inadvertently encourage negative body image in their partners in order to maintain power, enhance self-image, encourage a partner's efforts to maintain or improve appearance, or foster dependency. Further research is needed to evaluate these possibilities.

It is important to note that, in addition to the feedback of romantic partners affecting body image, body image disturbance may have deleterious effects on relationships. For example, as Wiederman's chapter on body image attitudes and sexual functioning reveals, negative body image is associated with fewer sexual experiences and lower sexual satisfaction, and body image self-consciousness and avoidance in sexual situations is related to lower sex drive for both men and women. The relationship between body image and sexual functioning is a good illustration of the reciprocal nature of interpersonal influences: Just as body image disturbance may negatively impact a couple's sex life, a poor sexual relationship may exacerbate body image anxiety in partners who interpret sexual difficulties as a reflection of their unattractiveness and undesirableness.

Strangers

The influence of strangers can be conceptualized as transmitting stereotypes of the appearance preferences of others. These stereotypes often emanate from sociocultural messages, so it is difficult to separate the effects of these influences on body image. Nonetheless, discrepancies between how individuals think they *should* look to be considered attractive to others and how they think they *actually* look can lead to significant body dissatisfaction.

Murray and colleagues examined the role of interpersonal influences in females with eating disorders and female and male controls. The researchers found that close to half of the total sample reported that members of the opposite sex, in general, affected their eating, exercise, and body satisfaction, with no significant differences between comparison groups. Women with eating disorders were most likely, and male controls were least likely, to report that members of the same sex influenced their body image and eating behavior. Interestingly, men were more likely to indicate desire to look attractive to the opposite sex.

In addition to the somewhat passive influence introduced by concerns about appearing attractive to others, strangers may more directly influence body image by providing feedback on physical appearance. A dramatic example of this point relates to an incident that happened to a woman whom one of us (S.T.-D.) treated for obesity and depression. After mustering the motivation to begin an exercise program, her confidence was shattered when teenage boys in a passing car yelled "Cow!" when she was taking a brisk walk through her neighborhood. This cruel act undermined much of her progress and became the focus of several therapy sessions. Although the client eventually returned to exercising, she would only ride a stationary bike in the privacy of her home and had resigned herself to being a "social outcast" until she lost weight.

Fortunately, strangers' appearance-related feedback is often less critical and much more subtle. Research on appearance-related feedback indicates that facial expressions, topics of conversation, and levels of friendliness and respect sometimes convey a great deal of information about how others evaluate one's physical appearance. Numerous studies suggest that people ascribe a variety of negative attributes to individuals they perceive as unattractive and/or overweight. They give preferential treatment to attractive individuals (including children) across many contexts, and this differential treatment can lead to differences in psychosocial adjustment. Thus strangers can affect body image, which in turn can impact social functioning.

IMPLICATIONS FOR ASSESSMENT

Increasing recognition that interpersonal factors play an important role in the development and sequelae of body image disturbance has led to creation of several assessment measures that tap into the extent to which peers, family members, and others, in general, influence body image. A wide variety of these instruments, thoroughly reviewed in Thompson and colleagues' 1999 text, are readily accessible and valuable for both research and clinical purposes. Researchers have employed measures such as the Feedback on Physical Appearance Scale, Perception of Teasing Scale, Peer Dieting Survey, and the PAIRS to investigate the significance of these factors individually and in relation to one another. Including interpersonal measures in body image research may further enhance our understanding of how relationships fit into the complex picture of many widely studied variables that have failed to fully explain body image disturbances. Construction of additional psychometrically sound measures that are more comprehensive (some questionnaires contain as few as one to four items) may facilitate increased research efforts in this area.

Although many of the available instruments are easily administered questionnaires, clinicians may yield the most valuable information by simply asking clients about their teasing history, familial influences on body image, and perceptions of how romantic partners contribute to their appearance-related concerns. Clients may inadvertently omit interpersonal aspects of their body dissatisfaction, sometimes because they have difficulty recognizing when appearance concerns reflect experiences in their relationships. Children typically do not tell adults about teasing incidents, and adults sometimes do not recall their influential childhood experiences. Involving clients' significant others to gain their perspectives and observe their interactions may also prove beneficial. Overall, including interpersonal questionnaires and/or interviews may be helpful in treatment planning and may increase the effectiveness of most body image therapies.

IMPLICATIONS FOR TREATMENT

Consideration of interpersonal factors leads us to approach not just assessment but also treatment from an interpersonal perspective. Interpersonal therapy (IPT) focuses primarily on helping clients identify and modify interpersonal problems and enhance their relationships rather than concentrating on overt symptoms of disturbance (e.g., body image concerns). Traditionally, cognitive-behavior therapy has been the treatment of choice for body image disturbances (see Cash and Strachan's chapter in this volume). Although the efficacy of IPT is yet to be determined, outcome research has yielded promising results of IPT treatment for eating disorders. As reviewed in Garner and Garfinkel's *Handbook of Treatment for Eating Disorders*, Fairburn and his colleagues have conducted several studies that compared IPT, cognitive-behavioral therapy (CBT), behavior therapy (BT), group therapy, and wait-list controls. The findings have sometimes favored CBT, but the research has generally demonstrated that IPT has a profound and sustained impact. In fact, in one study IPT patients surpassed those in CBT over a 12-month follow-up period, and another study showed no significant differences between CBT and IPT at posttreatment and follow-up. Therefore, using IPT as a primary or at least adjunctive therapy for body image disturbance may be beneficial, especially for clients whose social relationships clearly contribute to their negative body image.

Another implication of an interpersonal perspective on body image is the value of including significant others in treatment. From educating family members and romantic partners about their impact on a client's body image to clarifying misinterpreted feedback, broadening the focus to include others may be therapeutic for everyone involved. In addition, group therapy and the opportunity to enhance communication and relationship skills may be beneficial when issues such as lack of assertiveness are involved in clients' struggles with body image.

SUMMARY AND DIRECTIONS FOR FUTURE RESEARCH

Based on the research to date, we can say with relative certainty that interpersonal factors have a significant impact on the development of body image and on body image states in everyday life. In short, what others think and do matters; but perhaps more importantly, *perceptions* of what others think and prefer regarding physical appearance influence how we feel about our bodies. Despite the widely accepted premise that the opinions of others influence development of the self, research has largely been limited to understanding the importance individuals place on those opinions rather than exploring their actual impact. Whereas sociocultural and social comparison theories have been the subject of many investigations, more personally relevant interpersonal experiences have received relatively limited attention. Within a culture that contains pervasive, almost inescapable, messages that physical attractiveness is important and where unrealistic images of thinness and muscularity abound, we must investigate why some individuals develop body image disturbances and others do not. Do familial and peer subcultures transmit appearance-related beliefs, values, and behaviors that serve either to buffer or amplify media influences and other sociocultural pressures? To what extent do age, gender, and ethnicity mediate interpersonal influences? Do differences in cognitive processing account for differential responses to teasing and others forms of appearance-related feedback? Clearly, further research is needed to answer these questions and elucidate the processes by which interpersonal experiences impact body image. This knowledge holds the potential to enhance current approaches to treatment and prevention of negative body image.

INFORMATIVE READINGS

Cattarin, J., & Thompson, J. K. (1994). A three-year longitudinal study of body image and eating disturbance in adolescent females. *Eating Disorders: The Journal of Treatment and Prevention, 2,* 114–125.—A longitudinal investigation that examined the roles of teasing history, maturational status, and weight in the development of eating disorders.

Cattarin, J. A., Thompson, J. K., Thomas, C., & Williams, R. (2000). Body image, mood, and televised images of attractiveness: The role of social comparison. *Journal of Social and Clinical Psychology, 19,* 220–239.—An experiment that manipulated social comparison to test its role in negative outcomes associated with media exposure.

Crandall, C. S. (1988). Social contagion of binge eating. *Journal of Personality and Social Psychology, 55,* 588–598.—An examination of the relationship between social pressure and binge eating in sororities.

Garner, D. M., & Garfinkel, P. E. (Eds.). (1997). *Handbook of treatment for eating disorders* (2nd ed.). New York: Guilford Press.—An extensive overview of various treatment approaches, including IPT, as well as specific challenges for therapy and research on eating disorders.

Murray, S. H., Touyz, S. W., & Beumont, P. J. V. (1996). The influence of personal relationships on women's eating behavior and body satisfaction. *Eating Disorders: The Journal of Treatment and Prevention, 3*, 243–252.—A comparison of social pressures experienced by patients with eating disorders and a community sample.

Paxton, S. J., Schutz, H. K., Wertheim, E. H., & Muir, S. L. (1999). Friendship clique and peer influences on body image concerns, dietary restraint, extreme weight loss behaviors, and binge eating in adolescent girls. *Journal of Abnormal Psychology, 108*(2), 255–266.—An examination of the relationship between friendship variables and various dimensions of body image and eating behavior in a sample of 523 girls with a mean age of 16.

Ricciardelli, L. A., McCabe, M. P., & Banfield, S. (2000). Body image and body change methods in adolescent boys: Role of parents, friends, and the media. *Journal of Psychosomatic Research, 49*(3), 189–197.—An examination of the perceived effect and importance of family, friends, and the media on 12- to 17-year-old boys' body image.

Rieves, L., & Cash, T. F. (1996). Social developmental factors and women's body-image attitudes. *Journal of Social Behavior and Personality, 11*, 63–78.—Examines developmental precursors to women's body image such as teasing, social comparison, and modeling.

Rieves, L. C., & Cash, T. F. (1999). *Do you see what I see?: A study of actual and perceived physical appearance attitudes in romantic relationships.* Unpublished manuscript. Available from Jessica L. Gokee, Old Dominion University, Norfolk, Virginia.—Examines the interrelationships, correlates, and implications of romantic partners' self, other, and perceived-other body image evaluations.

Rosen, M.C., Orosan-Weine, P., & Tang, T. (1997) Critical experiences in the development of body image. *Eating Disorders: The Journal of Prevention and Treatment, 5*, 191–204.—Two studies that used open-ended interviews to identify body image influences in clinical and nonclinical participants and tested their ability to predict body image and psychological problems.

Tantleff-Dunn, S., & Thompson, J. K. (1995). Romantic partners and body image disturbance: Further evidence for the role of perceived–actual disparities. *Sex Roles, 33*, 589–605.—A study of romantic partners' ratings of self, partner, and ideal same- and opposite-sex figures and their relation to body image disturbance.

Thompson, J. K., Heinberg, L. J., Altabe, M., & Tantleff-Dunn, S. (1999). *Exacting beauty: Theory, assessment, and treatment of body image disturbance.* Washington, DC: American Psychological Association.—A comprehensive review of research findings, assessment measures, and treatment issues in body image disturbance.

Vincent, M. A., & McCabe, M. P. (2000). Gender differences among adolescents in family and peer influences on body dissatisfaction, weight loss, and binge eating behaviors. *Journal of Youth and Adolescence, 29*(2), 205–221.—Examined perceived influences of family and peers in a large sample of children ages 11–18.

14

Sexual Abuse and Body Image

PATRICIA FALLON
DIANN M. ACKARD

Abuse experiences can have a number of negative effects on survivors' quality of life, including emotional distress, cognitive distortions, and psychopathology. Little is known about the specific impact of childhood sexual abuse (CSA) on the development and stability of a positive body image, although there is substantial evidence that CSA has both short- and long-term deleterious effects on self-esteem, a factor correlated with positive body image. In this chapter we review the definitions of and relationship between body image and CSA, common body image problems of survivors of CSA, and suggestions for clinical interventions. In particular, we focus on cognitive and experiential treatment of body image disturbance related to sexual abuse.

Body image is a mental representation of the body that includes perceptions of appearance, feelings and thoughts about the body, how it feels to be inside the body, and the body's functions and capabilities. New information is continually incorporated into one's body image. As the information is processed, body image changes. For example, running a half-marathon may enhance body image as the runner feels competent about what his or her body can do, whereas hearing a teasing or derogatory comment may be detrimental. Body image evaluation can span a wide range, including body satisfaction, dissatisfaction, and the distortion and disparagement evident in body dysmorphic disorder. The development of body image is a fluid process, much like growth and aging over the lifespan; one is frequently adjusting to major or minor changes.

Defining and assessing the impact of childhood sexual abuse is a complex task. Definitions of what constitutes childhood sexual abuse range widely from sexual jokes and comments to covert sexual abuse (e.g., watching someone undress or peering into public showers) to overt sexual abuse (e.g., physical contact of a sexual nature, including touching, fondling, and penetration). Methods of collecting information about abuse range from the use of open-ended interviews to carefully constructed yes/no questions. Assessing the impact of CSA is complicated by the likelihood that the impact changes over time. Initial consequences may differ substantially from long-term sequelae. Another challenge to assessment is that sexual abuse can happen to a person of any age, can last from a moment to years, and can be committed by a friend, a relative, or a stranger. Epidemiological studies suggest that the prevalence of sexual abuse is higher for girls than for boys, and although several differences between men and women who have been sexually abused have been noted, none specific to body image has been reported. Compared to sexually abused girls, sexually abused boys are more likely to be subjected to accompanying physical abuse, to be abused forcefully, and to be younger at first abuse but older when forcefully abused. Additionally, sexually abused boys are less likely than sexually abused girls to tell someone about the abuse, thus increasing the likelihood that they will receive less social support, which has been correlated with isolation and lowered self-esteem. Furthermore, whereas some studies show no differences between sexually abused men and women on indicators of emotional stability and well-being, others suggest important differences. Findings suggest that sexually abused men are more likely to use externalizing coping strategies, such as aggression and avoidance, whereas sexually abused women are more likely to use internalizing strategies, such as repression and self-criticism.

In addition to characteristics related to sexual abuse, there are substantial differences between girls and boys regarding the process of body image integration. Body image development may be a greater challenge for sexually abused girls than boys, due to the manner in which abused girls process information: They tend to make more internal and personal attributions for negative events than girls not sexually abused, and they exhibit insecure attachments, a correlate of weight concerns. Girls subjected to CSA are more likely to have experienced early menarche and thus experienced an earlier exposure to potentially negative events related to the normal development of adipose tissue and body fat, such as peers commenting about changes in body size and shape. These experiences combine to propel them into dealing with body image issues at an earlier age. Additionally, due to their younger age, these girls are likely to have fewer cognitive coping strategies to help them deal with these complex body image issues.

Although both males and females can be victims of childhood sexual abuse and may struggle with their body image, girls are more likely than boys to be abused over their lifetime, to experience body image disturbance, and to suffer from eating disorders. Much of the material offered in this chapter relates to both sexes. However, to reflect the increased incidence of CSA among girls and for ease of reading, we will use the female pronoun.

A positive body image is difficult for girls and women in Western cultures to develop and maintain. Incorporation of the normal and appropriate physical changes (e.g., growing taller, breast development) is central to developing a stable body image. All girls must learn to contend with appearance-related cultural messages and peer inspections, comments, and comparisons. When this already challenging process of body image development is interrupted by a single or multiple intrusions of sexual abuse, the typical developmental pathway to a stable body image becomes a labyrinth that, at best, is difficult and, at worst, impossible to traverse.

COMMON BODY IMAGE PROBLEMS FOR SEXUALLY ABUSED INDIVIDUALS

Abuse that occurs at any point can have deleterious effects on body image development. However, when abuse occurs during critical stages of normal body image development, such as during puberty, it interferes with the individual's ability to attain a stable concept of self and body. The profound cognitive, physiological, emotional, and social changes that begin in early adolescence (ages 10–13) and continue through late adolescence (18–25) make the integration of body image into one's sense of self a central task of the teenage years. If sexual abuse occurs (most typically, abuse occurs during childhood or early adolescence), surviving the event with an integrated body image and a healthy sense of self is improbable. Survivors of sexual violence often have a disrupted view of the specific body part(s) violated during the abuse. This disrupted view may range from hating the abused body parts to bodily mutilation, such as cutting or burning.

Body image problems stemming from abusive experiences are not only specific to the abused body part but may be generalized to the entire body, resulting in overall body dissatisfaction, intense feelings of shame about the event and the body, and body distortion (e.g., perceiving the body as much larger than its actual size). An abuse survivor of normal weight and size, but laden with the burden of abuse, might describe her body as "fat and heavy." She may see her body as huge, disgusting, and ugly, and this change in cognitive schema may reflect how she views the abusive experience—as disgusting and ugly. In attempting to manage her discomfort with her body and her sexuality, in general, she may significantly restrict or increase her dietary intake. In her mind, altering her body to make it dramatically smaller or larger will make her unattractive to the sexual advances of others, and thereby decrease the risk of further abuse. For some individuals, the result is an eating disorder, particularly bulimia nervosa, as they attempt to reject the body's own physiological needs to eat. The feelings of loss of control over one's body inherent in binge eating may trigger particularly intense needs in the sexual abuse survivor to regain control through purging, exercise, or stringent dietary restriction.

Sexual abuse affects individual survivors as well as their relationships. For example, an abused woman who is uncomfortable in her body may not express her needs and opinions confidently. She may believe that her needs will not be respected, or will not matter—beliefs that mirror the helplessness experienced during the abusive event(s). Sexual functioning and intimacy in relationships may be compromised by feelings that the body is only a vessel for others' wants and desires. Girls who experience arousal during the abuse may believe that their body betrayed them. As adults they may refuse to engage in sexual intimacy, detach emotionally from sexual practices, or become more sexually active in an attempt to regain control. (See Wiederman's chapter on body image and sexuality in this volume.) Such responses can leave the survivor with a deflated sense of power and esteem, and potentially vulnerable to repeated victimization.

TREATMENT

Body image therapy with individuals who have been sexually abused needs to address the development of maladaptive schema resulting from the abuse as well as the visceral/affective aspect of the trauma. Often, this is a long and difficult process, as therapy attempts to undo long-held damaging beliefs and feelings. To achieve these aspects of healing, both cognitive and experiential interventions for body image disturbance with sexually abused individuals are often used.

Cognitive Therapy

Cognitive schemas are long-held organizing beliefs about self, others, the world, and the future. Similar to body image, schemas lie on a continuum and can incorporate both positive and negative beliefs. In some individuals, positive body schemas are never formed because their development was interrupted by early trauma. In other individuals, sexual abuse alters already-formed body schemas, such that the person replaces neutral or positive body schemas with negative ones. Schemas guide personal interactions and identity formation and can be resistant to change and intervention. Because schemas formed by CSA experiences are particularly powerful and deeply embedded, cognitive interventions are essential components of the therapeutic process and must be done with sensitivity and care on the part of the treatment provider. Cognitive interventions need to address specific schemas as well as thoughts and feelings related to the damage to body image inflicted by sexual abuse. Survivors are likely to hold beliefs similar to the following:

- "My body is a weapon that can be turned against me."
- "I cannot protect my body from harm by others."

- "My body betrayed me (I felt aroused during the abuse experience)."
- "No one will want me now. I am 'damaged goods.' "

General cognitive techniques specifically directed toward body image trauma include monitoring and replacing negative self-statements with positive self-statements, and making specific connections between the abuse and current body image functioning. (See chapter by Cash and Strachan in this volume.) Assigning a female patient the homework of observing a young girl and seeing how that girl seems to feel about her body can help the patient identify the difference between her body image, as a consequence of the abuse, and the "normal" body image of a child (it can be helpful to suggest that the girl chosen for observation be similar in age to when the survivor was abused). In addition, asking the sexual abuse survivor to respond to how she feels about the following questions is an important aspect of therapy:

- "What statements were made to me about my body before, during, or after the abuse?"
- "What types of comments or situations currently trigger my negative body feelings?"
- "What was the specific impact of the sexual abuse on my body image?"
- "What other positive or negative messages did I get from others about my body?"
- "Did the messages change after the abuse? If so, how or in what way?"

It is important for the clinician to understand how the timing of the sexual abuse interacted with and interrupted the developmental process of integrating body image into a sense of self. It can also be helpful for the survivor to understand and articulate the specific impact of the abuse on her peer interactions, self-esteem, and blossoming sexuality. Survivors should be reminded that developing such insight takes constant vigilance. We sometimes tell our patients that it is like learning to downhill ski after age 50—you can do it, but it may never feel completely natural or easy.

Experiential Treatments

Experiential therapies use approaches other than verbal expression to work through traumatic events. (See chapter by Rabinor and Bilich in this volume.) The purpose is to help patients amplify their feelings, perceptions, and thoughts about an event and, ultimately, to change their experience of the event. Common experiential approaches include such interventions as dance and movement therapy, guided imagery, art and music therapies, and sometimes written exercises. Patients who have been sexually abused typically describe feelings of shame, lack of control over the event and their body, and insecurity regarding interpersonal relationships. Experiential therapies offer opportunities to address the shame, regain their sense of control, and "rewrite" a different ending to the abuse story (see Fallon & Wonderlich, 1997, for examples of experiential techniques in CSA treatment). For example, patients may use sculpting or painting to portray two states: one of the body after the abuse, and the other of the body having healed from the traumatic experience. Seeing the two different renditions of the body may help clients put the experience into a visible format and move forward in reclaiming their body.

Others find that telling the story of the abuse and rewriting the ending can be helpful. For example, in the new version they confront the perpetrator in order to feel a sense of control, or they talk with a trusted individual about the abuse in an effort to progress in their journey of healing. Writing can also be a helpful tool in expressing affect that is uncomfortable, even frightening, to discuss out loud. The patient may choose to write an angry letter to the perpetrator, then ceremoniously destroy the letter to symbolize her choice not to let the experience destroy her and to move onward in her life.

Guided imagery techniques use scripted visualization exercises designed to help the patient address especially difficult aspects of the abuse, such as intense feelings of shame, or to create a more positive body schema. Typically, patients assume a comfortable position, close their eyes, and allow themselves to relax. Then the therapist verbally guides them through a difficult experience and into a new way of thinking about the body—that is, that their body is strong, protected, safe, respected. Examples of guided imageries for creating a new body schema can be found in Kearney-Cooke and Striegel-Moore.

Movement, dance, self-defense techniques, and relaxation therapies can be excellent interventions for survivors having a difficult time feeling safe within their body. These interventions provide opportunities to experience the body differently, for example, from weak and vulnerable, to strong and powerful. Patients can shift their body experience from one of passivity to activity; from one of allowing their body to control how they feel, to using the body to convey assertive messages to other people; and from one of mere form (how the body looks), to function (the power of the body that can be used for the purpose of healing). Learning to recognize and identify the various tension and relaxation states felt by the survivor can introduce new feelings of competence and help her identify different states within the body that can be used as a "radar" to guide future interactions with others. For example, when a patient learns to detect and respect anxious feelings within her body, she can then choose to seek safety by talking with a trusted individual, or to avoid the situation that is creating the uncomfortable and overwhelming feelings of anxiousness. She can develop the capacity to use the sensations in her body as information that guides her in everyday interactions.

Making Connections

An essential part of the therapeutic process is to establish a strong, secure, and trusting relationship between the therapist and patient that enables the patient to feel a new sense of personal power and control in close relationships and which experientially changes powerful schemas about safety and trust. (See chapter by Krueger in this volume.) Studies have shown that the amount of social support the survivor receives after the discovery of the abuse is a mediating factor in how well the survivor copes with the trauma. Individuals who received positive responses after the abuse from those close to them can adjust their schemas to "It wasn't my fault," whereas those who received no or negative social support believe "It was my fault."

In a good therapeutic relationship, the therapist persistently encourages the development of social support and connections in the patient's everyday life. Developing such a network serves several purposes. First, it continues the important process of schema change as the patient experiences other helpful, not harmful, relationships. Second, the experience of connection and support is counter to the typical abuse experience in which the victim is purposefully isolated in order to keep the abuse a "secret." Lastly, it can expose the individual to constructive mentors, an experience that has been related to an increase in self-esteem that can lead to increases in positive feelings about the body.

CONCLUSION

Childhood sexual abuse interrupts the normal and frequently difficult developmental process of incorporating a positive, stable body image that is central to facilitating the cultivation of important aspects of self: positive self-esteem, trusting and respectful relationships, and positive, stable cognitive schemas. The informed therapist is sensitive to issues that may arise in the therapeutic relationship during treatment and acknowledges the need to address both the affective and cognitive sequelae of the trauma. Future research needs to address the specific developmental impact of childhood sexual abuse on the various stages of body image development, and the differing impact of trauma on males and females. Treatment remains a complex and multifaceted process and must address both cognitive and affective sequelae. Healing from trauma creates new pathways for survivors; clinicians and researchers can work together to provide maps for this journey.

INFORMATIVE READINGS

Briere, J. N., & Elliott, D. M. (1994). Immediate and long-term impacts of child sexual abuse. *The Future of Children, 4*(2), 54–69.—Describes clinical psychopathology associated with childhood sexual abuse in males and females.

Connors, M. E. (2001). Relationship of sexual abuse to body image and eating disorders. In J. K. Thompson & L. Smolak (Eds.), *Body image, eating disorders, and obesity in youth.* Washington, DC: American Psychological Association.—Reviews the literature on associations between sexual abuse and body image and eating disturbances in children, adolescents, and adults.

Fallon, P., & Wonderlich, S. A. (1997). Sexual abuse and other forms of trauma. In D. M. Garner & P. E. Garfinkel (Eds.), *Handbook of treatment for eating disorders* (2nd ed., pp. 391–414). New York: Guilford Press.—Reviews the literature on sexual abuse and eating disorders and offers practical applications for the assessment and treatment of survivors of sexual abuse.

Goodwin, J. M., & Attias, R. (1999). *Splintered reflections: Images of the body in trauma.* New York: Basic Books.—Includes two chapters addressing body image disturbance in individuals with histories of incest and childhood sexual abuse.

Kearney-Cooke, A., & Ackard, D. M. (2000). The effects of sexual abuse on body image, self-image, and sexual activity of women. *Journal of Gender-Specific Medicine, 3*(6), 51–60.—Describes results from research comparing sexually abused and non-sexually abused women on measures of body image, self-image, and sexual practices.

Kearney-Cooke, A., & Striegel-Moore, R. (1997). The etiology and treatment of body image disturbance. In D. M. Garner & P. E. Garfinkel (Eds.), *Handbook of treatment for eating disorders* (2nd ed., pp. 291–306). New York: Guilford Press.—Provides a theoretical description and clinical illustrations of body image development and treatment of body image disturbance.

Rosenbaum, M. (1993). The changing body image of the adolescent girl. In M. Sugar (Ed.), *Female adolescent development* (2nd ed., pp. 61–80). New York: Brunner/Mazel.—Describes adolescent body image development in the context of pubertal changes, social influences, and cognitive organization.

Thompson, J. K., Heinberg, L. J., Altabe, M., & Tantleff-Dunn, S. (1999). Sexual abuse and sexual harassment. In J. K. Thompson, L. J. Heinberg, M. Altabe, & S. Tantleff-Dunn (Eds.), *Exacting beauty: Theory, assessment, and treatment of body image disturbance* (pp. 231–247). Washington DC: American Psychological Association.—Describes relevant research, theory, assessment, and treatment issues related to body image disturbance in sexually harassed and abused individuals.

Watkins, B., & Bentovim, A. (1992). The sexual abuse of male children and adolescents: A review of current research. *Journal of Child Psychology and Psychiatry, 33*(1), 191–248.—An extensive overview of the literature on many aspects of sexual abuse in boys.

Weiner, K. E., & Thompson, J. K. (1997). Overt and covert sexual abuse: Relationship to body image and eating disturbance. *International Journal of Eating Disorders, 22,* 271–284.—Describes findings from research that indicate the impact of both covert and overt sexual abuse on body image and eating disturbances.

III

Body Image Assessment

15

Body Image Assessment of Children

RICK M. GARDNER

Body size distortion and dissatisfaction are recognized as important in their own right as well as in the development of eating disorders. Previously, extreme body image dissatisfaction was believed to begin with the onset of pubertal development and adolescence. Recent evidence, however, suggests that many children as young as 8 years of age are already unhappy with their body size and that the origins of body size dissatisfaction begin to appear around grade 3. Typical findings reveal that nearly one-half of girls in the age range 7–13 years want to be thinner.

An important distinction is drawn between perceptual and attitudinal components of body image disturbance. Perceptual distortion involves inaccurate judgments of one's body size; individuals with eating disorders often overestimate their body size. The attitudinal component, also frequently observed in individuals with eating disorders, involves their dissatisfaction with the size or shape of their body. Of course, body image attitudes may pertain to particular physical attributes or overall appearance. Interestingly, the perceptual and attitudinal components function in a manner largely independent of each other. Most researchers today believe that body image is a multidimensional construct that requires the assessment of both perceptual and attitudinal components.

This chapter provides an overview of body image assessment in preadolescent children under the age of 12. The subsequent two chapters discuss assessment in postadolescent children and adults.

MEASURING THE PERCEPTUAL COMPONENT

Relatively little research has been conducted on perceived body size distortions in children; most studies on children's body image have used figural drawings, a technique that precludes the measurement of perceptual components per se. Although a variety of perceptual techniques has been used with children, the following discussion focuses on those most frequently employed.

Research in our laboratory has used a video projection technique with children between the ages of 6 and 14. A life-size video image of the child is projected on a screen, and the child adjusts the width of the image, either wider or thinner, by depressing buttons on a hand-held mouse. A computer measures the amount of over- or underestimations in the children's judgments. This technique allows precise measurement of perceived body size distortion to 0.01%. We have found that children are very accurate in estimating their body width. In one study, the average overestimations were less than 2% and decreased consistently with increasing age. No differences were found between boys and girls. We have successfully used a similar video distortion technique in children as young as 5 years old.

This technique allows researchers to use common psychophysical procedures that simultaneously measure attitudinal and perceptual aspects of body image. For example, in the method of constant stimuli, the experimenter distorts the width of the child's video image and then asks the child to judge whether the image is too wide or too thin. The resulting data—the point at which the child judges his or her projected image to be subjectively equal to his or her body size—can be used to compute the size distortion. This value, known as the "point of subjective equality" (PSE), is a good indicator of the amount of perceived distortion. In addition, this technique can be used to measure how much change must occur in the child's body size before the child can reliably detect such a change. This value, commonly known as the "difference threshold" or "just noticeable difference" (JND), is a good measure of how perceptually sensitive children are to changes in their body size. In our studies we found that 6-year-old children could reliably detect a change in body size of around 5% and that this amount of change consistently decreased as children became older. By age 14, children could reliably detect a change of about 2% in their body size.

Another useful psychophysical procedure used with the video distortion technique is the staircase methodology. Children are presented a video image of themselves that is initially distorted, either too wide or too thin. Immediately after it appears, the image is sequentially distorted in size, either wider or thinner, at a constant rate of change. Children indicate when the changing body size matches their perceived size. The direction of distortion then reverses, and the children indicate when the image, now being sequentially distorted in the opposite direction, corresponds to their perceived size. After several such sequences are completed, the perceived body size is taken as the average of the transition points. This fast-paced methodology quickly captures the attention of children as young as 5 years of age and allows a large number of data trials to be collected in a relatively short period of time.

Another perceptual measurement technique uses a distorting mirror. A pliable Mylar sheet is flexed to adjust a person's body size. Readings are then made of the amount of distortion present. Although this methodology has never been used with children, it should prove as useful as the video distortion technique.

Finally, Kevin Thompson and his colleagues developed an adjustable light beam apparatus to measure children's body size judgments. Children as young as 10 are asked to adjust the width of four light beams, projected onto a wall, to match the perceived width of their cheeks, waist, hips, and thighs.

MEASURING THE ATTITUDINAL COMPONENT

The most commonly measured attitudinal component of body image is body size dissatisfaction. Body dissatisfaction is most frequently defined as the discrepancy between a person's perceived size and the size they would like to be, ideally. The perceptual techniques outlined above allow for a precise measurement of this discrepancy. With the video distortion technique, children are asked to adjust the width of their image to both the size they perceive themselves to be and to their ideal size. The distorting mirror and adjustable light beams offer similar capabilities. Research in our laboratory has indicated that children as young as 6 have little difficulty in understanding instructions to adjust the video image to the size they would like to be.

Figural Scales

Schematic drawings or figures, sometimes referred to as silhouettes, also have been developed to measure body size dissatisfaction in children. These scales consist of a set of line drawings of children's bodies that range in size from very underweight to very overweight. Typically, the experimenter presents between seven and nine figures and asks the children to select the one figure that represents their current size and the one figure that depicts the size they would like to be, ideally. The difference between the two figures constitutes the discrepancy index and represents body dissatisfaction. Table 15.1 summarizes the figural scales most frequently used with children.

The most commonly used figural scale is the one developed by Collins. Its popularity is probably due to the large number of children used in the standardization sample and the high test–retest correlations obtained (see

Table 15.1). In addition, criterion-related validity coefficients have been demonstrated with this scale by comparing the figure selections with the child's actual weight (.36) and body mass index (.37).

In selecting a figural scale, preference should be given to those that provide stability of measurement. The test–retest reliability coefficients shown in Table 15.1 for each test are a good reflection of this stability. As a general rule, a coefficient of .70 or greater is preferred.

One limitation of children's figural scales is that they only measure body size dissatisfaction, not the accuracy of perceived body size. As noted earlier, body dissatisfaction is defined as the discrepancy between the figure selected to reflect their perceived size and the figure selected to depict their ideal size. The larger the absolute value of the discrepancy, the greater the dissatisfaction with body size. However, it is not possible to determine the extent to which this discrepancy reflects an accurate or distorted judgment of actual size.

There are several methodological issues related to the use of these scales. Figural scales are age-specific, and no single scale is appropriate for

TABLE 15.1. Figure Scales Used for the Assessment of the Attitudinal Component of Body Image in Children

Author(s)	Test name	Description of figures	Test–retest reliability	Standardization sample
Collins (1991)	None given	Seven male and seven female figure drawings	3 days: self = .71; ideal/self = .59; ideal/other child = .38	1,118 preadolescent children
Childress, Brewerton, Hodges, & Jarrell (1993)	Kids' eating disorder survey	Eight male and eight female figure drawings	4 months: .83 for entire survey; not given for figures only	3,178 children, grades 5–8
Veron-Guidry & Williamson (1996)	Body Image Assessment— Children	Two scales; nine silhouettes of male and female children and preadolescents	Immediate: current = .94; ideal = .93; 1 week: current = .79; current/ideal = .67	22 boys and girls, ages 8–10; 40 boys and girls, ages 8–10
Sands, Tricker, Sherman, Armatas, & Maschette (1997)	Body Image Scale	Seven side profiles of prepubescent boys and girls	3 months: current = .56; 6 months: current = .40	26 girls and 35 boys, ages 10–12
Tiggemann & Pennington (1990)	None given	Nine figure drawings of children and adolescents	Not given	34 girls and 37 boys, ages 9–10

all age ranges. None of the scales has been standardized for children under the age of 8. Furthermore, because the scales were drawn to represent Caucasian subjects, the ability to generalize their effectiveness to their use with different ethnic groups is largely unknown.

The method used to present the figural stimuli is important. Investigators often present all of the figures on a single sheet of paper, with the figures arranged in ascending size from left to right. Children then select the figures representing both their perceived and ideal sizes. Research in our laboratory has revealed that this procedure produces artificially high test–retest reliability coefficients because the children have little difficulty remembering which figure they selected previously. A recommended alternative is to place each figure on a separate card and arrange the cards randomly for each testing session. This procedure should be followed for measuring both the perceived size and the ideal size.

Finally, in quantifying self–ideal discrepancies, researchers must recognize that averaging signed scores can mask discrepancies that differ in direction. If half of a group desires to be much thinner and half desires to be much larger, averaging these positive and negative numbers would result in a number reflecting a desire for no change.

Questionnaires Measuring Appearance Dissatisfaction

Several questionnaires have been developed to measure appearance dissatisfaction in younger children. Table 15.2 lists the most commonly used instruments. Note that some of the scales provide a global, comprehensive evaluation of the child's body dissatisfaction, while others focus on body satisfaction with specific body sites. Most of these scales have acceptable psychometric properties, although some do not report any reliability measures. Of these scales, the Body Dissatisfaction Scale, contained in the Eating Disorders Inventory (EDI-2 and EDI-C), and the Body Esteem Scale have been used most frequently.

AGE CONSIDERATIONS

Investigators measuring either the perceptual or attitudinal components of body image need to be aware of the developmental limitations of younger children. Children under the age of 7 have limited attentional capacity that can make any lengthy procedure involving numerous measurements problematic. Although we have used the video distortion technique successfully with children as young as 5, we have frequently found it necessary to prompt these younger children to pay attention. In addition, it is necessary to break up any lengthy measurement procedure into shorter blocks in order to retain children's interest and attention.

TABLE 15.2. Questionnaires Measuring Appearance Dissatisfaction in Children

Author(s)	Questionnaire	Description of test	Reliability[a]	Standardization sample
Garner (1991)	Eating Disorder Inventory (EDI-2) Body Dissatisfaction Scale	Nine-item subscale assesses feelings about satisfaction with body size; items are 6-point forced choice; reading level is fifth grade	IC: females = .91; males = .72	109 boys and girls, ages 8–10
Garner (1991)	Eating Disorders Inventory for Children (EDI-C) Body Dissatisfaction Scale	Same nine-item subscale as EDI; wording was rephrased for grades 1–2 reading level	No data	None
Mendelson & White (1982)	Body Esteem Scale	Participants report their degree of agreement with various statements about their bodies	IC: Split-half reliability = .85	97 boys and girls, ages 8.5–17.4
Thelen, Powell, Lawrence, & Kuhnert (1992)	Body Image and Eating Questionnaire	14 items focusing on overweight concerns, dieting, and restraint. Items assessed by 4- or 5-point Likert scale or yes–no format	IC: All values ≥ .68	191 children, ages 7.8–13.6
Mintz & Betz (1986)	Body-Cathexis Scale	Participants rate satisfaction with 15 body characteristics or parts, using response scale ranging from 1 (extremely satisfied) to 7 (extremely dissatisfied)	No data	170 girls, ages 8.1–15.5
Shisslak et al. (1999)	McKnight Risk Factor Survey III (MRFS-III)	Five-item subscale assesses concern with body weight and shape	IC: fourth and fifth grades = .82 TR: fourth and fifth grades = .79	103 girls, fourth and fifth grades

[a]IC, internal consistency; TR, test–retest.

Complex tasks that are sometimes used with the perceptual measures may place unreasonable cognitive demands on some younger children. For example, in our research children were asked to make judgments about whether a projected video image of their body was distorted larger or smaller than their perceived size. For 6- and 7-year-olds, we had to explain the procedure several times and allow the children numerous practice trials to ensure that they understood the nature of the task.

In general, we have found that children take a genuine interest in procedures that measure the perceptual and attitudinal components of their body image. Conducting even complex psychophysical tasks lasting 30 minutes or longer was possible with children as young as 6, although the patience of the investigator was sometimes sorely tried. Verbal encouragement and support from the experimenter are often necessary to sustain the attention of younger participants.

INFORMATIVE READINGS

Childress, A., Brewerton, T., Hodges, E., & Jarrell, M. (1993). The Kids' Eating Disorders Survey (KEDS): A study of middle school students. *Journal of the American Academy of Child and Adolescent Psychiatry, 32,* 841–850.—Figural drawings assessing body dissatisfaction in children grades 5 to 8.

Collins, M. (1991). Body figure perceptions and preferences among pre-adolescent children. *International Journal of Eating Disorders, 10,* 191–208.—Figural drawings assessing body dissatisfaction in preadolescent children; most frequently used of all the children's figural drawing scales.

Gardner, R. M. (1996). Methodological issues in assessment of the perceptual component of body image disturbance. *British Journal of Psychology, 87,* 321–337.—Discussion of important methodological issues and advantages of various psychophysical techniques to measure perceptual and attitudinal components separately.

Gardner, R. M., Friedman, B. N., & Jackson, N. A. (1998). Methodological concerns when using silhouettes to measure body image. *Perceptual and Motor Skills, 86,* 381–395.—Describes shortcomings of existing figural drawing scales and suggests ways to construct a scale to overcome those shortcomings.

Gardner, R. M., Friedman, B. N., Jackson, N. A., & Stark, K. (1999). Body size estimations in children six through fourteen: A longitudinal study. *Perceptual and Motor Skills, 88,* 541–555.—Describes a longitudinal study using the video distortion technique to measure how accurately children estimate their body size.

Garner, D. M. (1991). *Eating Disorder Inventory for Children* (EDI-C). Odessa, FL: Psychological Assessment Resources.—A revision of the adult version of the EDI, with wording that is appropriate for younger children.

Mendelson, B. K., & White, D. R. (1982). Relation between body-esteem and self-esteem of obese and normal children. *Perceptual and Motor Skills, 54,* 899–905.—Commonly used attitudinal test to measure appearance dissatisfaction in children and older adolescents.

Mintz, L., & Betz, N. (1986). Sex differences in the nature, realism, and correlates of body image. *Sex Roles, 15,* 185–195.—Describes a questionnaire measuring children's satisfaction with 15 body characteristics or parts.

Sands, R., Tricker, J., Sherman, C., Armatas, C., & Maschette, W. (1997). Disordered eating patterns, body image, self-esteem, and physical activity in pre-adolescent school children. *International Journal of Eating Disorders, 21,* 151–166.—Figural drawings measuring body dissatisfaction in prepubescent boys and girls; differs from other figural drawing scales in that it uses side profiles of children.

Shisslak, C. M., Renger, R., Sharpe, T., Crago, M., McKnight, K. M., Gray, N., Bryson, S., Estes, L. S., Parnaby, O. G., Killen, J., & Taylor, C. B. (1999). Development and evaluation of the McKnight Risk Factor Survey for assessing potential risk and protective factors for disordered eating in pre-adolescent and adolescent girls. *International Journal of Eating Disorders, 25,* 191–214.—Includes a scale to measure concern with body weight and shape in fourth- and fifth-grade children; standardization sample included adolescent girls through 12th grade.

Thelen, M., Powell, A., Lawrence, C., & Kuhnert, M. (1992). Eating and body image concerns among children. *Journal of Clinical Child Psychology, 21,* 41–46.—Describes a questionnaire measuring appearance dissatisfaction in children.

Thompson, J. K., & Spana, R. E. (1988). The adjustable light beam method for the assessment of size estimation accuracy: Description, psychometric, and normative data. *International Journal of Eating Disorders, 7*(4), 521–526.—Describes a procedure for measuring perceived body size which has been used successfully with children.

Tiggemann, M., & Pennington, B. (1990). The development of gender differences in body-size dissatisfaction. *Australian Psychologist, 25,* 301–311.—Figural drawings to measure body dissatisfaction in children ages 9–10; also used with adolescents ages 15–16.

Veron-Guidry, S., & Williamson, D. (1996). Development of a body image assessment procedure for children and preadolescents. *International Journal of Eating Disorders, 20*(3), 287–293.—Describes a figure scale used to measure body dissatisfaction in children.

16

Measuring Perceptual Body Image among Adolescents and Adults

J. KEVIN THOMPSON
RICK M. GARDNER

Perhaps no other area of body image research has generated the controversy, mixed empirical findings, and overall confusion as the topic of perceptual disturbance. Additionally, interest and activity in this area has waxed and waned over the years, from an initial intense interest in the 1970s and early 1980s to a relative lack of focus in the 1990s. In recent years, however, a reconceptualization of the problem and new technological advances have regenerated enthusiasm for the research viability and clinical utility of the concept. In this chapter we review the history of research in this area and then summarize contemporary thought and methods.

THE PERCEPTUAL COMPONENT: A BRIEF HISTORY

Arguably, no other component of body image can be so clearly traced to its connection with clinical disorders, specifically eating disorders. Slade and Russell's seminal study in this area was conducted in 1973—one of the most widely cited and influential studies in the literature on eating disorders. In their investigation, an apparatus referred to as the "movable caliper technique" was used to gauge the ability of individuals with anorexia nervosa and non-eating-disordered controls to accurately estimate their body dimensions (such as the width of the waist, hips, and thighs). The apparatus had lights mounted on tracks that participants adjusted to approximate their conceptions of their width at various body sites. The experimenter assessed actual site dimensions using body calipers. The difference between the estimated and actual widths was used as the index of accuracy.

Slade and Russell found that individuals with anorexia nervosa overestimated their body sizes to a greater degree than individuals without this eating disorder. This finding stimulated a great deal of research and theorizing, primarily because the results intuitively suggested an explanation for the dominant symptom of anorexia—excessive dieting and pursuit of thinness in the absence of an elevated body weight and/or size. In essence, if anorexics saw themselves as larger than they really were (body size overestimation), perhaps this was the impetus for continuing to restrict caloric intake and increase exercise level. Slade and Russell also created an index of size accuracy and a terminology that would be used for many subsequent investigations. The Body Distortion Index (BDI) was computed using the formula of (estimated size/actual size) × 100. For instance, if a patient thought her waist was 40 cm in width but the actual width was 30 cm, the BDI index would be 133.

In the years following Slade and Russell's report, a wealth of research emerged on the perceptual component of body image, much of it confined to an examination of individuals with eating disorders. Researchers created numerous variations on the original movable caliper technique, such as the image marking procedure, body image detection device, and adjustable light beam apparatus. Such strategies were labeled single-site measurement techniques. In addition, a second category of methods was developed that allowed for the assessment of whole image accuracy. These methods usually allowed the participant to adjust the entire image via the experimental modification of a TV or photographic image, or by use of a distorting mirror. Many of these methods remain in use today, and the essentials of their construction and utilization have been reviewed in previous works by Cash, us, and our colleagues.

Several lines of research converged in the late 1980s that temporarily culminated in a general lack of interest in the perceptual aspect of body image. First, the entire focus of body image researchers began to move beyond the relatively narrow confines of the eating disorders field. Researchers were beginning to find that individuals without eating disorders reported a subjective unhappiness with their appearance, and the topic of body dysmorphic disorder began to appear with increasing frequency in the literature. Questionnaire measures of subjective disturbance could be administered to large groups of individuals, whereas the perceptual research methods were far more time consuming. Second, investigators were beginning to note that size overestimation and subjective disturbance were not highly correlated, and the variable of subjective unhappiness with appearance appeared to be a better predictor of psychological functioning (self-esteem, depression) than perceptual disturbance. Third, various experimental studies and review articles noted that the perceptual component, previously thought to be a static and rather unmalleable aspect of body image, was instead a dimension of body image affected by numerous contextual factors. For instance, in 1989 Thompson and Dolce found that estimates of size were larger if participants were asked to make an "affective" rating (i.e., "How large do you feel?") versus a "cognitive" rating ("How large do you think you look?"). Size estimates were also found to be affected by repeated testing, consumption of food during the testing session, lighting variations in the testing situation, and the type of clothing worn by participants. Fourth, studies found that the correspondence between the two methods of measuring size estimation (i.e., site-specific and whole image adjustment strategies) was often much lower than expected.

The bulk of interest shifted in the late 1980s from a focus on the perceptual aspect of body image to an examination of subjective disturbances. The emergence of the cognitive revolution in psychology also had an effect on body image work. Studies began to document cognitive aspects of disturbance (irrational beliefs and distortions regarding one's looks) and questionnaire measures of cognitive body image disturbance were developed. Notably, empirically supported methods of improving body image satisfaction, pioneered by Cash and Rosen, largely focused on the enhancement of subjective and attitudinal aspects of disturbance. (See Cash and Strachan's chapter in this volume.) Although there was a shift away from investigating the perceptual aspects of body image disturbance, some researchers maintained an interest in the perceptual component, challenged the existing methodologies, and offered a reconceptualization of previous theory and research strategies.

THE PERCEPTUAL COMPONENT: A RECONCEPTUALIZATION

Beginning in the late 1980s, researchers began to employ sophisticated psychophysical techniques that allowed for a separation of the *sensory* and *nonsensory* components of body size distortion, as summarized in Table 16.1. With respect to body size estimation, the sensory component refers to the responses of the visual system, including the retina and visual cortex, whereas the nonsensory components, sometimes characterized as the cognitive or affective factors, refer to the brain's *interpretation* of the visual input.

Signal Detection Theory

In the late 1980s Gardner and colleagues were the first researchers to use a signal detection theory approach for this purpose. With this methodology, individuals are presented with static video images of themselves that are distorted either too wide or too thin. Separate measures of sensory sensitivity and response bias are found by examining an individual's correct re-

TABLE 16.1. Methodologies for Measuring the Sensory and Nonsensory Components of Body Image Size Estimations

Methodology	Brief description	Dependent measures	Separate measures of sensory and nonsensory components	Examples of studies using methodology
Method of constant stimuli	A static video image is presented, with size distortion present or absent; subjects judge presence or absence of distortion.	Judgments of subjective size and sensitivity to detecting changes in body size	Nonsensory: point of subjective equality (PSE) Sensory: difference threshold (DL)	Gardner, Morrell, Watson, & Sandoval (1989)
Signal detection theory	A static video image is presented, with size distortion present or absent; subjects judge presence or absence of distortion.	Sensitivity to detecting body size distortion and response bias in judging body size	Nonsensory: response criterion (β) Sensory: sensitivity in detecting size distortion (d')	Gardner & Moncrieff (1988); Smeets, Ingleby, Hoek, & Panhuysen (1999)
Adaptive probit estimation	Video image presented at one of five levels of distortion; subjects judge whether perceived image is wider or thinner than their actual body size.	Judgments of subjective size and sensitivity to detecting changes in body size	Nonsensory: point of subjective equality (PSE) Sensory: difference threshold (DL)	Gardner, Jones, & Bokenkamp (1995); Gardner, Friedman, Stark, & Jackson (1999)

sponses and errors. *Sensory sensitivity* refers to the person's ability to detect correctly whether the image is distorted as too thin or too wide; *response bias* measures the person's tendency to overreport the body as too wide or too thin. Because these sensory and nonsensory factors function largely independently of each other, a person may correctly detect whether an image is distorted or not but still have a bias to report that his or her body is too wide or too thin.

In the earliest study (1988) to employ this technique, Gardner and Moncrieff demonstrated that anorexic subjects had no differential sensitivity in their ability to detect distorted images of themselves when compared to control subjects. However, anorexic subjects did show an increased response bias to report that their image was distorted in size. This study showed that the frequently reported perceptual size distortion in eating-disordered subjects is caused by nonsensory attitudinal factors. Several more recent studies have confirmed this conclusion. In other words, it is one's beliefs, attitudes, and thoughts that influence willingness to perceive body image as either normal or distorted, rather than any sensory deficit. Nevertheless, it is important to recognize that even though no sensory distortion is present, the image still appears distorted to the individual.

Method of Constant Stimuli

A variant of the psychophysical method of constant stimuli has also been used to measure judgments of body size. As with the signal detection methodology, a single static video image is presented, with size distortion present or absent; the person is asked to report the presence or absence of distortion. By using a range of discrete distortion levels, this technique allows calculation of the percent of body size distortion (if any) that corresponds to the subject's perception of his or her body size. This point is designated as the point of subjective equality (PSE). In addition, the procedure allows the investigator to ascertain how much distortion in body size beyond this PSE is necessary before the person detects the changes as a "just noticeable difference" (JND). This value is referred to as the difference threshold or difference limen (DL). However, the PSE and the DL operate largely independent of each other. The PSE reflects the attitudinal aspects of body size estimation, whereas the DL indicates the perceptual ability to detect size distortion.

Gardner and colleagues applied this methodology to examine body size estimations in obese and normal-weight subjects. Both weight groups were very accurate in judging their body size, with an average PSE of –.62%. This result indicated that the subjects judged an image that was slightly smaller than their actual size as being subjectively equal to their body size. The average DL of 7.27% across all subjects indicated that, on average, subjects who saw their bodies distorted an average of ±7.27% were able to detect that distortion 50% of the time. Both obese and normal-weight subjects showed equal accuracy in detecting size distortion. This particular methodology, unfortunately, requires numerous trials at several different levels of size distortion, which becomes time consuming and burdensome for both the subject and the experimenter.

Adaptive Probit Estimation

Gardner and colleagues have recently used a more efficient psychophysical technique, called "adaptive probit estimation," to measure separately the perceptual and affective aspects of body size estimations. Based on the method of constant stimuli, adaptive probit estimation also requires that subjects make a forced choice between two alternatives of body size. Individuals view a video image that is distorted too wide or too thin and are asked to report whether they judge the image to be too wide or too thin.

Because a detailed discussion of adaptive probit estimation is beyond the scope of this chapter, the interested reader is referred to the suggested readings that follow. Briefly, however, this methodology presents a static video image at one of five discrete levels of distortion. The range of distortion levels, both too wide and too thin, is set by the experimenter and is made sufficiently large to ensure that the subject's perceived body size is included. A computer interfaced with a video projector controls the amount of distortion. After a set of initial trials, the computer recalculates the subject's perceived body size (PSE) and adjusts the amount of distortion in subsequent trials around this value, based on the calculated difference threshold (DL) from the subject's data. This process continues for a total of eight blocks of 40 trials. At that point, the computer calculates (1) the subject's overall perception of PSE and (2) the difference threshold, or how much change in body size was needed to detect the change 50% of the time.

This technique derives both nonsensory (PSE) and sensory (DL) sensitivity values relative to body size perception in a far more efficient and rapid fashion than the method of constant stimuli. Stable measurements of PSE and DL are possible after approximately 20 minutes of data collection. This procedure requires a digital camera, a video projector, and a specialized computer program. Interested investigators should contact Rick Gardner to obtain a version of this program for use with personal computers.

Several studies have indicated the importance of both sensory and nonsensory factors in body image size estimation. Since these factors function largely independently, research methodology should employ measurement techniques that assess both components.

SUMMARY

The subfield of body image research that focuses on measurement of the perceptual component has evolved dramatically over the past 30 years. In a preceding chapter in this volume, Gardner discusses the use of perceptual assessments with children. A simple conception that size overestimation is specific to patients with eating disorders and reflective of a purely sensory dysfunction is no longer tenable. As scientists develop newer and more precise theoretical models and measurement tools, our understanding of the relative role of perceptual processes in body image is surely to expand.

INFORMATIVE READINGS

Cash, T. F., & Deagle, E. A. (1997). The nature and extent of body-image disturbances in anorexia nervosa and bulimia nervosa: A meta-analysis. *International Journal of Eating Disorders, 22,* 107–125.—A meta-analysis of studies utilizing perceptual and attitudinal measures.

Gardner, R. M., Friedman, B. N., Stark, K., & Jackson, N. A. (1999). Body-size estimation in children six through fourteen: A longitudinal study. *Perceptual and Motor Skills, 88,* 541–555.—Illustration of the use of method of adjustment and adaptive probit estimation techniques in measuring children's body size estimations.

Gardner, R. M., Jones, L. C., & Bokenkamp, E. D. (1995). A comparison of three psychophysical techniques for estimating body size perception. *Perceptual and Motor Skills, 80,* 1379–1390.—Comparison of method of adjustment, signal detection, and adaptive probit estimation as techniques for measuring body size estimations.

Gardner, R. M., Martinez, R., & Sandoval, Y. (1987). Obesity and body image: An evaluation of sensory and nonsensory components. *Psychological Medicine, 17,* 927–932.—Describes a signal detection analysis of body size estimation data with obese subjects.

Gardner, R. M., & Moncrieff, C. (1988). Body image distortion in anorexics as a nonsensory phenomenon: A signal detection approach. *Journal of Clinical Psychology, 44*(2), 101–107.—Illustration of how signal detection methodology is used with eating-disordered patients to measure separately the sensory and nonsensory components of body image.

Gardner, R. M., Morrell, J., Watson, D., & Sandoval, S. (1989). Subjective equality and just noticeable differences in body-size judgments by obese persons. *Perceptual and Motor Skills, 69,* 595–604.—Use of the method of constant stimuli to measure body size estimates in obese individuals.

Slade, P. D., & Russell, G. F. M. (1973). Awareness of body dimensions in anorexia nervosa: Cross-sectional and longitudinal studies. *Psychological Medicine, 3,* 188–199.—Seminal study in the assessment of the perceptual component of body image disturbance.

Smeets, M. A. M., Ingleby, D., Hoek, H. W., & Panhuysen, G. E. M. (1999). Body size perception in anorexia nervosa: A signal detection approach. *Journal of Psychosomatic Research, 46,* 465–477.—Illustration of signal detection procedure with a sample of individuals with anorexia nervosa.

Thompson, J. K. (1996). Assessing body image disturbance: Measures, methodology, and implementation. In J. K. Thompson (Ed.), *Body image, eating disorders, and obesity: An integrative guide for assessment and treatment* (pp. 49–81). Washington, DC: American Psychological Association.—A comprehensive overview of perceptual measures and the methodological issues relevant to their use.

Thompson, J. K., & Dolce, J. (1989). The discrepancy between emotional vs. rational estimates of body size, actual size, and ideal body ratings: Theoretical and clinical implications. *Journal of Clinical Psychology, 45,* 473–478.—Investigation that suggested that instructional protocol (i.e., affective vs. cognitive) would affect perceptual ratings of body size.

Thompson, J. K., Heinberg, L. J., Altabe, M., & Tantleff-Dunn, S. (1999). *Exacting beauty: Theory, assessment, and treatment of body image disturbance.* Washington, DC: American Psychological Association.—Broad overview of contemporary assessment and treatment methods, including a focus on perceptual aspects of body image.

17

Measuring Body Image Attitudes among Adolescents and Adults

J. KEVIN THOMPSON
PATRICIA VAN DEN BERG

Over the past 20 years, a wide range of measures has been developed for the assessment of various aspects of body image in adolescents and adults. The breadth of coverage provided by these strategies offers an impressive selection to researchers and practitioners interested in measuring body image disturbances. There is general agreement on the distinctions between the dimensions of the attitudinal component. Attitudinal body image is generally classified into the following four components:

1. Global subjective dissatisfaction or disturbance—refers to overall satisfaction–dissatisfaction with one's appearance.
2. Affective distress regarding appearance—refers to one's emotions about one's appearance, including anxiety, dysphoria, and discomfort.
3. Cognitive aspects of body image—refers to investment in one's appearance, erroneous thoughts or beliefs about one's body, and body image schemas.
4. Behavioral avoidance reflective of dissatisfaction with appearance— refers to avoidance of situations or objects due to their elicitation of body image concerns.

In contrast to the assessment of the perceptual dimension of body image, which is an area rife with methodological perplexity (see the preceding chapter by Thompson and Gardner), attitudinal body image measurement is relatively straightforward. Nevertheless, there are important issues and methodological concerns to consider when conducting attitudinal assessments. In this chapter we review the measures developed to index the above dimensions, and provide an overview of methodological issues relevant to the optimal selection of measures. Table 17.1 delineates many of these assessments, along with specific information for contacting their authors.

GLOBAL MEASURES OF BODY IMAGE SATISFACTION

A broad measure of body image satisfaction can be obtained in a variety of ways. *Satisfaction* itself must be further defined to reflect such components as weight satisfaction, shape satisfaction, and satisfaction with specific body sites and features. A very simplistic method of addressing weight satisfaction is to obtain a participant's actual weight and ideal weight. The discrepancy between the two indices quantifies as weight dissatisfaction. This concept of discrepancy (actual vs. ideal) is used widely in the assessment of attitudinal body image. Another relatively simple measure, which can be adapted to weight, size, shape, or specific body features, is a Likert-type scale (usually a five- or seven-point scale with endpoint descriptors of "strongly agree" and "strongly disagree") containing items such as "I am satisfied with the appearance of my body." Many researchers create Likert-type items to reflect specific theoretical or practical goals of their research. Another simple method in this category is the visual analogue scale, using a 100-mm line with endpoints defining ratings (i.e., from extremely dissatisfied to extremely satisfied) (see Thompson & colleagues). Participants make a slash at the point on the line that reflects their level of dissatisfaction.

Although the above measures have the advantages of efficiency and adaptability, they are necessarily limited in range and scope. More comprehensive methods may be amenable to extensive psychometric evaluation, indicating their suitability (vis-à-vis validity and reliability estimates) for widespread use with large-scale and potentially diverse samples.

Figural Ratings

Schematic figural methods of assessment represent a category of the global measures that provides a greater level of measurement complexity than do single-item indices. The common theme among the wide variety of these strategies is the use of a broad range of figures ranging in size from, for instance, very thin to very overweight. These figures can be schematic outlines or silhouettes of the human form. Participants select the figures representing their perceived current and ideal sizes. The discrepancy between the two

TABLE 17.1 Measures of Body Satisfaction and Related Concepts

Type and name of instrument	Author(s)[a]	Description	Reliability[b]	Standardization sample	Author address
Global satisfaction measures—figural ratings					
Body Image Assessment	Williamson et al. (1989)	Select from nine figures that vary in size from underweight to overweight	IC: NA TR: immediately to 8 weeks (.60–.93); bulimics—ideal (.74), current (.83); obese—ideal (NS), current (.88); binge eaters—ideal (.65), current (.81)	659 females, including bulimics, binge eaters, anorexics, normals, obese subjects, and atypical eating-disordered subjects	Donald A. Williamson, PhD, Pennington Biomedical Research Center, 6400 Perkins Rd. Baton Rouge, LA 70808 *williada@pbrc.edu*
Figure Rating Scale	1) Stunkard et al. (1983) 2) Thompson & Altabe (1991)	Select from nine figures that vary in size from underweight to overweight	1) IC: NA 2) TR: 2 weeks; ideal: males (.82), females (.71); self-think: males (.92), females (.89); self-feel: males (.81), females (.83)	1) 125 males, 204 females 2) 58 females, 34 males	Albert J. Stunkard, MD, University of Pennsylvania, Department of Psychiatry, 3600 Market St., Room 734, Philadelphia, PA 19104-2648; *stunkard@mail.med.upenn.edu*
Contour Drawing Rating Scale	Thompson & Gray (1995)	Nine male and nine female schematic figures, ranging from underweight to overweight	IC: NA TR: 1 week (.79)	40 male and female undergraduates	James J. Gray, PhD, American University, Department of Psychology, Asbury Building, Room 317, Washington, DC 20016-8062; *jgray@american.edu*
Somatomorphic Matrix	Pope et al. (2000)	Computerized: choose from 100 figures that vary on two axes: % body fat and muscularity	IC: NA TR: None reported	200 undergraduate college men	Harrison G. Pope, MD, McLean Hospital, 115 Mill St., Belmont, MA 02478

Global satisfaction measures—questionnaires

Body Esteem Scale	Franzoi & Shields (1984)	Modification of body cathexis scale with 16 new items; factor analysis yielded three factors for male and female samples	IC: females (.78–.87), males (.81–.86) TR: None given	366 females and 257 male undergraduates	Stephen Franzoi, PhD, Department of Psychology, Schroeder Health Complex, 454, Marquette University, P.O. Box 1881, Milwaukee, WI 53201-1881 *franzois@marquette.edu*
Body Esteem Scale for Adolescents and Adults	Mendelson et al. (2001)	23 Likert-type items on three subscales: attribution, appearance, weight	IC: appearance (.92), weight (.94) TR: 3 months; attribution (.83), appearance (.89), weight (.92)	IC: 1,308 (appearance), 1,283 (attribution), 1,312 (weight) ages 12–25 TR: 95 junior college students	Morton J. Mendelson, PhD, Department of Psychology, McGill University, 1205 Doctor Penfield Ave., Montreal, Quebec H3A 1B1, Canada; *mmendelson@psych.mcgill.ca*
Body Satisfaction Scale	Slade et al. (1990)	Indicate degree of satisfaction with 16 parts (three subscales: general, head, and body)	IC: range (.79–.89) TR: None given	Females: undergraduates, nursing students, volunteers, overweight subjects, anorexics, bulimics	P. D. Slade, PhD, Department of Psychiatry and Department of Movement Science, Liverpool University Medical School, P.O. Box 147, Liverpool, L69 3BX, England
Body Shape Questionnaire	Cooper et al. (1987)	34 items regarding concerns about one's body shape	IC: None given TR: None given	Bulimics, several control samples	Peter Cooper, PhD, Department of Psychiatry, University of Cambridge, Addenbrooke's Hospital, Hills Rd., Cambridge, CB22QQ, England

(continued)

TABLE 17.1 (*continued*)

Type and name of instrument	Author(s)[a]	Description	Reliability[b]	Standardization sample	Author address
Global satisfaction measures—questionnaires (*continued*)					
Eating Disorder Inventory—Body Dissatisfaction Scale	1) Garner et al. (1983) 2) Shore & Porter (1990) 3) Wood et al. (1996)	Rated degree of agreement with nine statements about body parts being large (seven items)	1) IC: anorexic participants (.90), controls (.91) 2) IC: adolescents (11–18), female (.91), male (.86) 3) IC: children (8–10), girls (.84), boys (.72)	1) 113 female anorexics, 577 female controls 2) 195 boys, 414 girls 3) 109 boys, 95 girls	David M. Garner, PhD, c/o Psychological Assessments Resources, Inc., P.O. Box 998, Odessa, FL 33556; *www.parinc.com*
Multidimensional Body Self-Relations Questionnaire—Appearance Scales	Brown et al. (1990)	Appearance Evaluation: overall appearance evaluation. Appearance Orientation: cognitive-behavioral investment in appearance. Body Areas Satisfaction Scale: satisfaction with specific areas of the body. Overweight Preoccupation: fat anxiety, dieting, and weight vigilance. Self-Classified Weight: rating weight from "very underweight" to "very overweight."	IC: AE: males (.88), females (.88) AO: males (.88), females (.85) BASS: males (.77), females (.73) OWP: males (.73), females (.76) SCW: males (.70), females (.89) TR: 1 month AE: males (.81), females (.91) AO: males (.89), females (.90) BASS: males (.86), females (.74) OWP: males (.79), females (.89) SCW: males (.86), females (.74)	IC:AE, AO, OWP: 996 males, 1,070 females BASS, SCW: 804 females, 335 males TR: 804 female, 335 male college students	Electronically available from the author for a nominal fee at *www.body-images.com*

146

Instrument	Source	Description	Psychometrics	Sample	Availability
Body-Image Ideals Questionnaire	Cash & Szymanski (1995)	11 items assessing self-ideal discrepancy and importance of ideals in 10 specific aspects of appearance and overall appearance	IC: males (.81), females (.76) TR: None reported	192 male, 896 female adults	Electronically available from the author for a nominal fee at *www.body-images.com*
Self-Image Questionnaire for Young Adolescents—Body Image Subscale	Peterson (1984)	Designed for 10–15 year-olds; 11-item body image subscale assesses positive feelings toward the body	IC: boys (.81), girls (.77) TR: 1 year (.60); 2 years (.44)	335 sixth-grade students who were followed through the eighth grade	Anne C. Peterson, PhD W. K. Kellogg Foundation, One Michigan Ave. East, Battle Creek, MI 49017-4058
Affective					
Physical Appearance State and Trait Anxiety Scale	Reed et al. (1991)	Rates the anxiety associated with 16 body sites (eight weight relevant, eight non-weight relevant); trait and state versions available	IC: Trait: .88–.92 State: .82–.92 TR: 2 weeks, .87		J. Kevin Thompson, PhD, Department of Pyschology, PCD, 4118G, University of South Florida, 4202 E. Fowler Ave., Tampa, FL 33620-8200 *Thompson@chuma1.cas.usf.edu; luna.cas.usf.edu/~jthomps1*
Situational Inventory of Body-Image Dysphoria	Cash (1994)	Measures how often one experiences negative emotions about body image across 48 situational contexts	IC: males (.96), females (.96) TR: 1 month, males (.80), females (.86)	IC: 1,207 females, 386 males TR: 30 males, 110 females	Electronically available from the author for a nominal fee at *www.body-images.com*

(continued)

TABLE 17.1 (*continued*)

Type and name of instrument	Author(s)[a]	Description	Reliability[b]	Standardization sample	Author address
Cognitive					
Appearance Schemas Inventory	Cash & Labarge (1996)	14 items assess dysfunctional appearance-related assumptions	IC: males (.82), females (.86) TR: 1 month, males (.76), females (.72)	IC: 332 males, 1,349 females TR: 30 males, 114 females	Electronically available from the author for a nominal fee at *www.body-images.com*
Attention to Body Shape Scale	Beebe (1995)	Seven items assess degree of focus on body shape	IC: males (.70–.82), females (.70–.83) TR: males (.87), females (.76)	IC: 22 males, 167 females in three samples TR: 22 males, 49 females	Dean Beebe, PhD, Children's Hospital Medical Center, 3333 Burnet Ave., Cincinnati, OH 45229-3039
Sociocultural Attitudes Towards Appearance Questionnaire—3; Sociocultural Internalization of Appearance Questionnaire—Adolescent	Thompson, van den Berg, Roehrig, Guarda, & Heinberg (in press); Keery, Shroff, Thompson, Wertheim, & Smolak (in press)	SIAQ-A: five items assess internalization of sociocultural appearance ideals from the media SATAQ-3: 13 items assess internalization of sociocultural ideals from the media	SIAQ-A: IC: females (.86) TR: females (.86) SATAQ-3: IC: females (.91) TR: None reported	SIAQ-A: IC: 187 middle school girls TR: 33 middle school girls SATAQ-3: IC: 150 female undergraduates	J. Kevin Thompson, PhD, Department of Psychology, PCD, 4118G, University of South Florida, 4202 E. Fowler Ave., Tampa, FL 33620-8200; *Thompson@cas.usf.edu; luna.cas.usf.edu/~jthomps1*
Behavioral					
Body Image Avoidance Questionnaire	Rosen et al. (1991)	Assesses the frequency with which one engages in avoidance behaviors related to body image	IC: .89 TR: 2 weeks, .87	145 female undergraduates	James C. Rosen, PhD, Department of Psychology, University of Vermont, Burlington, VT 05405; *j_rosen@deavey.uvm.edu*

[a]Full citations for these sources are found at the end of the chapter.
[b]IC, internal consistency; TR, test–retest

ratings is a measure of dissatisfaction. Paper and pencil schematic figures have also been developed for the measurement of muscularity satisfaction. (See Olivardia's chapter for a discussion of a computerized measure that allows for muscularity and overall size ratings.)

Questionnaire Measures

Questionnaire measures have also been developed to measure the subjective global satisfaction component of body image. For instance, Cash and colleagues (see Cash, 2000) developed the Body Areas Satisfaction Scale, in which participants rate their satisfaction with weight and other aspects of appearance. One widely used subscale of the Eating Disorder Inventory, developed by Garner and colleagues, is the Body Dissatisfaction Scale (EDI-BD), which measures satisfaction with several weight-relevant body sites (waist, hips, buttocks, etc.). Cash and colleagues (see Cash, 2000) developed the Body Image Ideals Questionnaire, wherein respondents rate 11 physical characteristics in relation to their degree of disparity with personal physical ideals. The personal importance of each ideal is also rated, and cross-products of the discrepancy and importance ratings are tabulated.

Generic body image satisfaction measures capture a more complex and broader notion of one's appearance rating. Such measures include items that might evaluate how one appears to others or one's sexual attractiveness. The Appearance Evaluation subscale of Cash's Multidimensional Body Self-Relations Questionnaire (MBSRQ) (see Cash, 2000) is one such measure; the Self-Image Questionnaire for Young Adolescents is another that captures this component. Still other scales tap a general satisfaction component of body image, although the authors use terms such as "body-esteem" or "body concern."

MEASURES OF AFFECTIVE, COGNITIVE, AND BEHAVIORAL COMPONENTS OF BODY IMAGE

Affective Measures

Measures discussed in this section were developed by researchers with the intent of specifically addressing a unique dimension of the attitudinal construct. Thompson and colleagues addressed the affective component by constructing the Physical Appearance State and Trait Anxiety Scale, which asks participants to rate the anxiety level associated with both weight-related and non-weight-related appearance features. Cash and colleagues (see Cash, 2000) developed the Situational Inventory of Body-Image Dysphoria to assess the presence of negative body image emotions in 48 widely divergent social and personal situations.

Cognitive Measures

Cognitive measures attempt to capture a very specific dimension of body image: the beliefs, thoughts, attributions, or other cognitive components of disturbance. The Appearance Schemas Inventory, for instance, contains 14 items that measure the degree of dysfunctional cognitive schema regarding one's appearance. This measure was developed by Cash and colleagues (see Cash, 2000) to address multiple domains, including self-attentional focus, emotional/identity investment in one's appearance, beliefs concerning historical or developmental influences regarding appearance, beliefs related to interpersonal issues, and internalization of social stereotypes regarding appearance. Also relevant to this category are scales that tap into the internalization of societal values regarding appearance. For instance, Thompson and colleagues developed the Sociocultural Attitudes Towards Appearance Questionnaire—3, which has a subscale measuring the internalization of appearance values.

Behavioral Measures

Behavioral measures have received limited analysis in the body image literature. Such a measure would encompass a rating by an observer of a participant's behavior related to body image, such as avoidance of mirrors or weight scales. It is perhaps understandable why researchers have not focused attention in this area: Body image is such an intrapsychic phenomenon that the more direct approach of asking participants about their experience is preferred. However, it is well documented that a central component of disturbed body image, especially in the form of body dysmorphic disorder, is behavioral avoidance; therefore, a global assessment of the attitudinal perspective should include such a method of assessment. Rosen and colleagues developed the Body Image Avoidance Questionnaire, which yields a self-report score of avoidance, such as avoidance of weighing or social activities, or wearing specific types of clothes (e.g., loose-fitting) to cover parts that produce discomfort. Importantly, this measure was validated by roommates' reports of such activities. Thus, even though it is a self-report measure, there is evidence that scores may validly reflect actual behaviors.

INTERVIEW METHODS

Two methods developed to measure eating-disordered behaviors are relevant to this discussion, because they also include an assessment component for body image disturbance (a necessary criterion for the diagnosis of eating disorders). The Eating Disorder Examination is a widely used interview method, revised 12 times since it was developed by Fairburn and Cooper. Two of its four subscales—shape and weight concerns—assess body image components. The Interview for Diagnosis of Eating Disorders-IV was developed by Williamson and colleagues (Netemeyer & Williamson, 2001)and also covers aspects of body image disturbance. Finally, as Phillips discusses elsewhere in this volume, there are structured interviews to assess body image experiences associated with the diagnosis of body dysmorphic disorder.

METHODOLOGICAL ISSUES

In several review articles Thompson and colleagues have noted that care should be taken when selecting and utilizing a body image assessment measure for research or clinical purposes. First, the assessor should have a clear sense of the body image topic of interest—that is, which *aspect* of body image is relevant (size, weight, muscularity) and which *dimension* is relevant (general dissatisfaction, affective, cognitive, behavioral). For some purposes, a broad multidimensional assessment, such as the MBSRQ, is indicated. In other cases, such as in an experimental investigation, a fine-grained analysis of cognitive bias or affective response is indicated. In a subsequent chapter in this volume, Cash discusses the assessment of body image states in specific contexts.

A second concern is the instrument's psychometric data on validation samples. Notably, this is a concern when considering a measure for younger or ethnic minority samples. Many measures are validated on adult samples only, typically composed of Caucasian college females. Research reports should be scrutinized and authors contacted for information regarding validation samples. Importantly, some measures (in Table 17.1) received extensive work with diverse samples of adolescents and adults of both genders, including the MBSRQ scales and the EDI-BD.

A third concern involves the insufficient psychometric evaluation of figural rating scales. For instance, most have unknown test–retest reliabilities, and some have reliabilities below .70. In addition, as Gardner has noted, many scales have a restriction of scale range, leading to a narrow range of selection of figures for most participants. Only two figural strategies have been developed to ensure that consistent size gradations exist from one figure to the next (see Table 17.1, Thompson and Gray; Gardner and colleagues). Finally, the instructional protocol is important when using figural scales. Asking for an affective rating (e.g., "Rate how you *feel*") may yield higher size ratings than requesting a cognitive rating (i.e., "Rate how you *think* you look").

SUMMARY

The array of attitudinal body image measures makes selection of a specific index or indices a daunting task, even for the experienced body image researcher or clinician. In this chapter, we reviewed various methods and issues. Giving care and attention to the specific dimensions of interest and scale development properties will well serve one's clinical or research goals.

INFORMATIVE READINGS

Cash, T. F. (1997). *The body image workbook: An 8-step program for learning to like your looks.* Oakland, CA: New Harbinger.—Practical guide to the assessment of multiple components of body image disturbance that is also applied to treatment methods.

Cash, T. F. (2000). Manuals for the Multidimensional Body-Self Relations Questionnaire, the Body-Image Ideals Questionnaire, the Appearance Schemas Inventory, and the Situational Inventory of Body-Image Dysphoria (available from the author at *www. body-images.com*).—The scales, instructions, and psychometric information regarding these scales can be downloaded from the author's website.

Fairburn, C. G., & Cooper, Z. (1993). The Eating Disorder Examination (12th ed.). In C. G. Fairburn & G. T. Wilson (Eds.), *Binge eating: Nature, assessment and treatment* (pp. 3–14). New York: Guilford Press.—Describes a widely used interview method.

Gardner, R. M. (2001). Assessment of body image disturbance in children and adolescents. In J. K. Thompson & L. Smolak (Eds.), *Body image, eating disorders, and obesity in youth: Assessment, prevention, and treatment* (pp. 193–213). Washington, DC: American Psychological Association.—Review of measures and methodological issues regarding assessment of body image in children and adolescents.

Gardner, R. M., Stark, K., Jackson, N., & Friedman, B. (1999). Development and validation of two new body-image assessment scales. *Perceptual and Motor Skills, 89,* 981–993.—Describes measures that improve on existing figural rating scale strategies.

Netemeyer, S. B., & Williamson, D. A. (2001). Assessment of eating disturbance in children and adolescents with eating disorders and obesity. In J. K. Thompson & L. Smolak (Eds.), *Body image, eating disorders, and obesity in youth: Assessment, prevention, and treatment* (pp. 215–233). Washington, DC: American Psychological Association.—Summarizes assessments of the psychological and behavioral characteristics of these populations.

Rosen, J. C., Srebnik, D., Saltzberg, E., & Wendt, S. (1991). Development of a body image avoidance questionnaire. *Psychological Assessment, 3,* 32–37.—Details a measure of body image avoidance.

Thompson, J. K. (1996). Assessing body image disturbance: Measures, methodology, and implementation. In J. K. Thompson (Ed.), *Body image, eating disorders and obesity: An integrative guide for assessment and treatment* (pp. 49–81). Washington, DC: American Psychological Association.—Reviews a wide variety of measures for the measurement of body image and its disturbance.

Thompson, J. K., Heinberg, L. J., Altabe, M. N., & Tantleff-Dunn, S. (1999). *Exacting beauty: Theory, assessment, and treatment of body image disturbance.* Washington, DC: American

Psychological Association.—Covers multiple aspects of body image, including assessment and application of assessment to treatment selection.

Thompson, J. K., Penner, L., & Altabe, M. N. (1990). Procedures, problems and progress in the assessment of body image. In T. F. Cash & T. Pruzinsky (Eds.), *Body images: Development, deviance, and change* (pp. 21–48). New York: Guilford Press.—Overview of body image measurements and methodological issues.

Thompson, M. A., & Gray, J. J. (1996). Development and validation of a new body-image assessment scale. *Journal of Personality Assessment, 64,* 258–269.—Reports a figural scale with equivalent gradations between adjacent figure selections.

CITATIONS FOR ASSESSMENT INSTRUMENTS IN TABLE 17.1

Beebe, D. W. (1995). The Attention to Body Shape Scale: A new measure of body focus. *Journal of Personality Assessment, 65,* 486–501.

Brown, T. A., Cash, T. F., & Mikulka, P. J. (1990). Attitudinal body image assessment: Factor analysis of the Body-Self Relations Questionnaire. *Journal of Personality Assessment, 55,* 135–144.

Cash, T. F. (1994). The Situational Inventory of Body Image Dysphoria: Contextual assessment of a negative body image. *The Behavior Therapist, 17,* 133–134.

Cash, T. F., & Labarge, A. S. (1996). Development of the Appearance Schemas Inventory: A new cognitive body-image assessment. *Cognitive Therapy and Research, 20,* 37–50.

Cash, T. F., & Szymanski, M. L. (1995). The development and validation of the body-image ideals questionnaire. *Journal of Personality Assessment, 64,* 466–477.

Cooper, P. J., Taylor, M. J., Cooper, Z., & Fairburn, C. G. (1987). The development and validation of the Body Shape Questionnaire. *International Journal of Eating Disorders, 6,* 485–494.

Franzoi, S. L., & Shields, S. A. (1984). The Body Esteem Scale: Multidimensional structure and sex differences in a college population. *Journal of Personality Assessment, 48,* 173–178.

Garner, D. M., Olmsted, M. P., & Polivy, J. (1983). Development and validation of a multidimensional eating disorder inventory for anorexia nervosa and bulimia. *International Journal of Eating Disorders, 2,* 15–34.

Keery, H., Shroff, H., Thompson, J. K., Wertheim, E., & Smolak, L. (in press). The Sociocultural Internalization of Appearance Questionnaire—Adolescent version. *Eating and Weight Disorders: Studies on Anorexia, Bulimia, and Obesity.*

Mendelson, B. K., Mendelson, M. J., & White, D. R. (2001). Body-Esteem Scale for Adolescents and Adults. *Journal of Personality Assessment, 76,* 90–106

Petersen, A. C. (1984). A self-image questionnaire for young adolescents (SIQYA): Reliability and validity studies. *Journal of Youth and Adolescence, 13,* 93–111.

Pope, H. G., Gruber, A. J., Mangweth, B., Bureau, B., deCol, C., Jouvent, R., & Hudson, J. I. (2000). Body image perception among men in three countries. *American Journal of Psychiatry, 157,* 1297–1301.

Reed, D. L., Thompson, J. K., Brannick, M. T., & Sacco, W. P. (1991). Development and validation of the Physical Appearance State and Trait Anxiety Scale (PASTAS). *Journal of Anxiety Disorders, 5,* 323–332.

Rosen, J. C., Srebnik, D., Saltzberg, E., & Wendt, S. (1991). Development of a body image avoidance questionnaire. *Psychological Assessment, 3,* 32–37.

Shore, R. A., & Porter, J. E. (1990). Normative and reliability data for 11- to 18-year-olds on the Eating Disorder Inventory. *International Journal of Eating Disorders, 9*, 201–207.

Slade, P. D., Dewey, M. E., Newton, T., Brodie, D., & Kiemle, G. (1990). Development and preliminary validation of the Body Dissatisfaction Scale (BSS). *Psychology and Health, 4*, 213–220.

Stunkard, A. J., Sorenson, T. I., & Schulsinger, F. (1983). Use of the Danish Adoption Register for the study of obesity and thinness. In S. Kety, L. P. Rowland, R. L., Sidman, & S. W. Matthysse (Eds.), *The genetics of neurological and psychiatric disorders* (pp. 115–120). New York: Raven Press.

Thompson, J. K. & Altabe, M. N. (1991). Psychometric qualities of the Figure Rating Scale. *International Journal of Eating Disorders, 10*, 615–619.

Thompson, J. K., van den Berg, P., Roehrig, M., Guarda, A., & Heinberg, L. J. (in press). The Sociocultural Attitudes Towards Appearance Questionnaire—3: Development and validation. *International Journal of Eating Disorders.*

Thompson, M. A., & Gray, J. J. (1995). Development and validation of a new body-image assessment tool. *Journal of Personality Assessment, 64*, 258–269.

Williamson, D. A., Davis, C. J., Bennett, S. M., Goreczny, A. J., & Gleaves, D. H. (1989). Development of a simple procedure for assessing body image disturbances. *Behavioral Assessment, 11*, 433–446.

Wood, K. C., Becker, J. A., & Thompson, J. K. (1996). Body image dissatisfaction in preadolescent children. *Journal of Applied Developmental Psychology, 17*, 85–100.

18

Projective Techniques to Assess Body Image

LISA M. RADIKA
BERT HAYSLIP, JR.

Body image theorists and researchers emphasize the multidimensionality of body experience and perception. At any point in time, an individual may simultaneously monitor body size, attractiveness, and/or variations in body part size. Body image has often been differentiated into perceptual and attitudinal components. Projective measures are particularly valuable for assessing perceptual aspects of body image empirically and qualitatively and can provide incrementally valid data distinct from that obtained from structured interview or self-report techniques.

Projective measures of personality assessment purport to assess the tendency of individuals to be influenced by their interests, needs, and psychological organization as they interpret ambiguous stimuli. Any stimulus not structured to elicit a specific class of responses can evoke projective responses. These responses reflect some aspect of the individual's personality, of which the person may not be consciously aware. This ability of projective instruments to circumvent respondents' conscious defenses allows access to unique information not available through structured and objective personality measures.

This chapter summarizes the literature on the projective assessment of body image and body experiences. Questions regarding the current status and utilization of projective methods, as well as the predominant views regarding specific projective techniques purporting to assess body experiences, are discussed. Although many projective techniques claim to assess body experiences, those that have been most frequently researched are emphasized here.

CONSTRUCTION TECHNIQUES

The most common construction-based projective techniques require respondents to construct a drawing or create a story about a specific picture. These include human figure drawings and the Thematic Apperception Test.

Human Figure Drawings (HFDs)

The earliest projective technique used to examine body experiences was the Draw-A-Person (DAP) test. Developed by Machover in the early 1940s, the DAP requires the respondent to construct a free-hand drawing of a human figure. The DAP is based on the "body image hypothesis," which assumes that the drawing is a projection of the respondent's body image. That is, the attributes of the figure are believed to correspond to the attributes the respondent ascribes to his or her body. However, there is considerable debate regarding the validity of the HFD's body image hypothesis.

Machover's method of interpreting HFDs involved evaluating three aspects of the drawings. The first was the drawing's content, such as details of the body, which is interpreted in terms of its functional significance. That is, the content of drawing reflects individuals' perceptions of their body attributes, which, via the mechanism of projection, index internal personality dynamics as well as their views of others. These views presumably mirror aspects of how they choose to present themselves to others, thus revealing how their body image views might impact the quality of their interpersonal relationships. Second, the formal and structural aspects of the drawing, such as the size of the figure and/or its placement, are also examined. Third, attention is given to any aspect of the drawing thought to reflect conflict related to that bodily area. However, attempts at validating Machover's method of interpretation have netted mixed results.

Representative HFD research suggests that the size of the drawing is related to the respondent's mental age, with mature respondents drawing figures more accurate in size. Shorter, more constricted, and less adequately centered figures are commonly produced by older respondents, believed to reflect age-related body image changes. Studies using the DAP with amputees suggest that such persons construct figures that realistically represent their bodies, except for those individuals judged to have adjusted poorly and who reportedly overemphasize the absent limb in drawings. Finally, respondents who have been diagnosed with schizophrenia predominantly draw heads, giving support to the idea that the body portion of the body image disintegrates as a function of psychosis.

Human figure drawings are one of the top 10 most widely used assessment measures in psychological clinics, most likely due to the ease and brevity of administration. However, despite existing for over 50 years, the reliability and validity of HFDs are still questionable. It may be impossible to assess the validity of HFD as a measure of body image due to the difficulty of operationally defining body image in terms of projective drawing variables. Moreover, finding a reliable scoring system that accounts for different levels of artistic ability and dexterity is another fundamental challenge in documenting the validity of HFDs.

Thematic Apperception Test (TAT)

The TAT requires that the respondent create stories in response to a series of pictures involving a person or persons in various ambiguous situations. The stimuli include 30 black-and-white picture cards, in addition to one blank card. An examiner usually selects 19 cards (in addition to the blank card), based on characteristics of the respondent and the assessment context. The basic assumption originally believed to underlie the TAT is that the stories produced reflect the respondent's internal needs and perceptions of the environment (needs-press approach). This information would then allow the clinician to develop hypotheses about the respondent's needs and how he or she copes with various perceived situations. However, the needs-press approach is not commonly used today; rather, the scoring and interpretation of TAT responses is more subjective.

Published case studies by Mundy have indicated that card 12 BG (rowboat scene) tends to elicit felt or unconscious body image attitudes by female respondents. It was concluded that this card symbolizes female body image and attitudes about interpersonal relationships. However, although clinical experience with this card may suggest a trend for its ability to "pull" body image material, there is a lack of empirical support for this interpretation.

The TAT has been ranked as the ninth most frequently used clinical assessment instrument. Although it is the third most frequently researched instrument, its reliability and validity are not well established. In addition, there appears to be substantial variability in the specific stimulus cards and scoring schemes used in TAT research, making it difficult to evaluate its actual validity.

ASSOCIATION TECHNIQUES

Association techniques ask the client to respond to an ambiguous stimulus with the first image or word that comes to mind. The most frequently used medium for this type of task is inkblot stimuli, such as the Rorschach or Holtzman inkblot test.

In the 1950s, Fisher and Cleveland developed the Barrier and Penetration index scores to assess body boundary definitiveness. They discovered that how people depict the boundaries of their inkblot responses mirrors how they feel about their body boundaries. Barrier responses are conceptualized in terms of the degree to which respondents experience the external boundary regions of their body as more definite and prominent than the interior regions. Such responses are considered percepts that emphasize the symbolic value of the body boundary and that ascribe either "containing" or "protective" qualities to such boundaries. These qualities covary with the extent to which a given individual responds with either a high Barrier or high Penetration score. The Penetration score represents percepts that ascribe vulnerability to the body image. Although it was originally believed that Barrier and Penetration scores measured opposite body image tendencies, research suggests that the Penetration score has little predictive validity and is actually correlated with the Barrier score. Barrier and Penetration scores were viewed as having the advantage of providing easily scored indexes of body image definitiveness on the basis of responses to the Holtzman and Rorschach inkblots. In each case, objectivity of scoring has been shown to be consistently high, and there is evidence of adequate test–retest reliability.

Rorschach

The Rorschach Inkblot Test consists of 10 cards, each containing one inkblot (five are black, five colored). After viewing each card individually, the respondent is asked to report what he or she sees in the inkblot. This procedure is then repeated during an inquiry phase to gather information and assist with the scoring of the client's response.

Research examining the Barrier score in Rorschach protocols has determined that it is correlated with the Body Prominence score, which is defined as the intensity of sensory awareness of various body areas, as when one feels more threat, for example, regarding the genital or breast area. It also has been found that the more definite the body image boundaries are, the more likely that individuals will manifest clear communication with others in a social context. Additionally, research has indicated that respondents with low Barrier scores tend to show psychosomatic disturbances in internal organs, whereas those with high Barrier scores show more sensorimotor dysfunction (i.e., higher reactivity in muscles and skin).

In addition to Barrier and Penetration indices, Rorschach scores that provide information about body experiences include the Anatomy (*An*) and X-Ray (*Xy*) content scores, which are included in Exner's comprehensive scoring system. Anatomy scores are given to responses in which anatomy is described (e.g., bone structure, stomach), whereas X-Ray scores are used when the content of the response reflects skeletal or internal organ structures. In general, it is suggested that if the value for the composite of *An* + *Xy* is 3 or more, an unusual body concern exists. If there is not a legitimate physical/medical cause for the body concern, then this response pattern, particularly the bony/skeletal and muscular/visceral areas, may be viewed as indicating a vulnerable body condition, a threatened body image, or the fear of self-disintegration. It has also been argued that human detail responses (e.g., eyes, ears, hair) may also suggest body image sensitivity. However, there is no empirical support for any of these claims.

In the recent past, the Rorschach has ranked in the top 10 of the most frequently used assessment instruments, while placing second among the most frequently researched. Despite this attention, many published research articles (not just those dealing with body image), evidence methodological problems, such as inappropriate or vague hypotheses, design problems, post hoc findings presented as a priori, failure to control for extraneous variables, and interpretive problems. Although Exner's comprehensive scoring system has become the most widely used, some critics feel that the norms are outdated and, moreover, inadequate, because they are based on small samples.

Holtzman Inkblot Technique (HIT)

The HIT is a projective assessment measure that uses inkblots to obtain personality data. It was initially developed to improve upon the Rorschach's reliability and increase the total number of responses produced, thus providing a more representative picture of the respondent's personality dynamics. It consists of two parallel forms (45 cards each) and has evidenced good reliability and validity. The respondent is asked to give only one response per card. Responses can be scored for 22 variables, two of which (Barrier and Penetration) have been found to relate to body image. Much research has included the Barrier score in its purview, especially focusing on individuals who score high on this dimension. Respondents with a high Barrier score have been found to experience themselves as psychologically well differentiated from their environment, whereas respondents with a high Penetration score are believed to be experiencing themselves as psychologically vulnerable to intrusion from the environment. Individuals scoring high on the Barrier dimension have also been found to be more people-oriented, independent, able communicators, and have a clear sense of identity, of self. The Barrier index has also been related to achievement motivation, with underachievers having lower Barrier scores.

Research examining Barrier and Penetrations scores in HIT protocols suggests that these scores do not distinguish between groups of healthy persons and those diagnosed with a physical condition or illness. However, administering such indices before and after surgery has produced results that indicate stability in organization of body experience. In a rare example of lifespan-focused research, Hayslip and colleagues demonstrated that scores derived from HIT are sensitive to the effects of age: Young adults scored higher on both Barrier and Penetration indices compared to middle-aged and older adults. These results suggest that young adults, relative to older adults, demonstrate more established body boundaries, while also experiencing more vulnerability in body boundaries.

In addition to Barrier and Penetration scores, Anatomy (*At*) scores have been examined in HIT protocols in relation to body experiences. Confirming that *At* responses reveal body preoccupation, anxiety, and thought disturbances, studies have found that restriction in intellectual drive increases *At* responses; high *At* scores are reported for brain-damaged individuals, respondents diagnosed with chronic schizophrenia, and those with mental retardation. However, research examining this variable is limited due to the relative infrequency with which *At* scores appear in the HIT protocols of normal respondents.

One clear advantage of the HIT over the Rorschach is the fact that standardized percentile norms are provided for the 22 inkblot scores on a variety of populations, adding to its interpretive validity. Parallel forms permit the use of test–retest paradigms and the study of stability and change in the individual. Practical advantages of the HIT include the fact that group administration is possible and that computerized systems can assist with scoring. However, although the HIT appeared to be a promising psychometric alternative to the Rorschach, it is not one of the most frequently used or researched assessment instruments. Due to the prevalence of the use of the Rorschach in clinical practice, the fact that most graduate programs do not include instruction in the administration and scoring of the HIT most likely contributes to the lack of clinical and research use.

Additionally, research based on Fisher and Cleveland's work using the HIT also has some shortcomings. For example, some of the normative data was gathered from small samples, some collected by group administration while others were individually gathered, and some studies used the Holtzman while others used the Rorschach. Additionally, in most of the early studies, response frequency was limited to 24 responses, and these data appear to have been based on a variety of scoring systems. Future research examining Fisher and Cleveland's Barrier and Penetration scores using individual administration of Rorschach protocols scored according to Exner's method hopefully will provide more information regarding body experience.

CONCLUSIONS

Any statements regarding the potential of projective techniques to assess body experiences have to be understood in light of views about the value of projective techniques in general. Ideally, some consensus regarding body image indicators and generalizable dimensions across projective assessment tools is desirable. However, the idiosyncratic nature of many scoring systems and the difficulty of defining body image in precise terms undermine this goal. Indeed, it would be desirable to derive variables from various techniques that assess the same underlying dimensions of body image, thus promoting generalizability across techniques. For future progress to be made in the projective assessment of body experience, there is a definite need for much more construct validity data and collection of normative data on specific clinical populations.

Nevertheless, there is much to be learned about body image and body experiences that perhaps may be inaccessible using other means of assessment. Projective assessment measures can be regarded more as clinical tools that may provide supplementary qualitative information that helps guide the interview process and clinical hypothesis testing. It has been suggested that their value as clinical tools is proportional to the skill level of the clinician utilizing them. Thus their unique value in assessing body image may be more likely to emerge when they are interpreted by clinicians and researchers who chose to utilize the qualitative data that projective techniques yield.

INFORMATIVE READINGS

Ben-Tovim, D., & Walker, M. (1990). Women's body attributes: A review of measurement techniques. *International Journal of Eating Disorders, 10*(2), 155–167.—A review of techniques measuring women's attitudes toward their bodies, including self-report questionnaires, projective tests, silhouettes, and interviews.

Exner, J. E. (1993). *The Rorschach: A comprehensive system. Vol. I: Basic foundations* (3rd ed.). New York: Wiley.—A basic introduction to the Rorschach with a focus on administration, scoring, and interpretation.

Fisher, S. (1986). *Development and structure of the body image* (Vol. 2). Hillsdale, NJ: Erlbaum.—Review and evaluation of major theoretical concepts related to body image, including organization of the body image boundary and distortions in body perception.

Fisher, S., & Cleveland, S. (1968). *Body image and personality* (2nd ed.). New York: Dover.—A classic review of research on the influence of an individual's body image on his or her behavior, using the Holtzman and Rorschach inkblot tests.

Hayslip, B., Cooper, C., Dougherty, L., & Cook, D. (1997). Body image in adulthood: A projective approach. *Journal of Personality Assessment, 68*(3), 628–649.—An examination of perceptual dimensions of body image in adulthood, using projective measures.

Hill, E. F. (1972). *The Holtzman Inkblot Technique.* San Francisco: Jossey-Bass.—A handbook for the clinical application of this technique, consisting of a comprehensive review of interpretive information concerning HIT scores.

Kahill, S. (1984). Human figure drawing in adults: An update of the empirical evidence, 1967–1982. *Canadien Psychology 25*(4), 269–292.—An examination of empirical literature on the reliability and validity of human figure drawings with adults.

Lilienfeld, S. O., Wood, J. M., & Garb, H. N. (2000). The scientific status of projective techniques. *Psychological Science in the Public Interest, 1*(2), 27–66.—A review of the current state of the literature concerning the psychometric properties of the Rorschach, TAT, and human figure drawings.

Machover, K. (1949). *Personality projection in the drawing of the human figure.* Springfiled, IL: Charles C Thomas.—A description of the principles and interpretation of human figure drawings with respect to the clinical significance of a drawing's attributes.

Mundy, J. (1971). Content analysis: TAT card 12 BG: The rowboat as a symbol for female body image and sexual activity. *Psychological Reports, 28,* 219–222.—A description of responses to TAT card 12 BG in female subjects.

Offman, H., & Bradley, S. (1992). Body image of children and adolescents and its measurement: An overview. *Canadian Journal of Psychiatry, 37*(6), 417–422.—An examination of body image as a multidimensional construct and the difficulties associated with using the human figure drawings to measure body image.

Beyond Traits
Assessing Body Image States

THOMAS F. CASH

As preceding chapters on body image assessment clearly reveal, researchers and clinicians have a plethora of measures from which to choose. To most effectively use these measures, however, precisely what facet or facets of the body image construct are of interest must be identified. Is the goal to evaluate the extent to which people hold distorted perceptions of their body size? Or is the goal to measure individuals' evaluative experiences of their physical appearance? Given a focus on evaluative experiences, is the goal to assess evaluative cognitions, such as body image thoughts or appraisals, or to assess the emotions associated with these cognitions? Is the goal to tap global evaluations, such as overall appearance satisfaction, or more specific evaluations of particular physical attributes, such as weight or shape satisfaction? Should satisfaction be measured directly, or as the degree to which individuals view these attributes as discrepant from their personal ideals? Given the objective of quantifying people's psychological investment in their appearance vis-à-vis their sense of self, the questions become: To what degree have they internalized appearance-related standards or ideals, and how subjectively important is their attainment of these ideals? Are there strongly held beliefs, assumptions, or schemas about the meaning and influence of their physical appearance in their lives? Finally, is the objective to assess behavioral patterns that reflect individuals' attempts to control not only their appearance but also their thoughts and feelings about their looks?

THE NEED FOR CONTENT-SPECIFIC ASSESSMENT
OF BODY IMAGE STATES

In reviewing the tools available for assessing the above facets of the body image construct, it becomes apparent that despite their important differences, they share one key feature. Nearly all assessments of body image focus on stable and dispositional or trait-like characteristics; they measure how people usually think, feel, or act. However, they seldom take into consideration the situational and temporal variations of body image experiences within individuals. A woman who is generally discontent with her weight is not constantly thinking or feeling upset about it. Certain situations or events activate her thoughts and emotions, while at other times these body image experiences are either absent or much more benign. Moreover, a man may be generally accepting of his balding pate yet feel somewhat self-conscious and uncomfortable about his visible hair loss in a particular situation.

In the concluding chapter of our 1990 volume, *Body Images: Development, Deviance, and Change*, Tom Pruzinsky and I lamented the scientific neglect of body image as a fluid and dynamic person–situation interaction (or transaction), and the overemphasis on body image as a static, cross-situational trait. Of course, this fluid versus static issue has long permeated much of psychology, especially the domain of personality theory. In contrast to centralist (intrapersonal) and peripheralist (situational) perspectives, an interactionist view maintains that we must consider both the person and the situation if we are to understand the complexities of human behavior.

Thus the scientific investigation of body image properly requires the measurement of evaluative or affective body image states *in specific contexts* or in response to *experimental manipulations*. One example of a contextual approach to body image assessment is the Situational Inventory of Body Image Dysphoria (SIBID) that I developed several years ago. The SIBID asks that respondents rate the frequency of negative body image emotions in each of 48 distinct situations (20 situations in the SIBID short form). These situations include both social and nonsocial contexts pertaining to eating, exercising, grooming, intimacy, physical self-focus or body exposure, social comparisons, and changes in appearance. The value of the SIBID, which has excellent reliability and validity, is that it captures body image experiences by having respondents consider their emotional reactions to particular contexts, events, or activities. However, its single mean score does not differentially weigh these situations with respect to how often they occur in the person's life or how psychologically important they are to the individual. These variables constitute potential weighting factors vis-à-vis the questionnaire assessment of the experience of body image emotions. Moreover, the SIBID does not assess positive body image affect, albeit by design. There is a need for the bipolar measurement of body image states that also includes positive experiences.

Another contextual assessment is my Body Exposure during Sexual Activities Questionnaire (BESAQ). My goal was to measure people's body self-consciousness (i.e., anxious self-focus) and avoidance of body exposure during sexual relations. The BESAQ asks respondents to indicate how often they think, feel, and behave in specific ways in such contexts. As Wiederman discusses in his chapter in this volume, these body image states can influence the quantity and quality of one's sexual experiences and functioning. Research with the BESAQ indicates that it predicts sexual functioning much better than do trait measures of body image satisfaction. Whereas the BESAQ zeroes in on sexual contexts in general, its instructions could also be adapted to assess body image states even more specifically—for example, during an individual's most recent sexual experience, or when having sex with a partner for the first time.

Experimental studies of the effects of informational stimuli, media images, and interpersonal events on body image require dependent measures of momentary body image experiences. To accomplish this difficult measurement goal, researchers often adopt or modify extant trait measures or fashion their own scale to meet a given study's needs, most likely because few validated tools have been published. Reed and colleagues constructed the Physical Appearance State and Trait Anxiety Scale (PASTAS). Their questionnaire averages the respondent's anxiety about 16 body parts (e.g., lips, wrist, feet, forehead, hips, weight, etc.). However, this anxiety measure does not assess broader affective experiences (e.g., shame or other dejective emotions) concerning one's *overall* appearance. This latter domain would seem to better reflect the construct and have greater potential utility. Indeed, Tiggemann's recent research suggests that assessing feelings about sundry body parts or features may be less sensitive to situational contexts than is desirable.

A more promising approach in measuring body image states asks people to rate their experiences on somewhat broader dimensions. For example, in their 1999 volume, *Exacting Beauty*, Thompson and his colleagues present a two-item Visual Analogue Scale (VAS) pertaining to body weight/size dissatisfaction and overall appearance dissatisfaction. Respondents mark their "level of disturbance" on a 100-mm line. Guided by this approach, Lavin and I successfully used an expanded six-item VAS measure in a study that we published in 2001. One potential shortcoming of the VAS is that it is affectively unipolar and ignores positive body image states. Scoring is also tedious, necessitating a precise metric measurement of each rating, from 0 to 100 mm. Whether respondents really need or can reliably use a 100-point scale to report their body image states is arguable.

THE BODY IMAGE STATES SCALE

Recently, to address these limitations, my students and I developed and published the Body Image States Scale (BISS) a six-item measure of momentary evaluative/affective experiences of one's appearance. Using a sample of 174 college women and men, we examined its internal consistency, test–retest reliability, relationships with body image traits, sensitivity to situational contexts, and construct validity in an experiment on individual differences in the lability of body image states. To evaluate the latter, we tested the hypothesis that people who are dysfunctionally invested in their appearance are especially susceptible to the contextual induction of negative body image states.

The BISS's items tap the following domains of current body image experience: (1) dissatisfaction–satisfaction with overall physical appearance, (2) dissatisfaction–satisfaction with body size and shape, (3) dissatisfaction–satisfaction with weight, (4) feelings of physical attractiveness–unattractiveness, (5) current feelings about one's looks relative to how one usually feels, and (6) evaluation of one's appearance relative to how the average person looks. Responses to each item are given on nine-point bipolar Likert-type scales, semantically anchored at each point. The instructions ask respondents to convey "how you feel right now at this very moment."

Our data confirmed the acceptable internal consistency of the BISS for both women and men, whether administered in a neutral context or in contexts that elicited either positive or negative body image states. Over a 2- to 3-week period, the BISS was moderately stable in the neutral context yet appropriately less so than a trait measure: The BISS was sensitive to contextual manipulations. Both sexes reported more favorable body image states in positive than negative contexts. Moreover, women responded more strongly to the negative contexts than men, but women were comparable to men in the positive contexts.

We examined the extent to which various body image trait measures would predict BISS scores in a neutral context. Indeed, significant modest-to-moderate correlations indicated that trait body dissatisfaction, body shame, body surveillance, and dysfunctional investment in appearance predicted less favorable body image states. Individuals with a heavier body mass also reported more negative body image states, especially women.

In our experiment to evaluate the construct validity of the BISS, women completed it either before or after answering questions about their actual, ideal, highest, and lowest weights. As hypothesized, and consistent with the proposition that Williamson and colleagues articulated elsewhere in this volume, we found that women who were more dysfunctionally invested in their appearance (on the Appearance Schemas Inventory) prior exposure to these questions produced less favorable body image states than were ob-

served either for the control subjects or for women who were less dysfunctionally invested in their appearance.

Collectively, our findings offer initial evidence of the reliability and validity of this new assessment for both sexes. The potential value of the BISS
is further evident in its brevity, its bipolarity (i.e., both positive and negative
experiences), and its content (i.e., not a specific affect about discrete body
parts). Furthermore, with modified instructions, this questionnaire can be
administered as a trait assessment. Beyond its utility as a research instrument, the BISS could be particularly useful as a clinical tool for monitoring
body image states in targeted situations over the course of treatment.

THE BODY IMAGE DIARY

Another approach to the contextual assessment of body image derives from
my body image treatment program, described in my later chapter with Melissa Strachan. Reflecting its cognitive-behavioral basis, this program teaches
clients to monitor their body image experiences systematically in the course
of their daily lives. Clients are instructed in the use of a structured Body Image Diary (Figure 19.1), which distinguishes three elements of body image
experiences, termed the "ABC Sequence":

1. *Activators* are those events or situations that precipitate distressing
   body image thoughts and feelings.
2. *Beliefs* include thoughts, interpretations, and evaluative beliefs about
   one's body in the situation.
3. *Consequences* refer to one's ensuing emotional and behavioral reactions in that context.

Let me illustrate the use of this clinical tool with a hypothetical person,
Karen. The activating context for Karen is attending a beach party, where
she wears a "revealing" swimsuit. Her beliefs entail self-evaluative social
comparisons in which she looks extremely fat, inferences that others at the
party notice how fat she is, and conclusions that they are "grossed out" and
ashamed to be seen with her. Karen's emotional consequences include feelings of socially based self-conscious anxiety and shame. The behavioral consequences include attempts to conceal her "offending" body shape with a
towel and loose garment, restriction of her social interactions, and leaving
before the party is over. Karen also makes diary entries in which she rates
the intensity of each of these body image emotions as a 9 on a scale from 0 to
10 and specifies the duration of this episode as 2 hours.

Individuals can complete the Body Image Diary in four basic ways.
First, after identifying those situations and events that are the most recurrent

Date: _____

ACTIVATORS (Triggering event or situation):

_____
_____
_____
_____

BELIEFS (Your thoughts and interpretations of the event/situation):

_____
_____
_____
_____

CONSEQUENCES (Your emotional and behavioral reactions):

Types of emotions you felt	Intensity of emotions (0 = not at all intense to 10 = extremely intense)	Duration of emotions
_____	_____	_____
_____	_____	_____
_____	_____	_____

Effects on your behavior (what you did):

_____
_____
_____

FIGURE 19.1. The Body Image Diary. Adapted from T. F. Cash (1997). *The Body Image Workbook*. Oakland, CA: New Harbinger Publications. Copyright 1997 by Thomas F. Cash. Adapted by permission

activators of body image dysphoria, clients complete diaries that capture these prototypical and troublesome body image states. For the therapist and client alike, this is clinically useful in the process of beginning to understand the essentially scripted nature of the client's experiences, which are often replete with common themes (e.g., contextual similarities, underlying cognitive distortions and schemas, specific emotions, and coping strategies). A second way to use the Body Image Diary is to complete it as soon as possible after an episode of body image distress, ideally while the thoughts and feelings remain experientially accessible. Third, clients may complete the diary prophylatically and therapeutically, by delineating the body image experiences that they aspire to have in specific contexts. Finally, later in therapy, clinicians may review with clients their earlier diary entries as a means of reinforcing the treatment gains that have occurred.

CONCLUSIONS

Understanding the dynamic interplay of person variables (e.g., body image traits, physical characteristics, and personality attributes) and contextual events is crucial to our appreciation of body image fluidity in everyday life. We have made more progress in measuring dispositional elements of body image than in assessing specific body image experiences in circumscribed situations. Nevertheless, several instruments are now available that may take researchers and practitioners beyond the trait perspective on body image. We must continue to develop innovative and accurate methods for assessing body image states—measures that reflect pertinent personal and social contexts.

INFORMATIVE READINGS

Cash, T. F. (1994). The Situational Inventory of Body Image Dysphoria: Contextual assessment of a negative body image. *The Behavior Therapist, 17,* 133–134.—Reports the initial development of this measure, available from the author's website: *www.body-images.com.*

Cash, T. F. (1997). *The body image workbook.* Oakland, CA: New Harbinger.—The author's cognitive-behavioral program for body image change, which incorporates the Body Image Diary.

Cash, T. F. (2000–2001). *Body image assessments.*—Available from the author's website (*www.body images.com*) from which his questionnaires and manuals can be downloaded for a nominal fee.

Cash, T. F. (in press). The Situational Inventory of Body Image Dysphoria: Psychometric evidence and development of a short form. *International Journal of Eating Disorders.*— Summarizes evidence concerning this assessment.

Cash, T. F., Fleming, E. C., Alindogan, J., Steadman, L., & Whitehead, A. (2002). Beyond body image as a trait: The development and validation of the Body Image States Scale. *Eating Disorders: A Journal of Treatment and Prevention, 10,* 103–113.—Details the psychometric characteristics of this new assessment of body image states evaluations, also available from the author's website (*www.body-images.com*).

Haimovitz, D., Lansky, L., & Reilly, P. (1993). Fluctuation in body satisfaction across situations. *International Journal of Eating Disorders, 13,* 77–83.—An empirical study demonstrating the role of contexts in body image experiences.

Lavin, M. A., & Cash, T. F. (2001). The effects of exposure to information about appearance stereotyping and discrimination on women's body images. *International Journal of Eating Disorders, 29,* 51–58.—Illustrates the use of a body image state measure in an experimental study.

Pruzinsky, T., & Cash, T. F. (1990). Integrative themes in body-image development, deviance, and change. In T. F. Cash & T. Pruzinsky (Eds.), *Body images: Development, deviance, and change* (pp. 337–349). New York: Guilford Press.—An overview of key issues concerning body image, including the need for state and contextual assessment.

Reed, D. L., Thompson, J. K., Brannick, M. T., & Sacco, W. P. (1991). Development and validation of the Physical Appearance State and Trait Anxiety Scale (PASTAS). *Journal of Anxiety Disorders, 5,* 323–332.—Presents a body image anxiety assessment with both state and trait forms.

Thompson, J. K., Heinberg, L. J., Altabe, M., & Tantleff-Dunn, S. (1999). *Exacting beauty: Theory, assessment, and treatment of body image disturbance.* Washington, DC: American Psychological Association.—A comprehensive volume that provides information on specific assessment of body image, including several contextual and state measures.

Tiggemann, M. (2001). Person × situation interactions in body dissatisfaction. *International Journal of Eating Disorders, 29,* 65–70.—An investigation that demonstrates the importance of the contextual assessment of body image states.

20

Assessing Body Image and Quality of Life in Medical Settings

THOMAS PRUZINSKY
THOMAS F. CASH

Many variables influence patients' evaluations of their health-related quality of life (HRQOL). Surprisingly, body image assessment has not been well integrated into the HRQOL literature, despite consistent observations that changes in physical appearance, function, and body integrity are central to the experience of illness and medical treatment (see Part VI of this volume).

In this brief chapter it is impossible to address fully the medical contexts and range of issues relevant to HRQOL and body image assessment. However, we can articulate the benefits of improving body image evaluation in HRQOL assessment and provide a general structure for planning body image assessment in the context of HRQOL issues.

BENEFITS OF IMPROVED HRQOL BODY IMAGE ASSESSMENT

More Effective Screening for Body Image Distress

To provide the most effective and efficient clinical services that maximize patients' HRQOL, we must readily distinguish between patients who do, and do not, have body image concerns. Currently, we have limited data regarding the epidemiology of body image concerns in specific medical populations. However, it appears safe to conclude that of all individuals experiencing any particular medical problem, only a minority report body image concerns. These findings are consistent with Fisher's observations in his 1986 comprehensive review, *Development and Structure of the Body Image.*

Similarly, Susan Harter in her 1999 book, *The Construction of the Self*, describes a number of studies in which children with disfiguring medical conditions do not report appearance concerns. Thus one should not assume all people with a certain medical condition have body image problems; rather, one should assess individual experience.

Specifying Body Image Concerns

HRQOL assessment must account for the unique body image effects specific to a particular disease or treatment process. Below, we briefly review HRQOL body image assessment in the oncology, burn injury, and dermatology contexts to exemplify the need to specify body image assessment according to particular medical conditions.

Craig White (in this volume) and others emphasize the need for improved body image evaluation in the subfield of psycho-oncology. Traditional approaches to HRQOL in oncology have often grouped body image assessment with sexuality issues. Although the connection between sexuality and body image is critical (see Wiederman's chapter in this volume), each form of cancer is likely associated with additional specific body image concerns.

Fortunately, a number of new scales has been described and effectively utilized, including the Body Image Scale by Hopwood and colleagues, and The Body Image After Breast Cancer Questionnaire (used by Andrade et al., 2001). Similarly, Dropkin describes assessing functional and disfigurement-related concerns in patients with head and neck cancer.

Researchers at Johns Hopkins have been developing a burn-specific quality-of-life scale. Fauerbach and colleagues recently published the Satisfaction with Appearance Scale (SWAP) designed to detect the minority of patients who experience body image concerns following burn injuries. Recent research with the SWAP found that body image dissatisfaction identified early in treatment had significant and unique effects on HRQOL. Such important findings about the role of body image in burn-related HRQOL are not possible without such a burn-specific measure.

A review of the dermatology literature by Halioua and colleagues notes the unique approaches to quality-of-life assessment of patients with psoriasis, acne, atopic dermatitis, or genital herpes. In his recent review of androgenetic alopecia in men and women, Cash identified the foci of the condition's impact on body image and psychosocial functioning and developed the Hair Loss Effects Questionnaire to measure this impact. Similarly, Cash reviewed the literature on the quality-of-life impact of unwanted facial hair in women.

Currently, few researchers consider the obvious observation that body image concerns vary according to medical condition. Future research will greatly benefit from specifying the exact nature of these concerns and addressing these specific measurement challenges.

Refining the Measurement of Health Outcomes

A critical HRQOL assessment goal is to measure treatment outcomes. If one specific treatment goal is improved body image, as is true in so many medical contexts, then it seems we should measure this outcome variable more adequately. For example, Sarwer (in this volume) as well as Pruzinsky have argued that quality-of-life outcomes following plastic surgery are intimately related to body image. Nevertheless, little integration of body image measurement into the plastic and reconstructive surgery outcome literature has occurred. However, when body image is adequately evaluated in the plastic surgery context, using psychometrically sound and sensitive measures, the results are informative. For example, in 1997 Walden and colleagues evaluated the body image effects of removing silicone gel-filled breast implants and found important changes on the Breast Size Rating Scale, Body Image Automatic Thoughts Questionnaire, Multidimensional Body Self-Relations Questionnaire, and the Body Image Avoidance Questionnaire. In our own collaborations (Bolton et al., in press) with Yale Medical School researchers in plastic surgery, we have found such measures to be very useful in documenting outcomes in facial trauma and abdominoplasty.

Similar outcome issues need to be addressed in relation to certain types of dental treatment, short stature in children, and many other medical conditions. Evaluating the costs and benefits of specific treatments with specific reference to body image would seem to be a productive research direction.

Pharmaceutical companies and governmental regulatory agencies increasingly recognize that the efficacy of a drug or device depends on more than "objective" biophysical or clinician-rated criteria. Such products must demonstrably improve quality of life from patients' perspectives. For example, a new drug for treating androgenetic alopecia that produces significantly greater hair growth relative to a placebo must also differentially improve patients' perceptions of, and satisfaction with, their hair density and growth. What is the value of greater hair growth if patients cannot, or do not, perceive a satisfying change?

For this reason, in the third phase of clinical trials with new drugs and devices, carefully prevalidated measures of patients' experiences are often included to assess treatment efficacy. These measures focus on ascertaining "disease-relevant" dimensions of patients' experiences that should change if the product is to be experienced as efficacious. Defining specific dimensions for constructing assessments based on qualitative and quantitative methodologies is a challenging task. For example, consider a topical drug for the treatment of excessive facial hair in women. One must ask, what precisely are the psychosocial sequelae of this condition and what constitutes the desired changes patients want and expect? The answer is unlikely to be some global or distal construct, such as unhappiness, low self-esteem, a negative body image, or lack of confidence in social settings. It is more likely to be a very focused and proximal experience, such as self-conscious discomfort with facial appearance in particular social contexts, and/or the discomfort or bother associated with facial hair removal or concealment. If the new drug is efficacious with regard to quality-of-life experiences, it should improve these concerns. Assessing such changes with omnibus body image or self-concept measures would fail to detect the actual psychosocial outcomes of drug treatment.

Developing Empirical Bases for Influencing Health Policy

HRQOL evaluations are partially designed to influence health policy (see books by Dimsdale & Baum, and Drotar). In 2001 Cella stated that "the end user of a QOL questionnaire will not be a psychometrician or social scientist; it will be a health care provider making individual treatment decisions, a policy analyst deciding on resource allocation, or a health care payer deciding whether or not to cover a given therapy" (p. 63).

Documenting the efficacy of medical interventions to improve body image outcomes can help ensure that the maximum number of patients obtains the best treatment possible. Patients experiencing clinically significant body image distress may benefit further from body image rehabilitation interventions. One potentially effective method of improving current treatment standards is to provide consistent empirical documentation of the overall quality-of-life effects of body image distress in medical populations.

Improved Understanding of General Body Image Functioning

Improved understanding of body image adaptation in medical contexts can undoubtedly inform our understanding of general body image functioning. For example, improved explanations of why only some individuals experience body image distress when confronted with illness-related body changes can inform us about body image resilience. What factors predict adaptation to major negative changes in physical appearance and functioning?

Similarly, improved body image assessment in the medical context will inform us about the nature of body image distortion. Abbott and colleagues' 2000 study of females with cystic fibrosis found that they "perceive body shape optimistically as slimmer than it actually was" (p. 512). This finding contrasts with the more common misperception of being overweight evident in many women, especially those with eating disorders. Similar issues exist with respect to children with short stature. Wicklund and colleagues asked children to estimate future height attainment in response to growth hormone treatment and found that they often had completely unattainable expectations. How common is body image distortion? Is it ever adaptive? Improved understanding of body image with respect to HRQOL can shed light on such issues.

SPECIFIC MEASUREMENT ISSUES

Effectively assessing relationships between body image and HRQOL requires considering the psychometric characteristics of available instruments and the following issues.

General versus Disease-Specific Assessment

The HRQOL assessment literature invariably addresses whether general measures are more effective than disease-specific measures. In oncology, Cella notes that a combination of general and disease-specific approaches is standard. This usage also appears to be true in dermatology and other areas.

Similarly, it is important to ask if general measures of body image are as sensitive to the important domains of body image functioning and change in specific patient populations as disease-specific measures. Is it more informative to combine general and disease-specific measures?

Measures of body image evaluation and affect, such as the Multidimensional Body Self-Relations Questionnaire, Situational Inventory of Body Image Dysphoria, and Body Esteem Scale, are very effective in determining general body image functioning. They have been effectively used in studies of breast implant removal, facial trauma, multiple forms of cosmetic surgery, and other medical contexts. However, is it also best to include evaluations of body image specific to each disease and treatment process? This question has yet to be addressed adequately.

Multidimensional Assessment

Body image and HRQOL are best conceptualized as multidimensional. Clearly, there are many possible domains relevant to HRQOL body image assessment—for example, appearance evaluation, appearance investment, perceptions of bodily functions, sensations, and sense of body integrity. It is difficult to know how many different dimensions of assessment are needed to assess adequately the full range of potentially important areas of body image concern in any specific patient population.

Determining Clinical Significance

Defining clinically significant body image distress scores on specific measures for specific populations is essential. In oncology HRQOL research, Cella notes that even though clinical significance is the one issue that "ultimately determines whether people pay close attention to change in QOL over time" (p. 63), it is still inadequately researched.

Many challenges exist in determining clinical significance. For example, should the definition be categorical or dimensional? Do we combine scores on a series of measures (or dimensions) or use only scores from one specific measure? Are all dimensions weighted equally? Do we consider patients' weighting of domain importance?

The HRQOL assessment literature is beginning to incorporate "patient preferences regarding domain functioning." There is growing awareness of the utility of asking patients to define which dimensions are important to them. For patients who weight each dimension as equal, such preferences are not informative. However, Grobatenko-Roth and colleagues point out that there are very "large gains" in discriminative ability for patients who express important distinctions among specific domains. For example, the body image effects of disease on sexual functioning may be central to some patients and irrelevant to others.

Another method of determining clinical significance of HRQOL body image is to assess discrepancies in patients' perceptions of the effects of their illness. For example, White (in this volume) recommends defining a "clinically significant body image disturbance" in terms of patients' perceived discrepancies (e.g., between actual and ideal appearance of a particular physical feature) and assessing the degree to which any one individual is "invested" in this discrepancy. In this context, White notes the usefulness of Cash's Body Image Ideals Questionnaire.

Very little has been done to evaluate the utility of these approaches (i.e., differential weighting of domains, assessment of patient-perceived discrepancies) for defining clinical significance in HRQOL body image assessment. Currently, each researcher or clinician makes these determinations in light of the measures chosen for specific patient populations. These decisions are also determined by the application of the data, such as for treatment planning versus informing health policy development.

In the June 1999 issue of the *Journal of Consulting and Clinical Psychology*, a series of six articles addressed the topic of clinical significance in treatment outcomes, particularly in mental health contexts. Two articles, one by Kendall et al. and one by Jacobson and his colleagues, describe strategies for determining clinically meaningful outcomes. Gladis and her colleagues specifically discuss clinical significance and quality of life. Unfortunately, few, if any, of these measures tap body image.

Cash and Fleming recently developed and validated the Body Image Quality of Life Inventory (BIQLI), a questionnaire in which respondents rate the extent to which body image has negative-to-positive effects on 19 aspects of their lives, such as day-to-day emotions, eating, self-esteem, sexuality, and social relations. Thus, the BIQLI does not assess body image per se; rather, it assesses the impact of one's body image experiences on various psychosocial domains of life.

Pediatric Assessment

Many of the goals and challenges facing assessors of adult and pediatric body image HRQOL are similar. However, assessing pediatric patients is different, especially in terms of the developmental issues inherent in pediatric evaluation. Sensitivity to developmental and treatment stages may be particularly informative when evaluating a child's ability to adapt his or her body image to medical conditions.

For example, in their study of body image, disability, and disfigurement, Ben-Tovim and Walker noted that chronic illness beginning in adolescence may have more negative body image effects than illness beginning in childhood or adulthood. Additionally, Varni and colleagues, using the Harter Self-Perception Profile for children, found that perceived appearance was correlated with higher self-esteem and lower depression and anxiety scores in children with newly diagnosed cancer. Similar findings exist for children with limb deficiencies.

Drotar notes that there is only a "short history" of pediatric HRQOL assessment, and measurement instruments of body image in this context are even more limited. However, new measures exist, such as Kopel and colleagues' 1998 Body Image Instrument, which contains five subscales (general appearance, body competence, others' reactions to appearance, value of appearance, and body parts) and has good preliminary psychometric characteristics and clinical utility. This kind of progress in body image evaluation will surely lead to improved understanding of pediatric HRQOL.

Cultural Sensitivity

Several chapters in this book clearly document significant cultural variations in body image experience. There is every reason to believe that these differences are also important when evaluating HRQOL body image, though they have yet to be systematically documented.

CONCLUSION

The body image effects of medical conditions and their treatment have profound quality-of-life consequences for millions of people. As health-care providers, our responsibility is to better understand these effects in order to design effective and efficient treatment programs that enhance quality of life. There is little question that our ignorance about the influence of body image on quality of life helps perpetuate untold amounts of human suffering. It is a noble and pressing challenge to understand and attempt to relieve this suffering.

INFORMATIVE READINGS

Abbott, J., Conway, S., Etherington, C., Fitzjohn, J., Gee, L., Morton, A., Musson, H., & Webb, A. K. (2000). Perceived body image and eating behavior in young adults with cystic fibrosis and their healthy peers. *Journal of Behavioral Medicine, 23*, 501–517.—A clear illustration of how body image variables are influenced by the specific medical condition of the individuals being assessed.

Andrade, W. N., Baxter, N., & Semple, J. L. (2001). Clinical determinants of patient satisfaction with breast reconstruction. *Plastic and Reconstructive Surgery, 107*, 46–54.—This study demonstrates the importance of measuring body image variables specific to particular medical conditions via use of The Body Image After Breast Cancer Questionnaire.

Ben-Tovim, D. I., & Walker, M. K. (1995). Body image, disfigurement and disability. *Journal of Psychosomatic Research, 39*, 283–291.—This study demonstrates the potential importance of considering the influence of developmental stage at the time of acquiring one's medical condition on body image functioning.

Bolton, M. S., Pruzinsky, T., Cash, T. F., & Persing, J. (in press). Measuring psychological outcomes in aesthetic surgery: Body image and quality-of-life in abdominoplasty patients. *Plastic and Reconstructive Surgery.*—This study documents the need to precisely measure postoperative changes in body image, in contrast to assessing more general psychological outcomes (e.g., self-concept) when evaluating aesthetic surgery patients.

Cash, T. F. (1999). The psychological consequences of androgenetic alopecia: A review of the research literature. *British Journal of Dermatology, 141*, 398–405.—An illustrative review of the utility of using body image concepts and scales in dermatology.

Cash, T. F., & Fleming, E. C. (2002). The impact of body image experiences: Development of the Body Image Quality of Life Inventory. *International Journal of Eating Disorders, 31*, 455–460.—A newly developed and relatively brief measure specifically designed to evaluate the effects of body image experiences on quality of life.

Cella, D. (2001). Quality-of-life measurement in oncology. In A. Baum & B. L. Andersen (Eds.), *Psychosocial interventions for cancer* (pp. 57–76). Washington, DC: American Psychological Association.—Informative overview of the critical issues in HRQOL assessment in oncology, applicable to other medical specialties.

Dimsdale, J. E., & Baum. A. (Eds.). (1995). *Quality of life in behavioral medicine research.* Mahwah, NJ: Erlbaum.—Compendium of articles addressing the full range of issues regarding HRQOL assessment in medical populations.

Dropkin, M. J. (1999). Body image and quality of life after head and neck cancer surgery. *Cancer Practice: A Multidisciplinary Journal of Cancer Care, 7*, 309–313.—A review of specific body image concerns of head and neck cancer patients.

Drotar, D. (Ed.). (1998). *Measuring health-related quality of life in children and adolescents: Implications for research and practice.* Mahwah, NJ: Erlbaum.—Thorough review of issues regarding HRQOL assessment in pediatric psychology.

Fauerbach, J. A., Heinberg, L. J., Lawrence, J. W., Munster, A. M., Palombo, D. A., Richter, D., Spence, R. J., Stevens, S. S., Ware, L., & Muehlberger, T. (2000). Effect of early body image dissatisfaction on subsequent psychological and physical adjustment after disfiguring injury. *Psychosomatic Medicine, 62*, 576–582.—An illustration of how medical condition-specific assessment (i.e., use of the Satisfaction with Appearance Scale) results in documentation of important quality-of-life outcomes.

Gladis, M. M., Gosch, E. A., Dishuk, N. M., & Crits-Christoph, P. (1999). Quality of life: Exapnding the scope of clinical significance. *Journal of Consulting and Clinical Psychology, 67*, 320–331.—Very thorough review of quality-of-life issues in mental health.

Gorbatenko-Roth, K. G., Levin, I. P., Altmaier, E. M., & Doebbeling, B. N. (2001). Accuracy of health-related quality of life assessment: What is the benefit of incorporating patients' preferences for domain functioning? *Health Psychology, 20*, 136–140.—Illustrates usefulness of asking patients to report which domains of HRQOL are particularly relevant to them as a method to obtain the most clinically significant patient assessment.

Halioua, B., Beumont, M. G., & Lunel, F. (2000). Quality of life in dermatology. *International Journal of Dermatology, 39*, 801–806.—A review of the current state of the art of HRQOL issues in dermatology.

Harter, S. (1999). *The construction of the self: A developmental perspective*. New York: Guilford Press.—An extensive review of the research on the development of self-concept, including use of the authors's own measure, which assesses self-perceived appearance in addition to other variables.

Hopwood, P., Fletcher, I., Lee, A., & Al Ghazal, S. (2001). A body image scale for use with cancer patients. *European Journal of Cancer, 37*, 189–197.—A 10-item scale developed for evaluating quality-of-life outcomes in European clinical trials.

Kopel, S. J., Eiser, C., Cool, P., Grimer, R. J., & Carter, S. R. (1998). Brief report: Assessment of body image in survivors of childhood cancer. *Journal of Pediatric Psychology, 23*, 141–147.—Provides preliminary psychometric data on a body image measure designed to clinically identify patients with adjustment difficulties.

Lawrence, J. W., Heinberg, L. J., Roca, R., Munster, A., Spence, R., & Fauerbach, J. A. (1998). Development and validation of the Satisfaction With Appearance Scale: Assessing body image among burn-injured patients. *Psychological Assessment, 10*, 64–70.—This study describes an excellent example of how body image measurement must take into account specific characteristics of the medical population being assessed—in this case, burn survivors.

Pruzinsky, T. (1996). The psychology of plastic surgery: Advances in evaluating body image, quality of life, and psychopathology. *Advances in Plastic Surgery, 14*, 11–24.—Specifies critical role of body image variables in plastic surgery.

Varni, J. W., Katz, E. R., Colegrove, Jr., R., & Dolgin, M. (1995). Perceived physical appearance and adjustment of children with newly diagnosed cancer: A path analytic model. *Journal of Behavioral Medicine, 18*, 261–278.—Examines the many variables that may affect body image in children with cancer, and how the stage of the disease may influence body image experience.

Walden, K. J., Thompson, J. K., & Wells, K. E. (1997). Body image and psychological sequelae of silicone breast explantation: Preliminary findings. *Plastic and Reconstructive Surgery, 100*, 1299–1306.—An excellent example of how psychometrically sound body image measures can document the quality of life of patients who have had breast implants surgically removed.

Wicklund, I., Erling, A., & Albertsson-Wikland, K. (1998). Critical review of measurement issues in quality-of-life assessment in children with growth problems. In D. Drotar (Ed.), *Measuring health-related quality of life in children and adolescents: Implications for research and practice* (pp. 255–271). Mahwah, NJ: Erlbaum.—Reviews the range of measures, some of which specifically assess body image variables, used for evaluating children with growth-related problems.

IV

Individual and
Cultural Differences

21

Body Image Issues among Girls and Women

RUTH H. STRIEGEL-MOORE
DEBRA L. FRANKO

Over 15 years ago, Rodin and her colleagues coined the phrase "normative discontent" to describe the pervasive negative feelings that girls and women experience toward their bodies. Sadly, this term continues to convey the experience of the majority of females in this culture today. This chapter explores the body image challenges women face across the lifespan and offers commentary on current thinking about body image as a gendered construct.

Body image is a multidimensional concept that encompasses perceptual, attitudinal, and affective components. Disturbances in these components are termed "body image concerns." These disturbances may entail a negatively distorted view of one's appearance, body image dissatisfaction, or overvaluation of one's appearance in defining sense of self. Body image concerns can adversely affect psychological well-being and quality of life.

BODY IMAGE CONCERNS ACROSS THE LIFESPAN

Females are much more likely than males to experience body image concerns, regardless of age. Indeed, body image concerns are so widely seen as a "woman's issue" that many studies include females only, on the (implicitly or explicitly stated) assumption that these issues are not relevant for males. Methodological limitations are evident in much body image research. With the exception of recent studies of large and representative samples of adolescent girls, most studies rely on relatively small samples of convenience or fo-

183

cus on clinical samples of girls or women with eating disorders. Research on ethnic minority groups has been limited to small samples and studies that collapse different ethnic groups into one "minority group"—even though studies have shown that body image concerns vary across ethnicity (possibly because ethnic groups may differ in terms of certain determinants of body image concerns, such as acculturation, immigration status, socioeconomic status, and cultural acceptance of larger body sizes). Many studies report results by age groups (children, adolescents, adults). The groupings vary markedly, making it difficult to pinpoint when body image concerns arise, peak, or level off during development. The most commonly studied component of body image concern is weight dissatisfaction. Overvaluation of weight or shape has been studied in only a few studies, and only among adolescent girls and adult women. The complex assessment issues are well documented in Part II of this volume. Much of the literature is based on cross-sectional studies and does not permit conclusions about secular trends (e.g., have body image concerns become more common?) and developmental changes, or predictions about the clinical significance or prognostic utility of body image concerns.

Negative attitudes toward overweight emerge very early; indeed, stigmatization of overweight children is already present in 3-year-olds. It is estimated that as many as half of all girls ages 6–8 want to be thinner. However, experts caution that measures of body image concerns in children have not been validated conclusively, and further research is needed to address this important issue.

As girls enter puberty, body image concerns become more common; by midadolescence, it is normative for girls to report weight dissatisfaction, fear of further weight gain, and preoccupation with losing weight. In a large cohort study, Field and colleagues found that among 9-year-old girls, 20% reported trying to lose weight; among 14-year-old girls, the number exceeded 40%. Prospective studies have shown that this rise in body image concerns during adolescence is due, in part, to the weight gain associated with puberty. Weight dissatisfaction is correlated significantly with adiposity: The heavier the girl, the more likely she is to report weight dissatisfaction. It is of note, however, that most girls who report feeling fat and wanting to lose weight are within the normal-weight range.

A large body of literature documents the pervasiveness of body image concerns in female college students. Concern about weight gain is fueled by the widely discussed phenomenon of a significant weight gain during the first year in college. In a longitudinal study of female college students by Heatherton and colleagues, 82% of college women reported that they wanted to lose weight, though very few (1.4%) were statistically overweight; a decade later, 68% of those women still wanted to lose weight.

Findings from a recent study by Tiggemann and Lynch suggest that women (ranging in age from 20 to 84) continue to struggle with issues related to changing shape and size throughout the life cycle. Consistent with earlier studies, body dissatisfaction was found to remain relatively stable across the lifespan. However, the *meaning* of weight did not remain constant across age groups. Relative to younger women, older women reported larger ideal body shapes and less body monitoring, anxiety about appearance, and dieting to lose weight. These data suggest that although body dissatisfaction remains high, the psychological impact of this body dissatisfaction decreases as women age.

WHY ARE BODY IMAGE CONCERNS IMPORTANT?

Psychologists have long been interested in body image as an important component of self-image, and disturbances in body image have been linked to low self-esteem. In the past two decades, with the advent of research on eating disorders (especially bulimia nervosa), studies have focused more specifically on the relationship between body image concerns and eating behavior. Sociocultural models of bulimia nervosa assign body image concerns a causal role in the development of disordered eating (see Stice's chapter in this volume). These models describe the following etiological pathway: Internalizing the thin beauty ideal results in the experience of a discrepancy between the ideal and one's actual self and prompts body dissatisfaction for most girls, because the ideal is impossible to attain for all but very few. Weight dissatisfaction, in turn, motivates behavioral efforts to lose weight or prevent weight gain. Some girls resort to more extreme efforts because maintaining a low weight is biologically impossible, and these extreme efforts increase the risk of developing binge eating, a biological response to starvation.

As Stice discusses in his chapter, several prospective studies report evidence indicating the clinical significance of body image concerns. The data show that adolescent girls respond to their weight concerns by dieting and more severe weight control efforts, such as purging. Population surveys indicate that four of five adolescent girls diet at least once during their teenage years, and up to two-thirds of teenage girls are "on a diet" at any given time—even though most of these dieters are not overweight. Studies have shown that body dissatisfaction prospectively predicts the onset of dieting over and above the effects of other risk factors, including actual body mass. Weight dissatisfaction also predicts the onset of purging behaviors. In turn, dieting has been found to be a significant predictor of binge eating. Dieting has also been shown to contribute to the *increase* in adiposity and obesity—a relationship mediated by the link between dieting and binge eating. Hence, body image concerns may actually contribute to an increased risk for further weight gain. These findings have led researchers to conclude that body dissatisfaction is one of the most potent risk factors for eating disturbances.

The pervasiveness of body image concerns in adolescent girls has been hypothesized to contribute to the emergence of the gender disparity in depression during adolescence. Prospective data by Stice and his colleagues indicate that body dissatisfaction contributes to depression in adolescent girls. This finding suggests that the impact of body image concerns reaches beyond eating behavior.

In a provocative paper, Leslie Heinberg and her colleagues suggest that, contrary to the current zeitgeist, body dissatisfaction may not be entirely maladaptive. They argue that some degree of body image concern, particularly in the overweight and obese, may be beneficial and perhaps even necessary to motivate individuals to engage in healthy dieting and exercise behaviors. Calling upon numerous studies highlighting the connection between distress and behavior change, these authors hypothesize that *some* degree of worry about body image may be an important predictor of health behaviors. We wonder whether this potential relationship between body image concerns and healthy dieting behavior might hold true for adult women more so than for adolescent girls. For the adolescent, any degree of body image concern appears to be related to potentially negative consequences (lower self-esteem, disordered eating), whereas for the older woman whose weight is likely to increase with age, some body dissatisfaction may provide motivation for healthy eating and exercise. These questions await future research.

WHY ARE WEIGHT CONCERNS UBIQUITOUS IN GIRLS AND WOMEN?

Numerous theories have been developed to explain why weight concerns are normative experiences in females. Evolutionary explanations are based on the assumption that a culture's beauty ideal connotes health and that beautiful females enjoy an advantage in the process of mate selection, with the long-term outcome for the species of survival of the healthiest individuals. Social psychological studies have provided ample support for the interpersonal advantage enjoyed by females who fit a culture's beauty standard. Although there is considerable cross-cultural agreement about facial beauty, pronounced cultural differences exist for body weight/shape ideals. Cultures where food supplies are not consistently available for a majority of the population favor larger body sizes than cultures where famine or starvation is uncommon. In Western industrialized nations, the female beauty ideal has become increasingly thin. Due to globalization, individuals in non-Western countries increasingly have been exposed to Western ideals and behavioral practices. Cross-cultural studies have found that, in most cultures, at least some females aspire to the thin ideal even when the predominant preference is a more endowed female body. In light of the well-established health risks caused by severe emaciation, especially infertility, the evolutionary advantage of the contemporary female beauty ideal of is not immediately apparent.

Sociocultural explanations of weight concern have focused on three factors: the stigma associated with obesity, idealization of thinness in females, and the role of physical appearance as a core aspect of femininity (see chapters by Jackson and McKinley in this volume). In a series of studies on the prejudice against obese individuals, Crandall has shown that "antifat" attitudes are part of a social ideology that holds individuals responsible for their life outcomes and is correlated with attributions of controllability of life events. Obesity is seen as a "voluntary" condition that results from a person's inability to control his or her urges. Hence, obesity is seen not only as a cosmetic flaw but as a character defect as well.

Complementing the negative stereotype about obesity is the positive stereotype regarding physical attractiveness; for females, being thin is a hallmark of contemporary beauty. In the broader cultural context of viewing the body as infinitely malleable, pursuit of thinness has become a social norm for females. Increasingly drastic means of body modification are now presented as "normal," including the use of cosmetic surgery to remove unwanted body fat. Pursuit of thinness is imbued with the "myth of transformation": Losing weight holds the promise of changing more than just one's body size; it promises to change one's social status, both economically and interpersonally. This emphasis on thinness is in stark contrast to the rising rates of obesity. Indeed, several cultural changes make it increasingly difficult to maintain a low weight, including the decrease in physical activity, the increase in sedentary leisure activities, the rise in fast-food consumption, and the introduction of "super-sized" food portions.

To understand the powerful influence of the beauty myth on girls and women, we need to appreciate that beauty is a central component of the female gender role stereotype. Experiencing herself as beautiful serves to affirm a girl's or woman's identity as female. Looking beautiful affirms to others that a girl or woman complies with social expectations regarding femininity. As McKinley discusses in her chapter, objectification theory describes a fundamental gender difference in the conceptualization of the body. Females' bodies are more likely than males' bodies to be regarded in a way that is evaluative—and therefore objectifying. When males' bodies are evaluated, it is in terms of functionality more than aesthetics. Early on, girls are exposed to the societal expectations to pursue physical attractiveness. They gradually internalize the objectifying gaze, thereafter engaging in self-monitoring and self-improvement behaviors aimed at meeting the cultural beauty standard.

As Tiggemann reviews in this volume, a growing number of studies has begun to examine the role of the media as a major conveyor of these social norms about the female gender stereotype, the stigma of obesity, and the beauty ideal of thinness. The data suggest that thin females are over-represented in all visual media, and that certain media, especially video and computer games and music videos (which are used particularly by adolescents), have highly gender stereotypic content. This literature has produced somewhat mixed results regarding the hypothesis that media trends predict body image concerns. In one study, Becker and her colleagues investigated the impact of newly introduced Western television programming on ethnic Fijian schoolgirls; they found increased disordered eating and reports of self-induced vomiting in the group that experienced prolonged television exposure.

Researchers have begun to explore the role that cultural and ethnic diversity may play in the development of body image concerns (see Part IV of this volume). The major research questions address whether there are ethnic differences in the ideal female body size, and whether body weight concerns are less common in ethnic groups wherein the body ideal is less extreme in terms of thinness. In the United States, no epidemiological study of body image has been conducted with a representative sample that includes women from all ethnic minorities. Many studies have examined body image in black and white female samples and have found remarkably similar results. Compared to white adolescent and adult females, black adolescent and adult females (1) endorse a body ideal that is slightly heavier, (2) are less likely to report weight dissatisfaction and dieting to lose weight, and (3) report less social pressure to be thin. Studies of body image concerns in Latina girls and women suggest rates that are comparable to, or even greater than, those found in white females. In the few studies that sampled Asian girls living in the United States, body dissatisfaction was found to be a prevalent concern. Within each ethnic group, greater body dissatisfaction has been shown to be associated with symptomatic eating behaviors and low self-esteem, suggesting that when a female from any minority group experiences body image concerns, she may be at increased risk for adverse outcomes.

As Kearney-Cooke discusses in this volume, families can exacerbate body image concerns by amplifying the cultural pressures to aspire to the beauty ideal of thinness. Studies have shown significant correlations between parents' concerns about their own and/or their children's weight and body dissatisfaction in girls. Indeed, girls whose mothers attempted to control their daughters' food intake reported lower body satisfaction and self-esteem. Prospective studies are needed to examine whether parents' attitudes about their children's body weight contribute to the internalization of the thin ideal and the development of body image concerns.

Several personal vulnerability factors have been hypothesized to increase risk of developing body image concerns. Across the age spectrum, studies consistently find that body image concerns increase with increasing body weight. Overweight girls are at greater risk because their actual body size makes attaining the thin ideal difficult. Not surprisingly, body weight is the strongest predictor of weight dissatisfaction. Perfectionism also has been implicated as a risk factor, because pursuit of a thin body may represent one way of pursuing perfection. Prospective studies are needed to determine whether there is a causal relationship between perfectionism and body image concerns.

CHALLENGES ACROSS THE LIFESPAN

It is clear from the literature that body image concerns occur throughout development but that the challenges faced by girls and women differ over time. Although body image concerns are least likely to occur in childhood, the age at which such concerns begin to emerge appears to be decreasing. Indeed, experts recently have noted an increase in treatment referrals of children with anorexia nervosa or related eating problems. In the absence of epidemiological data, it remains unclear whether the rise in child referrals reflects a true increase of eating disorders in children or improved detection of such cases. Typically, body image concerns have been regarded as an adolescent phenomenon, yet children as young as 9 report weight dissatisfaction and dieting. Possible explanations for this trend include the decreasing age of menarche/puberty, the higher prevalence of childhood obesity, and media marketing to "tweens" (ages 8–11).

The emergence of body image concerns is most pronounced during adolescence. Data suggest that a confluence of developmental factors may account for this increase, including pubertal weight gain, greater academic demands, and increased social challenges. Although colleges have been regarded as "breeding grounds" for body image concerns and disordered eating, few studies have compared women who do and do not attend college. Therefore, it is unclear whether the pervasive body image concerns reported by college students reflect their particular challenges or are part of the developmental experience of young adulthood. Although seeming to carry fewer challenges, adulthood nevertheless casts its own unique impediments to women's sense of satisfaction with their size and shape. Several studies have found that pregnancy, and particularly the postpartum year, are times of increased body image concerns (see Heinberg and Guarda's chapter in this volume). As a woman enters menopause, concerns about femininity and sexuality may pose further challenges to her body esteem (see Whitbourne and Skultety's chapter in this volume).

CONCLUSIONS

For many women, body image concerns begin early and continue throughout the lifespan. Some interventions have been successful in reducing body image dissatisfaction in college-age women (see Cash and Strachan's chapter in this volume). However, prevention efforts with younger girls are needed to diminish body image concerns and decrease the risk of developing eating disorders during adolescence. Chapters in this volume by Levine and Smolak and by Winzelberg and colleagues discuss the promise of such prevention programs.

INFORMATIVE READINGS

Becker, A. E., Burwell, R. A., Gilman, S., Herzog, D. B., & Hamburg, P. (in press). The impact of television on disordered eating in Fiji. *British Journal of Psychiatry.*—A naturalistic experiment that examined the effects of the introduction of Western television programming on the eating behaviors of adolescent Fijiian girls.

Crandall, C. (1994). Prejudice against fat people: Ideology and self-interest. *Journal of Personality and Social Psychology, 66,* 882–894.—A series of studies comparing weight prejudice with symbolic racism that found parallels on all dimensions studied; the author concludes that "fatism" is similar to racism, though without the negative social desirability that is inherent in racism.

Field, A. E., Camargo, C. A., Taylor, C. B., Berkey, C. S., Frazier, A. L., Gillman, M. W., & Colditz, G. A. (1999). Overweight, weight concerns, and bulimic behaviors among girls and boys. *Journal of the American Academy of Child and Adolescent Psychiatry, 38,* 754–760.—A population-based study of 9- to 14-year-olds that reported the common occurrence of misperceived overweight and undue concern with weight.

Franko, D. L., & Orosan-Weine, P. (1998). Prevention of eating disorders: Empirical, methodological, and conceptual considerations. *Clinical Psychology: Science and Practice, 5,* 459–477.—A critical evaluation of risk factor research and prevention programs, with an emphasis on environmental, familial, and behavioral risk factors, including body image concerns.

Heatherton, T. F., Mahamedi, F., Striepe, M., Field, A. E., & Keel, P. K. (1997). A 10-year longitudinal study of body weight, dieting, and eating disorder symptoms. *Journal of Abnormal Psychology, 106,* 117–125.—Although disordered eating and body dissatisfaction decreased over time, this study found that body image concerns and the desire to lose weight remained relatively high.

Heinberg, L. J., Thompson, J. K., & Matzon, J. L. (2001). Body image dissatisfaction as a motivator for healthy lifestyle change: Is some distress beneficial? In R. H. Striegel-Moore & L. Smolak (Eds.), *Eating disorders: Innovative directions in research and intervention* (pp. 215–232). Washington, DC: American Psychological Association.—A comprehensive chapter arguing that some degree of body dissatisfaction may provide motivation to engage in healthy dieting and exercise behaviors.

Ricciardelli, L. A., & McCabe, M. P. (2001). Children's body image concerns and eating disturbance: A review of the literature. *Clinical Psychology Review, 21,* 325–344.—A review paper that summarizes and evaluates research on body image concerns in children ages 6–11 years old.

Rodin, J., Silberstein, L. R., & Striegel-Moore, R. H. (1985). Women and weight: A normative discontent. In R. Sonderegger (Ed.), *Nebraska Symposium on Motivation* (pp. 267–307). Lincoln, NB: University of Nebraska Press.—This now classic paper offers a comprehensive biopsychosocial model of body image concerns in females and exhaustively reviews the relevant empirical literature; its conclusions still hold today.

Striegel-Moore, R. H., Schreiber, G. B., Lo, A., Crawford, P., Obarzanek, E., & Rodin, R. (2000). Eating disorder symptoms in a cohort of 11- to 16-year-old black and white girls: The NHLBI Growth and Health Study. *International Journal of Eating Disorders, 27,* 49–66.—A large community sample examining ethnic differences in body image of black and white girls, which reported that white girls showed greater body dissatisfaction than black girls.

Tiggemann, M., & Lynch, J. E. (2001). Body image across the life span in adult women: The role of self-objectification. *Developmental Psychology, 37,* 243–253.—A study of 322 women between the ages of 20 and 84 found that body image dissatisfaction remains stable across the ages, although the negative correlates decrease with age.

22

Body Image Issues among Boys and Men

PATRICIA WESTMORELAND CORSON
ARNOLD E. ANDERSEN

There are many indications that body dissatisfaction in boys and men is becoming an increasingly common source of much suffering. Citing trends from three *Psychology Today* surveys over the last three decades on male body dissatisfaction, Pope and colleagues provide a rationale for heightened concern about male preoccupation with physical appearance. Although interpreting these epidemiological data is complicated (see Cash's chapter in this volume, there is no question that male body image problems across all age ranges demand increased attention by researchers.

A heightening awareness of male eating disorders is also occurring. Historically, shame and fear of public humiliation drove men with body image dissatisfaction and eating disorders "underground." Clearly, however, women are no longer alone in succumbing to the seduction of the gods of thinness and sacrificing their emotional well-being and productivity in the process.

In this brief review, we elucidate factors contributing to male body image development, distortion, and dissatisfaction. We also explore historical and social perspectives on this burgeoning cultural phenomenon and attempt to provide useful suggestions for identifying and treating male eating disorders and body image problems.

CULTURAL STANDARDS AND BODY IMAGE DEVELOPMENT

Western cultures are blamed for placing extreme value on physical beauty. However, in her seminal book *Survival of the Prettiest: The Science of Beauty*, Nancy Etcoff reports that cross-cultural research reveals that some residents of non-Western countries emphasize appearance as much as U.S. residents. Interestingly, Thompson notes that each race, culture, and socioeconomic level sets its own standards and is of "great influence" in determining body size satisfaction. Indeed, studies have found that the drive for thinness is dissimilar among different racial groups: black schoolchildren apparently select significantly larger "ideal sizes" than white schoolchildren, and when black schoolchildren desire to be thinner, their chosen ideal size is larger than that chosen by white schoolchildren. In 1996 Thompson reported that adolescent black males differed from their white male peers by selecting a larger body size as ideal, dieting less often, giving fewer subjective reports of being overweight, and selecting females with higher body mass indices as girlfriends. (See Smolak's and Smolak and Levine's chapters in this volume for related discussions.)

The incidence of body image disturbance is strikingly similar in countries of similar socioeconomic status. For instance, in 1997 Rolland and colleagues documented that U.S., Israeli, and Australian schoolchildren reported a similar drive for thinness, with approximately 50% of girls and 33% of boys wanting to be thinner, and 40% of girls and 24% of boys having attempted to lose weight. The cultural variations in appearance preferences likely have their origins in childhood and continue into adolescence. According to Pope and colleagues, many of the earliest messages a child receives regarding physical attractiveness standards come not only from television and movies but also from the toys with which they play. To investigate associations between societal concepts of desired male body image and how this message is relayed to children, Pope and colleagues collected children's popular action figures spanning three decades. They found that the "GI Joe" from the 1960s was significantly less muscular than the 1990s figure: If the former were 5 feet 10 inches tall, his "chest" would measure 44 inches and his biceps would measure 12 inches; the latter, however, would have a 55-inch chest and 15-inch biceps! Similar progressive enlargements of body size were found for other popular action toys (e.g., "Luke Skywalker"). Whereas "Barbie" seems to have gotten thinner (thus promoting the ideal of thinness in females), "GI Joe" and other male action figures have grown larger but leaner, conveying the value of extreme leanness and muscularity—and thereby setting the stage for muscle dysmorphia in males. (See Olivardia's chapter in this volume.)

The hypothesis that some male schoolchildren actually select a body ideal mimicking "GI Joe" seems to apply into late adolescence, with college-age men generally aiming for more muscular bodies. This goal appears to encourage body image distortion, as males want to be heavier but see themselves as lighter, and females wish to be lighter but see themselves as almost 10–15 pounds heavier than they really are. Whatever the "direction" of body image distortion, the motivating factors appear to be the same: concern with physical appearance, popularity, and attractiveness to the opposite sex.

SOCIAL EVOLUTION?

According to Nancy Etcoff, male appearance is important, from an early age onward, in establishing dominance hierarchies. Research has shown that, for example, participants at boys' camps select the "best looking, most athletic boy who shows the most mature physique" as pack leader. This pattern continues into adulthood. Etcoff cites Mazur's 1984 study of West Point cadets, which demonstrated the role of "facial dominance" (as evidenced by prominent chin, heavy brow ridges, deep set eyes, and ears close to the head) in predicting advancement through the military ranks and eventual success in later career.

Success, in turn, ensures a man's continued attractiveness to women. David Buss's 1994 study of transcultural mating preferences indicates that women rate ambition and financial success as crucial factors in determining male attractiveness. Favoring these attributes is said to be an evolutionary strategy that focuses females' mate choice on males who will promote stability and financial security. Sometimes the attributes of success and achievement override that of physical attractiveness when it comes to women's choice of mates. Indeed, Buss's findings suggest that physical attractiveness is less influential when it comes to women's evaluation of men. However, it may also be the case that male sociocultural roles have evolved to make attractive physical appearance an important prerequisite for success. As Faludi pointed out in 1999, this may be due partly to the shift from the Industrial Age to the Information Age, wherein being successful is about *appearing* successful and adorning oneself with the trappings of success.

This evolutionary shift may also have come about, as Etcoff suggests, in response to sexual competition: As women spend time around other men in the workforce, their mates feel compelled to enhance their own attractiveness in the face of this ongoing competition. Kimmel notes that some researchers go so far as to state that men are no longer necessarily the "breadwinners" and that current male interest in male appearance results from the fact that the workplace is no longer necessarily the place for men to test and prove their masculinity.

Another explanation for the modern generation's obsession with fitness and appearance is the concept of the "supermale." Pope and colleagues blame this media-endorsed creation as instrumental in infecting millions of young men with an "Adonis complex."

If we are to believe Etcoff's hypothesis that couples tend to be closely matched in terms of appearance (the more attractive the individual, the greater the chance his or her partner will be equally attractive), then the increasing prevalence of "lookism" in the male population should be no surprise. With Miss Americas becoming thinner and thinner (thus encouraging impossible standards of beauty and thinness), the image of the supermale as leaner, more muscular, and more handsome makes these male icons increasingly remote from what average men can possibly attain.

"NO PAIN, NO GAIN": APPEARANCE AT WHAT PRICE?

Many men are motivated to achieve the prowess and "physicality" that have become the essential ingredients of male attractiveness—whatever the cost. Pope and colleagues report that, when asked how many years of their lives they would trade to achieve their weight goals, 17% of males surveyed by a popular magazine said that they would sacrifice more than 3 years, and 11% answered 5 years. These figures are strikingly similar to those obtained from women.

Men are susceptible to a greater variety of weight concerns than females because the ideal to which men aspire is much more complex than the thinness norm women embrace. According to Pope and colleagues, men want to change their weight, as do women, but are often even more preoccupied with body shape and muscularity. Andersen and colleagues note that body shape concerns, lack of exercise versus compulsive exercise, and "appearance obsession" are common problems faced by today's man.

To what lengths will today's man go in order to achieve "appearance success"? In tallying the distance, we focused on eating disorders, compulsive exercising, and appearance obsession. However, muscle dysmorphia and body dysmorphic disorder, both of which are very pressing contemporary problems, are also critical to consider. These problems are addressed in detail in the chapters by Olivardia (on muscularity) and Phillips (on body dysmorphic disorder) in this volume. The bottom line is that the desire to meet current appearance standards leads many men to spend excessive amounts of time attempting to change their appearance—and often at considerable physical risk (e.g., using steroids, undergoing multiple cosmetic surgeries).

Eating Disorders and Compulsive Exercising

In 1986 Crisp and colleagues described common susceptibility characteristics for eating disorders in males and females: These individuals are perfectionists, driven to succeed, have low self-esteem, have an upper-middle-class upbringing, and come from families with a high degree of unexpressed emotion. Strober and colleagues noted that patterns of familial aggregation for males with eating disorders are akin to those reported in females. Additionally, Woodside and colleagues reported that the pathophysiology of men with eating disorders apparently does not differ significantly from females, a fact that suggests a similar biological etiology.

However, it is somewhat more difficult to diagnose eating disorders in males for several reasons: First, men are reluctant to admit having a "women's problem." Second, DSM-IV criteria for eating disorders are biased toward family-related characteristics (e.g., the menstruation criterion) and do not mention "body shape" (which, as Andersen points out, is apparently more of a concern to men than actual body weight). Third, practitioners often mistake male bingeing behavior for a hearty appetite (supposedly typical "guy behavior") and dismiss thinness as either the hallmark of a "health nut" or as secondary to another medical or psychiatric disorder.

The fact remains that anorexia and bulimia nervosa are no less serious in males. Siegel and colleagues suggest that males may have additional medical complications secondary to difficulties in establishing diagnosis and delays in seeking treatment. Compulsive exercise is as dangerous for males with eating disorders as it is for females. Although amenorrhea is obviously not a consideration when assessing males, it is essential to evaluate the possibility of testosterone depletion and the presence of dangerous electrolyte imbalances.

One troubling finding is that the premorbid tendency toward obesity appears to be greater in eating-disordered males than in females. Additionally, uncontrolled binge eating in men appears to be more common than either anorexia nervosa or bulimia nervosa. This finding may be directly related to the somewhat higher prevalence of binge eating disorder in males—3.3% for males versus 3.2% for females, as reported by Garfinkel and colleagues in 1995. The "night eating syndrome"—in which individuals restrict daytime eating, only to get up during the night and binge eat more than half of their total daily calories, with only a vague memory of the event—is another male-dominated form of eating disorder. Obesity (reportedly found in 63% of men and 55% of women over the age of 25) is often the sorry side effect of a life built around "food angst" and yo-yo dieting.

TREATMENT: STRIVING FOR IMPERFECTION IN A PERFECT WORLD?

Treatment of male body image concerns requires a comprehensive evaluation, including a longitudinal history, cross-sectional mental status exam, supplemental histories from significant others, and selected psychological tests. As noted, detecting an eating disorder or body dysmorphic disorder in males can be challenging. Clinicians should be especially tuned to listening for telltale phrases (e.g., "I don't like my body," "I want to change the way I look," "I can't stand the way I look," "I want to be thinner," or " . . . more muscular," or " . . . better defined") expressed by boys and men with varying degrees of body image disturbance.

Body image distress, which might appear to be no more than a culture-driven, overvalued belief, may also trigger obsessional patterns (such as restricting food intake, bingeing, overexercising) that result in a state of un-remitting existential angst and a full-blown eating disorder or body dys-morphic disorder. The most common form of body image distress emerges in young men as a vague sense of concern regarding body weight or shape, which abates when they are with friends and which does not find expression in significant weight or shape-changing activities or profound mood and self-esteem consequences. This symptomatology seldom (if ever) requires formal treatment, with the vast majority of young men going on to develop more of an interest in their career aspirations and social plans than in their body and eating habits.

A more serious situation arises when weight or shape-changing activities interfere with daily life to the extent that the man focuses exclusively on weight or shape and actively engages in weight or shape-changing activities that actually undermine physical, social, and emotional health. By the time such behavior has culminated in an eating disorder or body dysmorphic disorder, professional help is needed to avert serious bodily and psychological harm. Referral to a mental health professional who is well versed in treating these disorders is recommended at this stage. In a recent article on male eating disorders, Woodside and colleagues also concluded that alcoholism and depression are frequent comorbid conditions that should be screened at relevant intervals during treatment.

Treatment of eating disorders (and some cases of muscle dysmorphia) requires mandatory medical management to ensure survival and initiate healing. Extreme weight loss, electrolyte imbalances, and cardiac or other organ damage necessitate inpatient treatment where cautious refeeding can be instituted and a controlled environment disallows compensatory behavior (such as purging and compulsive exercising). While males and females suffer comparable degrees of osteopenia in anorexia nervosa, recovery for males entails rebalancing testosterone levels, whereas for females, the focus is estrogen.

Antidepressants (such as the selective serotonin reuptake inhibitors [SSRIs]) are helpful for treating individuals who have achieved (or are at) goal weight: however, they are not typically used to treat depression resulting from starvation and/or weight loss associated with anorexia nervosa. (See Allen and Hollander in this volume for a description of medication treatment in eating disorders.) In addition, the use of antidepressants in males with anorexia nervosa is not well studied, though Pope and colleagues note that SSRIs (alone or in combination with cognitive-behavioral therapy) have been successful in treating body dysmorphic disorder and muscle dysmorphia.

While the body heals, the psychopathology of the eating disorder should also be explored. Cognitive-behavioral therapy can be instrumental in this regard. At the core of most men's eating disorders are overidealized beliefs. The excessive value placed on thinness or muscularity has significant mood and behavior consequences. At the time of first assessment, a value system laden with "impossible dreams" and sustained by the persevering and self-critical traits of the individual may already be in place. Until the psychological sequelae of starvation (well documented by Key's landmark study) have been reversed, patients do not usually have the energy and attention to "untwist" their cognitive distortions or to properly "devalue" their overidealized beliefs.

CONCLUSION

What is the "take-home message" for addressing the body image concerns of the "new millennium male"? It cannot be overemphasized that the world in which we live plays a pivotal role in "setting men up for failure," with its perpetuation of the supermale myth and the apparent ease with which attainment of this ideal is purported to be within the reach of the average male. Men are thrust into thinking about body image before they are cognizant of what this term means, and before they are aware of the inherent danger of the "starve–eat–purge" charade. As Mark Twain once said, "The worst loneliness is not to be comfortable with yourself." In a world flush with the unparalleled opportunity to be "the best of the best," it is a loneliness men can ill-afford.

INFORMATIVE READINGS

Andersen, A. E., Cohn, L., & Holbrook T. (2000). *Making weight: Men's concerns with food, weight, shape and appearance*. Carlsbad, CA: Gurze Books.—The first book for men about weight, shape, and appearance.

Andersen, A. E., Watson, T. L., & Schlechte, J. (2000). Osteoporosis and osteopenia in men with eating disorders. *Lancet, 355,*1967–1968.—Establishes the fact that osteoporosis is a severe medical complication for males with eating disorders.

Buss, D. M. (1994). *The evolution of desire: Strategies of human mating*. New York: Basic Books.—This book details features that make men attractive to women and vice versa.

Carlat, D. J., Camargo, Jr., C. A., & Herzog, D. B. (1997). Eating disorders in males: A report on 135 patients. *American Journal of Psychiatry, 154*, 1127–1132.—A thorough, systematic study of clinic-based eating-disordered males.

Crisp, A. H., Burns, T., & Bhat, A. V. (1986). Primary anorexia nervosa in the male and female: A comparison of features and prognosis. *British Journal of Medical Psychology, 59*, 123–132.—This study compares features present in male and female eating disorders.

Etcoff, N. (1999). *Survival of the prettiest: The science of beauty.* New York: Doubleday.—A book detailing why being attractive leads to success in life; also thoroughly reviews the "science" of beauty and what attracts humans and animals to one another.

Faludi, S. (1999). *Stiffed.* New York: Morrow.—Details the struggle of the modern man in terms of learning to survive in a feminist culture.

Keys, A. B. (1950). *The biology of human starvation.* Minneapolis: University of Minnesota Press.—Absolutely essential reading on the physical, social, and psychological consequences of starvation in volunteers.

Kimmel, M. (1996). *Manhood in America.* New York: Free Press.—Examines the changing role of men in society.

Mazur, J., & Keating, C. (1984). Military attainment of a West Point class: Effects of cadets' physical features. *American Journal of Sociology, 90,* 125–150.—Did you know the shape of your chin and face can determine your leadership future?

Pope, Jr., H. G., Phillips, K. A., & Olivardia, R. (2000). *The Adonis complex: The secret crisis of male body obsession.* New York: Free Press.—A best-seller on body dysmorphia and men's obsession with fat-free muscularity.

Rolland, K., Farnill, D., & Griffiths, R. A. (1997). Body figure perception and eating attitudes among Australian schoolchildren aged 8 to 12 years. *International Journal of Eating Disorders, 21,* 273–278.—A study of eating disorder issues among young children.

Siegel, J. H., Hardoff, D., Golden, N. H., & Shenker, I. R. (1995). Medical complications in male adolescents with anorexia nervosa. *Journal of Adolescent Health, 16,* 448–453.—Reviews physical findings in eating disorder patients.

Strober, M., Freeman, R., Lampert, C., Diamond, J., & Kaye, W. (2001). Males with anorexia nervosa: A controlled study of eating disorders in first-degree relatives. *International Journal of Eating Disorders, 29,* 263–269.—This study demonstrates the familial and genetic contributions to eating disorders in males.

Thompson, S. H. (1996). Weight-related attitudes and practices of black and white adolescent males. *The Physical Educator, 53,* 102–112.—Compares cross-racial attitudes regarding eating and body image.

Thompson S. H., Corwin, S. J., & Sargent R. G. (1997). Ideal body size beliefs and weight concerns of fourth-grade children. *International Journal of Eating Disorders, 21,* 279–284.—This paper establishes the very young age at which weight concerns appear and notes racial differences.

Wolf, N. (1990). *The beauty myth: How images of beauty are used against women.* London: Vintage.—A provocative, seminal work that conveys a feminist perspective on society's use of beauty to undermine women's self-worth and power.

Woodside, D. B., Garfinkel, P. E., Goering, P., Kaplan, A., Goldblum, D. S., & Kennedy, S. H. (2001). Comparisons of men with full or partial eating disorders, men without eating disorders, and women with eating disorders in the community. *American Journal of Psychiatry, 158,* 570–574.—The first community study establishing the high prevalence of eating disorders in males in the general population.

Obesity and Body Image

MARLENE B. SCHWARTZ
KELLY D. BROWNELL

HOW DO OBESE INDIVIDUALS FEEL ABOUT THEIR BODIES?

It is widely assumed that obese individuals must feel bad about their bodies—after all, they are obese. This assumption reflects the powerful societal stigma against obese people: They should feel ashamed because their excess weight represents character flaws such as laziness, gluttony, lack of control, and self-indulgence. Research on this issue, however, reveals a more complex picture. Obesity is linked to poor body image, but not all obese people are affected, and among those who are, severity varies considerably.

It is important to understand the role of poor body image in the lives of obese individuals. Not only does poor body image cause psychological distress, it may also be a negative prognosis for treatment because it can persist in the face of weight loss and may increase the chances of relapse. Although the medical consequences of obesity are well documented, the psychological consequences remain unclear.

Friedman's and Brownell's meta-analysis on the psychological correlates of obesity found few consistent differences that distinguish obese individuals from their normal-weight peers, and concluded that the obese population is psychologically heterogeneous. The first generation of studies in this field simply compared overweight and normal-weight groups, usually using superficial forms of measurement. Friedman and Brownell suggest that the second generation of researchers seek to identify clusters of risk factors that predict which obese individuals are more likely to experience psychological difficulty. This chapter summarizes research that helps identify who is most at risk for poor body image and proposes new avenues for research and clinical intervention.

RISK FACTORS ASSOCIATED WITH BODY IMAGE DISTRESS

Binge Eating Disorder

Binge eating disorder (BED) is a diagnostic category identified as needing further research by the American Psychiatric Association in the DSM-IV. A consistent finding is that individuals with BED appear to be a distinct subgroup of the obese population that experiences more psychological distress (i.e., depression, anxiety, substance abuse, and personality disorders) than obese individuals who do not binge eat.

Diagnostic criteria for BED focus exclusively on eating behavior and feelings about binge eating. Unlike anorexia nervosa and bulimia nervosa, BED does not include consideration of body image distortion or distress. However, research suggests that individuals with BED have greater body dissatisfaction and concerns about weight and shape than obese individuals without this disorder. Wilfley, Schwartz, Spurrell, and Fairburn found patients with BED had similar levels of shape and weight concerns as those with anorexia nervosa and bulimia nervosa, and higher levels than obese people who do not binge eat. In a study by Milkewicz and Cash, higher levels of binge eating were related to a more negative body image and to poorer psychosocial adjustment for overweight women, as well as for those who have never been overweight. Controlling for body image reduced some, but not all, of the relationships between binge eating and psychological functioning. It appears, therefore, that individuals who binge eat are at increased risk of body image disturbance and poor psychological functioning.

Age of Obesity Onset

Clinicians have noted important differences between individuals who became overweight as children and those who gained weight as adults. This clinical impression has received mixed empirical support. In a case-controlled risk-factor study, Fairburn and colleagues found that childhood obesity was a specific risk factor for BED. Grilo and colleagues divided a sample of obese women seeking treatment into groups of childhood- versus adult-onset obesity. Although the groups did not differ in weight, women who also were obese as children reported higher levels of body dissatisfaction. This study supports the link between early onset of obesity and poor body image.

In contrast, Jackson and colleagues examined a sample of obese women with BED and found that all three groups (child-, adolescent-, and adult-onset obesity) were remarkably similar in current level of body dissatisfaction, eating pathology, and general psychological functioning. Adami and colleagues studied formerly severely obese people who had lost weight through surgery, and currently severely obese individuals. They found that among currently obese people, similar levels of body dissatisfaction were reported by those with childhood and adult-onset obesity. However, among the surgery patients, those with childhood-onset obesity had poorer body image than their adult-onset counterparts. This finding suggests that the onset of obesity at an early age increases the durability of poor body image following weight loss but does not predict a worse body image among severely obese people or those with BED.

One possible explanation for the conflicting findings is that body dissatisfaction may be consistently higher among certain groups (i.e., those with BED and surgery candidates) and therefore there are no body image differences due to age of obesity onset. Hence, although early onset of obesity may be a risk factor for body image problems in the entire range of obese individuals in the population, it will not emerge when studying particular subgroups of obese individuals.

Stigma and Discrimination

There is growing awareness of the social oppression obese individuals face. In a recent literature review, Puhl and Brownell argued that the stigma against obesity makes it the last socially acceptable form of discrimination. Because many people believe that individuals have control over their weight (as compared to their race and sex), there is a willingness to blame. Obese individuals may internalize these feelings and blame themselves for others' negative reactions to them.

Milkewicz and Cash recently studied body image, psychosocial adjustment, and the experiences of weight-related stigmatization in overweight women and found that the woman's history of stigmatization (i.e., during childhood, adolescence, and/or adulthood) was consistently associated with a currently negative body image. Greater stigmatization was predictive of greater social anxiety, depression, lower self-esteem, and less life satisfaction. Controlling for body image attenuated some, but not all, of these relationships.

Myers and Rosen measured the frequency and type of stigmatizing experiences that a sample of obese individuals had endured and the coping mechanisms they employed. There was a significant relationship between the amount of their stigmatization and the severity of their negative body image, even when controlling for obesity levels. Individuals who used more maladaptive coping strategies (e.g., "negative self-talk," "cry," "isolate myself," and "avoid or leave situation") were more dissatisfied with their bodies. Those using positive coping strategies (e.g., "see situation as others' problem," "refuse to hide body, be visible," and "self-love, self-acceptance") reported higher self-esteem but no improvement in body image. This research points to two important avenues for intervention: At the individual level, treatment can help obese people develop positive coping strategies to replace maladaptive ones; on the societal level, such research can raise awareness about the array and frequency of stigmatizing experiences faced by obese individuals.

History of Childhood Teasing and Parental Criticism about Weight

A specific type of stigmatization is childhood teasing about appearance. Research by Jackson and colleagues examined how childhood teasing about general appearance, as well as weight and size, is related to current body image, self-esteem, and depression in a clinical sample of women with BED. The findings suggest that childhood teasing is significantly related to poor self-esteem and depression. Interestingly, only general appearance teasing (not shape and weight teasing) related to current body dissatisfaction.

Stigmatization of obese children also can occur at home where parents' criticism of a child's weight can have potentially damaging effects. Fairburn found that people with BED were more likely than psychiatric controls to report negative comments by the family about shape, weight, and eating behavior.

History of Weight Cycling

Weight cycling (the experience of losing and regaining weight repeatedly over time) is prevalent among obese individuals. The research findings on the medical and psychological consequences of this behavior have been mixed, and two research design problems have emerged: First, there is no standard definition and measurement of weight cycling; second, analyses used in some studies assume that someone who loses and regains twice as much weight (i.e., 100 vs. 50 pounds) should have twice as much distress. This assumption is probably untrue. Recent work by Friedman, Schwartz, and Brownell (1998) distinguishes between the subjective experience of oneself as a weight cycler (i.e., endorsing "I am a yo-yo dieter") and the degree of weight fluctuation (i.e., the number of times a specific number of pounds was lost and regained). This approach has yielded a more reliable way of identifying individuals at higher risk of body dissatisfaction. People with a subjective view of themselves as weight cyclers are more likely to be dissatisfied with their bodies, have lower self-esteem, and lower levels of life satisfaction. In contrast, the number of pounds lost and regained is not linked to degree of psychological distress.

Degree of Obesity

Unlike normal-weight people with bulimia nervosa or body dysmorphic disorder, obese individuals are not simply imagining that they differ from societal ideals. This reality raises the possibility that as one's level of obesity increases, so does one's body dissatisfaction. Wilfley and colleagues addressed this question in a study of psychopathology in patients with BED. They found no differences in weight and shape concerns at different levels of obesity. Thus greater obesity in patients with BED does not necessarily cause more body dissatisfaction.

In a study by Eldredge and Agras of a primarily female sample from a commercial weight loss program, individuals with BED reported greater weight and shape concern than non-eating-disordered individuals, and this concern was not linked to weight category. The researchers suggested that in obese individuals, degree of overweight does not contribute independently to the importance of weight and shape in self-evaluation. Similarly, Sarwer and colleagues studied women seeking treatment (whose binge eating was not reported) and found no relationship between body mass index and body dissatisfaction.

Strong Investment in Appearance

Another potential risk for body image distress is the degree to which individuals are invested in physical appearance. Cash examined individuals engaged in a very low calorie diet program and compared them to age- and weight-matched control subjects. Individuals seeking treatment were more strongly invested in their appearance and level of fitness and had more body image distress. The finding that those who seek weight loss treatment are distressed by their body image suggests the importance of addressing body image in weight loss programs.

Gender

Adolescent and adult women across the weight spectrum are consistently more dissatisfied with their bodies than adolescent and adult men. This risk is magnified for obese women, and there is evidence that they are even more likely to feel dissatisfied with their bodies than their normal-weight peers. The association between obesity and body image for males has received less empirical attention, but there is evidence that overweight men may not necessarily experience body image distress in the same way as overweight women. Cash and Hicks found that overweight men who labeled themselves as overweight were less dissatisfied with their bodies than normal-weight men who labeled themselves as overweight. The authors hypothesized that heavier males may see themselves as "big and strong" rather than "fat." In contrast, truly overweight women who labeled themselves as overweight were less happy with their bodies than normal-weight women who also labeled themselves as overweight.

BODY IMAGE DISTORTION

There are mixed findings on the perceptual dimension of body image in obese individuals. One problem is that the method of recruiting subjects may have a dramatic impact on the results. For example, Brodie and Slade assessed body fat, body size estimation, and body dissatisfaction in female volunteers. There was no relationship between body fat and accuracy of body size estimation, despite a significant relationship between increasing body fat and body dissatisfaction. Gardner and colleagues examined mirror feedback and judgments of body size using obese and normal-weight community volunteers. Again, there was no difference between the groups in their body size estimates. A study of overweight female dieters by Collins and colleagues found that all participants overestimated their body size; however, the errors were greatest among the most obese individuals.

Kreitler and Chemerinski recruited obese and normal-weight females from weight control clinics and universities and measured the degree to which obese individuals misjudged their body size. Absolute difference scores were used to account for both over- and underestimation. The absolute difference scores were significantly correlated with psychopathology on various measures of the obese individuals, but not for the normal-weight individuals; the authors concluded that the body image of obese individuals is on a developmentally lower level. However, the authors did not specify if the obese individuals were recruited solely from weight control sites, nor did they consider the fact that clinical samples differ from community controls in ways other than weight status. Therefore, these findings may reflect a difference between clinical and community populations rather than between obese and normal-weight individuals.

Valtolina assessed the accuracy of body size estimation by obese individuals with a mean body mass index of 36, who were currently hospitalized for a weight reduction program. The subjects significantly underestimated their actual body dimensions. The author did not say how long they had been in the hospital or how much weight they had lost, but it is likely that one's body experience while rapidly losing weight is not representative of the experiences of average obese individuals in the community.

In sum, studies of perceptual body image in the obese variously report that they overestimate, underestimate, and are accurate regarding body size estimation, relative to normal-weight individuals. The conflicting conclusions may be due to different methods of subject recruitment and varying weight status (whether individuals were currently gaining, losing, or maintaining weight).

LIMITATIONS OF CURRENT RESEARCH

Need for Population Studies

One limitation of existing research is that most studies used women recruited from treatment programs. Only a small subgroup of the obese population seeks treatment, and the psychological characteristics of the subgroup may not represent those who do not seek treatment. Treatment seekers may experience more psychological distress than similarly overweight people who do not seek treatment. Therefore, research with obese people from the general population would provide a clearer picture of the nature and degree of body image disturbance that occurs.

Causality Still Unknown

Most studies used correlation analyses and retrospective self-report; hence, we cannot infer causal relationships between body image and the other variables under study (i.e., teasing, stigmatization, weight cycling). Although childhood teasing precedes adult body dissatisfaction, an alternate explanation is that people with poor body image are more likely to remember and report experiences of being teased. Longitudinal studies are needed to ascertain causality among these variables.

IMPLICATIONS FOR INTERVENTION RESEARCH

Two significant risk factors worthy of intervention are binge eating and coping with discrimination and stigma. Due to the apparent co-occurrence of binge eating and body dissatisfaction, it would be useful to understand how these two variables interact. A study comparing cognitive-behavioral treatment for BED with Cash's body image treatment would help identify how body image and binge eating are related, and how treating one might affect the other. Other research strategies include examining how pretreatment body image and its changes over the course of treatment predict response to treatment for BED. Another question is whether adding a body image component to cognitive-behavioral treatment for BED would improve outcome; our prediction is that it would. Body image treatment may become a standard component of therapy for BED.

The impact of discrimination and stigma on obese individuals is also an important area for further study. The finding that certain types of coping with stigmatization are linked to poorer psychological outcomes suggests the importance of developing interventions to teach overweight children and adults positive coping strategies to replace maladaptive ones. Positive coping strategies do not necessarily protect against poor body image; however, future research should seek to identify resiliency factors that protect some individuals from clinical levels of body image distress.

Finally, research on obesity and body image must move beyond individual experience and treatment to focus on how society stigmatizes obese people and permits discrimination. Changes made at the societal level (as have occurred, to some extent, with some minority groups) may help obese individuals find it easier to accept their bodies.

INFORMATIVE READINGS

Adami, G. F., Gandolfo, P., Campostano, A., Meneghelli, A., Ravera, G., & Scopinaro, N. (1998). Body image and body weight in obese patients. *International Journal of Eating Disorders, 24*, 299–306.—Compared severely obese patients to formerly obese patients (who had obesity surgery) and found that childhood onset of obesity predicted poorer body image among the formerly obese patients.

Brodie, D. A., & Slade, P. D. (1988). The relationship between body-image and body-fat in adult women. *Psychological Medicine, 18*, 623–631.—A study of a community sample using multiple assessment methods of body fat and body size estimation.

Cash, T. F. (1993). Body-image attitudes among obese enrollees in a commercial weight-loss program. *Perceptual and Motor Skills, 77*, 1099–1103.—Provides evidence the obese individuals who seek weight loss treatment through very low-calorie diets have different body image concerns than obese people who are not seeking treatment.

Cash, T. F. (2002). The management of body image problems. In K. D. Brownell & C. G. Fairburn (Eds.), *Eating disorders and obesity: A comprehensive handbook* (2nd ed., pp. 599–603). New York: Guilford Press.—A review of body image treatment issues and an outline of an empirically validated treatment approach.

Cash, T. F., & Hicks, K. F. (1990). Being fat versus thinking fat: Relationships with body image, eating behaviors, and well-being. *Cognitive Therapy and Research, 14*, 327–341.—Provides evidence of the importance of self-classification as normal weight or overweight as a variable that predicts level of body image in a sample of men and women.

Cash, T. F., & Roy R. E. (1999). Pounds of flesh: Weight, gender, and body images. In J. Sobal & D. Maurer (Eds.), *Interpreting weight: The social management of fatness and thinness* (pp. 209–228). Hawthorne, NY: Aldine de Gruyter.—A review of the literature on culture and body image in normal weight and overweight men and women.

Collins, J. K., McCabe, M. P., Jupp, J. J., & Sutton, J. E. (1983). Body percept change in obese females after weight reduction therapy. *Journal of Clinical Psychology, 39*, 507–511.—Used a video-image method of body size estimation with a sample of female dieters and found that all subjects overestimated their size, and the greatest errors were by the most obese subjects.

Eldredge, K. L., & Agras, W. S. (1996). Weight and shape overconcern and emotional eating in binge eating disorder. *International Journal of Eating Disorders, 19*, 73–82.—

Presents evidence that overconcern for weight and shape should be considered a diagnostic feature of BED, and that the degree of weight and shape concern is not correlated with level of overweight in people with BED.

Fairburn, C. G., Doll, H. A., Welch, S. L., Hay, P. J., Davies, B. A., & O'Connor, M. E. (1998). Risk factors for binge eating disorder: A community-based, case-control study. *Archives of General Psychiatry, 55*, 425–432.—This study compares a sample of patients with BED to patients with bulimia nervosa, general psychiatric patients, and a control group. The primary risk factors that emerge for BED are childhood obesity and exposure to negative comments about shape, weight, and eating.

Friedman, M. A., & Brownell, K. D. (1995). Psychological correlates of obesity: Moving to the next research generation. *Psychological Bulletin, 117*, 3–20.—This meta-analysis of the obesity field suggests a generational approach that moves from comparing obese to normal-weight individuals to identifying risk factors for psychological distress and to understanding causal relationships between risk and pathology.

Friedman, M. A., Schwartz, M. B., & Brownell, K. D. (1998). Differential relation of psychological functioning with the history and experience of weight cycling: Psychological correlates of weight cycling. *Journal of Consulting and Clinical Psychology, 66*, 646–650.—A study of a large sample of community dieters that examines the psychological correlates of viewing oneself as a weight cycler.

Gardner, R. M., Gallegos, V., Martinez, R., & Espinoza, T. (1989). Mirror feedback and judgments of body size. *Journal of Psychosomatic Research, 33*, 603–607.—Assessed the accuracy of body size perception using a video TV method with obese and normal-weight subjects and found that both groups similarly overestimated their body size.

Grilo, C. M., Wilfley, D. E., Brownell, K. D., & Rodin, J. (1994). Teasing, body image, and self-esteem in a clinical sample of obese women. *Addictive Behaviors, 19*, 443–450.—Examines a sample of 40 obese women seeking treatment (15 adult-onset and 25 early-onset) and finds that being teased as a child may be a risk factor for body dissatisfaction.

Jackson, T. D., Grilo, C. M., & Masheb, R. M. (2000). Teasing history, onset of obesity, current eating disorder psychopathology, body dissatisfaction, and psychological functioning in binge eating disorder. *Obesity Research, 8*, 451–458.—Examines a sample of 115 women with BED and assesses the influence of general appearance teasing, weight and shape teasing, and age of obesity onset on several measures of psychopathology and body image.

Kreitler, S., & Chemerinski, A. (1990). Body-image disturbance in obesity. *International Journal of Eating Disorders, 9*, 409–418.—Examined a sample of obese and normal-weight women on a battery of projective tests, and arrived at questionable conclusions due to their use of an inappropriate control group.

Milkewicz, N., & Cash T. F. (2000, November). *Dismantling the heterogeneity of obesity: Determinants of body images and psychosocial functioning.* Poster presented at the convention of the Association for Advancement of Behavior Therapy, New Orleans.—Compares three groups of women—never overweight, formerly overweight, and currently overweight—on multiple facets of body image and psychosocial adjustment.

Myers, A., & Rosen, J. C. (1999). Obesity stigmatization and coping: Relation to mental health symptoms, body image, and self-esteem. *International Journal of Obesity, 23*, 221–230.—A two-part study that created a comprehensive inventory of stigmatizing experiences and coping strategies.

Puhl, R., & Brownell, K. D. (2001). Bias, discrimination, and obesity. *Obesity Research, 9*, 788–805.—A comprehensive review of the literature documenting substantial stigma experienced by obese individuals.

Rosen, J. C. (2002). Obesity and body image. In K. D. Brownell & C. G. Fairburn (Eds.), *Eating disorders and obesity: A comprehensive handbook* (2nd ed., pp. 399–402). New York: Guilford Press.—A literature review that points out the importance of establishing a standard definition of body image disorder for obese individuals.

Sarwer, D. B., Wadden, T. A., & Foster, G. D. (1998). Assessment of body image dissatisfaction in obese women: Specificity, severity, and clinical significance. *Journal of Consulting and Clinical Psychology, 66*, 651–654.—Assessed a sample of obese women seeking treatment and found that greater body image dissatisfaction was associated with higher levels of depression and lower self-esteem, but not body mass index.

Valtolina, G. (1998). Body-size estimation by obese subjects. *Perceptual and Motor Skills, 86*, 1363–1374.—Examined the accuracy of body size estimation in a sample of obese patients who were voluntarily hospitalized for weight reduction and found that they underestimated the size of their bodies significantly more than the normal-weight control subjects.

Wilfley, D. E., Schwartz, M. B., Spurrell, E. B., & Fairburn, C. G. (2000). Using the Eating Disorder Examination to identify the specific psychopathology of binge eating disorder. *International Journal of Eating Disorders, 27*, 259–269.— Presents findings on the severity of eating disorder psychopathology in a sample of patients with BED and presents evidence that level of distress is independent of degree of obesity.

Body Image and Muscularity

ROBERTO OLIVARDIA

MUSCULARITY AND MASCULINITY

Many men today suffer from an "Adonis complex." Adonis was the Greek half-man, half-god who represented the ideal masculine body image—the V-shaped, muscular body. Unlike many women who strive to lose weight and achieve thinness, many men are in a pursuit of losing body fat while maintaining lean muscle mass. Dutton maintains that muscles symbolize health, dominance, power, strength, sexual virility, and threat. Because muscular men are perceived to embody these traditionally masculine traits, they may feel or aspire to feel more respected, admired, attractive, and confident.

"Threatened masculinity" theory, first discussed by Mishkind and colleagues, posits that the growing parity of women in Western culture has placed men in a crisis, leaving them to define their masculinity through the one thing that will forever distinguish them from the opposite sex—their bodies. As feminism has changed females' perceptions of themselves and their gender roles, the definition of masculinity and the way men view their maleness has also changed in the process. According to Gillet and White, men's quest for a muscular body is an attempt to establish dominance and reassert a social patriarchy among men and women. Because women are achieving more power and financial independence, they can be more selective in the mates they choose. Thus men are in a position of having lost many of their traditional bases for feeling masculine. As Klein argues in his book *Little Big Men*, the desire for a hypermasculine body may arise from men's growing insecurity about their gender role. Muscularity may be an attempt to preserve the traditional notion of the male role. In short, the relative importance of men's bodies in Western cultures seems to be changing.

CHANGING IMAGES OF MUSCULARITY

Although the "threatened masculinity" theory has yet to be proven scientifically, substantial evidence attests that societal standards and ideals for muscularity have changed dramatically. In our book, *The Adonis Complex*, Pope, Phillips, and I observe that contemporary actors, such as Arnold Schwarzenegger and Sylvester Stallone, dwarf Hollywood actors of yesteryear, such as James Cagney and Jimmy Stewart. Advertisers such as Calvin Klein use male models with perfect physiques to model clothes and underwear. Men's bodies are increasingly used in advertisements for products unrelated to the body. The proportion of undressed women in popular women's magazines (such as *Cosmopolitan*) has remained fairly steady over the last 30 to 40 years, while the proportion of undressed men has skyrocketed—from as little as 3% of ads in the 1950s to as high as 35% in the 1990s. Even male mannequins now possess larger genital bulges and more defined muscular builds. In 2000, in the *International Journal of Eating Disorders*, Leit and colleagues calculated that the average *Playgirl* centerfold man had lost 12 pounds of fat while gaining approximately 27 pounds of muscle over the last 25 years.

The socialization of these new muscular standards is evident in images aimed at children and adolescents. In 1999 Pope and colleagues documented trends over time in the muscularity of male action figures such as G.I. Joe. Like the Barbie doll, which is an unrealistic and unattainable female body image, today's G.I. Joe figure is just as unattainable by boys. A G.I. Joe figure in 1964 would have a 32-inch waist, 44-inch chest, and a 12-inch bicep if he were a man 5 feet 10 inches tall. This is a reasonable, attainable physique, similar to that of an ordinary man in reasonably good physical shape. G.I. Joe's 1998 counterpart, however, would have a 55-inch chest, a 27-inch bicep, and a 36-inch waist. Note that the bicep is almost as big as the waist—and bigger than that of the greatest body-builders of all time.

Researchers caution that media messages should not be underestimated in the impact they can have on how men feel about their bodies and general appearance. Men who fall short of these ideals often feel more dissatisfied with their appearance.

PERCEPTION, PREFERENCE, AND PERSONAL CONSEQUENCES

Silhouette figures, developed in 1983 by Stunkard and his colleagues, have often been used in assessing body image perception and ideals. (See Thompson and Gardner's chapter in this volume.) This measure appears reasonable for most women, but it is not effective with men: Figures reflect a thin-to-fat scale without any account for muscularity. Investigators and their participants must discern what is meant when a larger male figure is chosen: Is the figure chosen because it is perceived as fatter, more muscular, or both?

To remedy this problem, Gruber and colleagues recently developed the somatomorphic matrix (SMM), a computer instrument that measures male body image perceptions using separate axes for fat and muscularity. Men are first presented with a "median" body image and may then click on one of four "buttons" on the screen to make the image more or less fat and more or less muscular. Men are asked to create the image that best represents their own body, their ideal body, the body of an average person their age and sex, and their perception of that most desired by the opposite sex.

My study of 154 heterosexual college men using the SMM found that satisfaction with appearance depends on satisfaction with muscle mass. Men perceived themselves to be fatter than they actually were and chose an ideal body with 25 pounds more muscle and 8 pounds less body fat. Muscle belittlement (believing that one is less muscular than is actually true) was significantly positively correlated with scores on depression and eating disorder scales. Self-esteem was significantly negatively correlated with muscle belittlement, muscle displeasure, dissatisfaction with bodily proportions, feeling out of shape, and not liking one's body.

In a 1985 study in the *Journal of Obesity and Weight Regulation*, Harmatz and colleagues reported that underweight men were comparable to, or even worse off than, overweight women in terms of negative self-view and low self-esteem. Underweight men were more dissatisfied with their build, felt less handsome, felt that they had less sex appeal, and felt lonelier. This body dissatisfaction was attributed to a lack of musculature.

In his chapter on the epidemiology of body dissatisfaction in this volume, Cash summarizes the results of *Psychology Today* surveys from 1972, 1985, and 1996. Over time, men's discontent with their chest and muscle tone seems to have increased substantially. Muscle dissatisfaction or muscle belittlement can lead to serious body image disorders, such as muscle dysmorphia, and to anabolic steroid use.

MUSCLE DYSMORPHIA

In her chapter in this volume, Phillips discusses the severe body image disturbance called "body dysmorphic disorder" (BDD). In 1993 Pope and colleagues described a specific type of BDD characterized by a preoccupation with body build or musculature, which initially labelled "reverse anorexia nervosa." They described nine men who suffered from this condition, out of a sample of 108 body-builders. These men became obsessed with weight-lifting; all nine used anabolic steroids to achieve the opposite effect of anorexia nervosa—to be extremely muscular. In 1997 my colleagues and I described this condition in more detail and proposed formal diagnostic criteria. Noting that it was not truly an eating disorder, we renamed it "muscle dysmorphia."

The first criterion of muscle dysmorphia is a preoccupation that one is too small and not sufficiently lean or muscular, even though one may be extremely muscular. Associated behaviors include long hours of lifting weights, excessive mirror checking, and excessive attention to diet. My colleagues and I studied men with muscle dysmorphia who reported spending an average of 5½ hours per day thinking about their perceived lack of size. By comparison, ordinary weightlifters spent about 40 minutes daily thinking about such things.

Secondly, this preoccupation causes clinically significant distress or impairment in social, occupational, and other important areas of daily functioning. Men with muscle dysmorphia sacrifice activities because of a compulsive need to maintain their workout and diet schedules. Indeed, they are so consumed by working out that they may miss an important event, such as a final exam or job interview. They may try to adhere to a strict diet—for example, never eating in restaurants because the caloric content of the food is unknown. Some men have reported giving up promising careers because their jobs did not accommodate their obsessive need to work out.

These intrusive preoccupations also interfere with relationships. One man avoided sex with his wife, for fear that he would waste energy better used in workouts. Another man abstained from kissing his girlfriend, concerned that she might transmit calories through her saliva. Many men with muscle dysmorphia report sexual and intimacy problems due to their negative body image—feeling they are too ugly and weak looking.

Avoiding situations where the body is exposed to others or enduring such situations with marked anxiety is another symptom of muscle dysmorphia. Some men may not take their shirts off when at the beach, feeling that they look too small. Others wear layers of clothing to appear more muscular. Some men may become housebound for days because they feel so out of shape.

Men with muscle dysmorphia may continue to work out, diet, or use performance-enhancing substances despite knowledge of adverse consequences. For example, they exercise compulsively despite pain and injuries, or they continue to abide by their ultra-low-fat, high-protein diets even when hungry. Many take potentially dangerous anabolic steroids and other drugs to bulk up, because they think they do not look big enough.

Causes of muscle dysmorphia likely include a combination of genetic, psychological, and sociocultural contributions. Viewed as part of the spectrum of obsessive–compulsive disorders (OCD), muscle dysmorphia is hypothesized to share an underlying biological or genetic predisposition. BDD and OCD share common phenomenological features and may run in families. Psychologically, men with muscle dysmorphia typically have low self-esteem and may have issues with gender identity. Psychosocial experiences such as having been teased may have some impact. Society likely plays a powerful role by increasingly broadcasting messages that "real men" have big muscles and that a lack of muscles reflects a lack of masculinity, of virility.

The sport of body-building or weightlifting should not be pathologized. In a paper in the *Harvard Review of Psychiatry*, I differentiate the many factors that distinguish muscle dysmorphia from ordinary weightlifting. Such factors include the value an individual assigns to his appearance, the presence of body image distortions, and engaging in any unhealthy behaviors associated with the exercise routine, such as bulimic behavior or anabolic steroid use.

ANABOLIC STEROIDS

Pope and Brower describe androgenic–anabolic steroids (hereafter referred to simply as *steroids*) as including testosterone and a series of synthetic analogs of testosterone. These hormones promote lean muscle growth and strength. First used only by elite, competitive body-builders, steroids have now spread to other groups of men and boys. Pope, Phillips, and I estimate that 2–3 million men have used steroids. In a 1988 study in the *Journal of the American Medical Association*, Buckley and colleagues found that more than 6% of high school boys admitted having used steroids before turning 18. Other studies have produced similar statistics. Many males in these studies disclosed that they used steroids purely for body appearance ideals rather than for athletic ideals or goals.

Physical side effects of steroids can include acne, breast enlargement, and liver cancer. A significant side effect is arteriosclerosis, a chronic disease in which thickening and hardening of arterial walls interfere with blood circulation and may lead to heart attacks and strokes. Psychological side effects include mood disturbances, psychotic symptoms, and severe aggressiveness, also known as "roid rage." Research on muscle dysmorphia and steroid use is in its infancy; however, preliminary studies suggest that men with body dissatisfaction (particularly muscle belittlement), low self-esteem, perfectionistic personality traits, and a traditional masculine gender ideology may be more at risk for developing these problems.

GAY MEN AND MUSCULARITY

Previous studies have reported that gay men are overrepresented in samples of men with body image disorders. This may lead to the inaccurate conclusion that body image disorders hardly affect heterosexual men. Most of these studies have utilized clinical versus community samples. Pope and colleagues have noted that although most of the patients and research participants they have encountered were heterosexual, the majority of them had never sought treatment. The percentage of men who seek treatment for these problems is thought to be considerably lower than what is seen in women who suffer from similar issues. Gay men may be more willing to discuss such body image concerns and seek treatment. One study by Pope and colleagues, using the SMM, found a larger discrepancy between actual body and ideal body in heterosexual men than homosexual men.

As Rothblum documents in her chapter in the present volume, gay men do have body image concerns, specifically concerns about muscularity. In his book *Life Outside*, Signorile discusses how the pursuit of muscle has become common in gay communities. He notes that many gay men who experience internalized homophobia may seek a large, muscular build in an effort to appear masculine—and, more importantly, heterosexual. Although this motivation for muscularity is also held by heterosexual men, the gender identity of gay men is almost always called into question. Developing a large, tough exterior may be an effort to lay to rest all questions regarding one's sense of masculinity. Signorile also points out that gay men become invested in building a more muscular body to distance themselves from the image of the wasting syndrome associated with AIDS. As previously mentioned, muscularity symbolizes health and sexual virility. Thus, in the gay community, a fit and muscular body may convey HIV-negative status. Signorile observes that the use of steroids has become a problem among gay men who, like many heterosexual men, try to prove their masculinity through their muscularity.

RESEARCH AND CLINICAL IMPLICATIONS

Since the issue of body image and muscularity in men has emerged in the last two decades, a multitude of questions remain unexplored. Etiological factors for muscle dysmorphia must be analyzed more carefully, paying attention to family histories of psychiatric illness, peer experiences, and cultural exposure. Further research should examine the association between muscle dysmorphia and personality disorders as well as gender ideology and behaviors. The degree to which muscularity concerns transcend, or do not transcend, cultural, ethnic, sexual orientation, and socioeconomic groups remains unclear. Most current studies have been comprised of Caucasian heterosexual males from 15 to 30 years old.

Although this chapter has discussed body image and muscularity in relation to men, new research indicates that women are not immune to muscularity concerns. This finding should come as no surprise; more women are entering the athletic arena, and the pressure to be fit and toned is gaining as much popularity as the pressure to be thin. In 1999 Gruber and Pope reported in *Comprehensive Psychiatry* that a history of rape was common in a sample of women who were compulsive weightlifters and steroid users. Research with female athletes, body-builders, and nonathletes will be helpful in understanding the impact these concerns may have on women.

In clinical settings, we must recognize the association between muscle belittlement, depression, and eating disorders. Indeed, muscle belittlement may serve as a diagnostic signal to assess for depression or eating pathology in men, much as fat exaggeration may alert the clinician to eating disorders in women.

Treatment studies on muscle dysmorphia, per se, are lacking. The vast majority of men with these symptoms never presents for treatment. Consumed by their obsessions, they spend much of their time at the gym or worrying about their appearance. They also experience an enormous sense of shame and embarrassment about having this disorder. Therefore, it is important for clinicians to emphasize the patient's courage in seeking help and reassure him that he is not "vain," "narcissistic," or a "sissy" for having these feelings.

Pope, Phillips, and I hypothesized that since muscle dysmorphia is a form of BDD, it would be likely to respond to treatments previously found to be effective for other forms of BDD, such as cognitive-behavioral therapy and use of certain antidepressants. Psychotherapy should consider other contributing issues, such as gender identity, low self-esteem, and peer experiences. Psychoeducation is a necessary part of treatment and prevention, including information on proper nutrition, healthy exercise, the dangers of steroids, and the distortion in media images that espouse an inaccurate representation of what people look like or should aspire to attain, appearance-wise.

Concerns over muscularity are expected to continue to increase. Research on the prevention and treatment of muscle dysmorphia is essential to enhance our scientific and clinical understanding of this phenomenon.

INFORMATIVE READINGS

Buckley, W. A., Yesalis, C. E., Friedl, K. E., Anderson, W., Streit, A., & Wright, J. (1988). Estimated prevalence of anabolic steroid use among male high school seniors. *Journal of the American Medical Association, 260*, 3441–3445.—A study estimating the percentage of boys using steroids before turning eighteen.

Dutton, K. R. (1995). *The perfectible body: The Western ideal of male physical development.* New York: Continuum.—A historical and sociopolitical look at the evolution of the male body.

Gillet, J., & White, P. G. (1992). Male bodybuilding and the reassertion of hegemonic masculinity: A critical feminist perspective. *Play and Culture, 5*, 358–369.—A theoretical paper discussing body-building as a means of reestablishing gender order.

Gruber, A. J., & Pope, Jr., H. G., (1999). Compulsive weightlifting and anabolic drug abuse among women rape victims. *Comprehensive Psychiatry, 40*, 23–27.—A study assessing the relationship between steroid use and history of rape in women.

Gruber, A. J., Pope, Jr., H. G., Borowiecki, J. J., & Cohane, G. (1999). The development of the somatomorphic matrix: A bi-axial instrument for measuring body image in men and women. In T. S. Olds, J. Dollman, & K. I. Norton (Eds.), *Kinanthropometry VI.* Sydney, Australia: International Society for the Advancement of Kinanthropometry.—Describes the need for, and creation of, a more valid tool for assessing male body image.

Harmatz, M. G., Gronendyke, J., & Thomas, T. (1985). The underweight male: The unrecognized problem group of body image research. *Journal of Obesity and Weight Regulation, 4*(4), 258–267.—Discusses the body dissatisfaction among men who perceive themselves to be underweight.

Klein, A. M. (1993). *Little big men.* Albany: State University of New York.—An ethnographic look at the bodybuilding subculture, with an emphasis on gender and masculinity.

Leit, A., Pope, Jr., H. G., & Gray, J. J. (2001). Cultural expectations of muscularity in men: The evolution of *Playgirl* centerfolds. *International Journal of Eating Disorders, 29*(1), 90–93.—A study chronicling the increasing muscularity of Playgirl centerfolds over the decades.

Mishkind, M. E., Rodin, J., Silberstein, L. R., & Striegel-Moore, R. H. (1986). The embodiment of masculinity: Cultural, psychological and behavioral dimensions. *American Behavioral Scientist, 29*(5), 545–562.—A literature review of male body image studies discussing the association between appearance concerns in men and the growing parity of women.

Olivardia, R. (2001). Mirror, mirror on the wall, who's the largest of them all? *Harvard Review of Psychiatry, 9*, 254–259.—A paper detailing the phenomenology of muscle dysmorphia.

Olivardia, R., Pope, Jr., H. G., Borowiecki, III, J. J., & Cohane, G. H. (2002). *Male body image assessment and the somatomorphic matrix: The clinical importance of muscle belittlement.* Manuscript submitted for publication.—A large study assessing body image in 154 college students, using a newly developed instrument.

Olivardia, R., Pope, Jr., H. G., & Hudson J. I. (2000). Muscle dysmorphia in male weightlifters: A case-control study. *American Journal of Psychiatry, 157*(8), 1291–1296.—The first empirical study of muscle dysmorphia, comparing weightlifters with and without muscle dysmorphia on a variety of measures.

Pope, Jr., H. G., & Brower, K. J. (1999). Anabolic–androgenic steroid abuse. In B. J. Sadock & V. A. Sadock (Eds.), *Comprehensive textbook of psychiatry* (7th ed., pp. 1085–1096). Baltimore, MD: Williams & Wilkins.—Reviews various facets of anabolic steroid use.

Pope, Jr., H. G., Gruber, A. J., Choi, P., Olivardia, R., & Phillips, K. A. (1997). Muscle dysmorphia: An underrecognized form of body dysmorphic disorder. *Psychosomatics, 38*, 548–557.—The first paper describing the phenomenology of this new body image disorder.

Pope, Jr., H. G., Katz, D. L., & Hudson, J. I. (1993). Anorexia nervosa and "reverse anorexia" among 108 male bodybuilders. *Comprehensive Psychiatry, 34*(6), 406–409.—Describes nine cases of men who were extremely preoccupied with feeling too small, although they were very muscular.

Pope, Jr., H. G., Olivardia, R., Gruber, A. J., & Borowiecki, J. (1999). Evolving ideals of male body image as seen through action toys. *International Journal of Eating Disorders,* *26,* 65–72.—Study documenting the trend of increasing muscularity in action figures over the decades.

Pope, Jr., H. G., Phillips, K. A., & Olivardia, R. (2000). *The Adonis complex: The secret crisis of male body obsession.* New York: Free Press.—Reviews male body image and the manifestations of body image disorders (including eating disorders, body dysmorphic disorder, muscle dysmorphia, and anabolic steroid use) in various groups of men.

Signorile, M. (1997). *Life outside: The Signorile report on gay men: Sex, drugs, muscles and the passages of life.* New York: HarperCollins.—A book commenting on various aspects of contemporary gay male culture, including anabolic steroid use and the pursuit of muscularity.

25

Body Image and Athleticism

CAROLINE DAVIS

Because we marvel at the physical accomplishments of high-performance sport, and regard the elegance and finesse of a classical ballet with admiration, we also assume that the men and women who execute these skills are highly satisfied with their bodies. However, the research linking subjective body image perceptions and athleticism suggests that the relationship between the two is far from simple, nor is it always positive. Instead it is influenced and moderated by a number of factors, such as the *type* of activity, the *gender* of the participants, their degree of *commitment*, and a host of *psychological* characteristics. Another consideration—and one that provides the framework for this chapter—is the distinction between body image in the context of competitive athletics and (semi)professional dance, and that relating to recreational sport and exercise activities.

The impression we hold of our body is usually the complex outcome of factors that foster satisfaction, offset by those that create dissatisfaction. Whether we examine the sporting arena, the dance studio, or the health club, it is clear that each environment can exert both positive and negative influences, albeit they may affect different individuals in different ways. This chapter describes the most consistent findings in the area of body image and athleticism and considers how body image can impact a variety of health-related behaviors such as dieting and other weight loss methods.

COMPETITIVE SPORT AND PROFESSIONAL DANCE

Most competitive athletes recognize the important relationship between optimal performance and low body weight, since weight greater than a healthy minimum tends to limit agility and speed and contributes to increased fatigue. A high power-to-weight ratio also confers a performance advantage in activities that require jumps, tumbles, and lifts. In sports where performance is not determined by objective criteria but rather by judges' subjective ratings—for example, in gymnastics and figure skating—there is an added advantage to achieving an ultraslender body shape, given the aesthetic standard of a thin and petite figure for women in these sports. Furthermore, in these "lean body" sports, female athletes are required to perform in scant and revealing clothing, intensifying the focus on their body shape. In addition to our cultural preference for a thin female body shape, these sport-specific factors create a particularly strong aversion to fatness and strong incentives to reduce body fat to very low levels. Adding to the problem, training regimes and performance expectations have become progressively more stringent over recent decades, increasing the potency of weight and shape concerns for many female athletes.

While the motivation for female athletes to engage in assiduous—even extreme—weight loss methods is clear, it has been suggested that such behaviors are even *encouraged* among high-performance athletes because an imperative of the competitive sport ethic is to overcome any impediments to success even if this requires training through illness, pain, and injury. It is not surprising, therefore, that two large-scale studies—one in the United States and the other in Norway—found that as many as 15% to 20% of high-level competitive female athletes regularly engage in clinically significant weight loss methods such as severe food restriction, self-induced vomiting, and laxative use in order to conform to the body-shape standards of their sport. Moreover, these percentages may be conservative estimates since a number of researchers have described the tendency of competitive athletes to underreport their psychological difficulties, lest they be deemed unfit for competition and lose their place on the team. Indeed, in our own research, we recently found that the average Drive-for-Thinness and Body Dissatisfaction scores (on the Eating Disorders Inventory) were close to zero for a group of elite female artistic gymnasts—a finding that is highly unlikely, both statistically and intuitively!

In the general population, weight and diet concerns are strongly correlated with poor body esteem, leading to the conclusion that body dissatisfaction is the primary motive for dietary restriction. It appears, however, that the correlation between these two factors is not found in all female athletes. In a recent meta-analysis of 34 studies that sampled a variety of sports, Smolak and her colleagues concluded that although athletes tended to report a high drive for thinness, they fared substantially better than age-matched women in the general population in terms of body dissatisfaction. Very similar results were found in two studies not included in the meta-analysis. One was a study of elite figure skaters, and the other pertained to female members of varsity long-distance and cross-country running teams. Although a large proportion of these athletes were very satisfied with their body and general physical appearance, a relatively high prevalence of dieting and other pathogenic weight loss methods was reported by both groups, despite the fact that 85% of the skaters were below the 50th percentile in body mass index for weight by age. Because their dieting behavior was not linked to self-perceptions of being overweight, it was concluded that the unique and demanding pressures of these sports motivated the athletes' attempts at weight loss.

However, such findings are not consistent across all sports. For example, among elite female field hockey players, the pattern described above was actually reversed. Dissatisfaction with body shape tended to be a greater issue for these women than was a preoccupation with thinness. In another study, a strong positive relationship, similar to that found in the general population, was observed between body dissatisfaction and concerns about weight in elite heavyweight female rowers. It seems, therefore, that the dissociation between body dissatisfaction and a drive for thinness occurs mainly in sports that emphasize a lean and slender body build. Perhaps this occurs because a prerequisite to achieving success in these sports is the body type that matches the thin ideal. Nevertheless, recognition that one possesses the ideal body shape does not eliminate a preoccupation with weight. Indeed it may foster and even exacerbate this concern if the athlete strongly overvalues the degree to which her success is dependent on her slenderness.

Many researchers have drawn parallels between the demands placed on competitive athletes and those experienced by dancers in full-time training or professional ballet troupes, because the extreme pressure to maintain a body weight well below average and the long hours of physical training are common to both. Some claim that female dancers, particularly ballet dancers, are a self-selected, genetically lean group; the inference is that they are less prone to exigent weight loss pressures, since their slender body shape has occurred "naturally." However, if the body of a dancer were a wholly natural and therefore easily maintained shape, we would not find, as we do, that a significant proportion reports symptoms of anorexia nervosa. In fact, in the meta-analytic study described earlier, dancers were found to be at *greatest* risk for eating disturbances. Additionally, in our own recently reported work with eating-disordered patients who were identified as "elite athletes" prior to diagnosis, we found that 28% had been professional dancers or in full-time ballet training—a representation greater than we found for any other sport.

Gender comparisons on measures of body satisfaction among athletes are generally consistent in reporting lower levels of dissatisfaction in male athletes. Such results are consistent with the gender differences repeatedly found in the general population. However, similar to the research carried out with female athletes, the degree of body satisfaction seems to be moderated by the type of sport in which the male athlete participates. For example, studies have found that body satisfaction is higher among football players and body-builders—sports characterized by a muscular body build—than in those participating in sports such as cross-country and distance running, where upper-body strength is a disadvantage. Because the current masculine body image ideal is a lean but very muscular form, it is not surprising that athletes who mirror this ideal would be more satisfied than those who do not.

There is also agreement that male athletes, in general, have greater body satisfaction than age-matched nonathletes. However, in most cases the athletes also have a more favorable body composition—in particular, a lower body fat content—so it is not possible to determine whether their enhanced body satisfaction derives from appearance-related factors or from greater feelings of physical competence and skill.

RECREATIONAL EXERCISE

Clearly, the exigencies of elite sports can exact a cost from their athletes. This is sometimes reflected in the athletes' neglect of healthful behaviors and sometimes in the compromise of their psychological well-being. In contrast, recreational sport and exercise are generally associated in people's minds with a myriad of positive outcomes—what one might describe as the "exercise halo." For example, it is commonly believed that the more we exercise, the better we feel about our bodies. However, the research suggests that the association between body esteem and physical activity is more complex than we might expect, and that several factors mitigate a generalizable dose–response relationship. (Elsewhere in this volume, Martin and Lichtenberger discuss the effects of fitness-enhancing exercise programs on body image change.)

Both the age and the gender of the exercise participant are important considerations, as illustrated by a recent study. In young women (16–21 years), level of exercising was *negatively* associated with body satisfaction, and the commonly expected positive association was found only in men and older women. We are also beginning to learn that people's motivation for exercising is connected to their attitudes about weight and diet and to their degree of body esteem. Some people feel driven to exercise by a desire to maintain a fit and healthy body; for others, exercising is a social activity; and for many others, exercise is motivated by the hope that it will enhance their appearance. In a study of regularly exercising young women, Hubbard and her colleagues found that those who exercised to work off the food they had eaten had scores on the Eating Disorders Inventory that were almost double those who did not exercise for this reason. The former also expressed a greater investment in their appearance and greater feelings of physical unattractiveness, even though there was no significant difference between the two groups in body size. Additionally, it is significant that in Hubbard's study, twice as many women were classified as "food-related" exercisers compared to the number of "non-food-related" exercisers.

Personality also plays a role in the relationship between physical activity and body image. In particular, women who are characterized by high levels of anxiety and perfectionism are more likely to exercise for appearance-related reasons than for reasons associated with health and fitness. These are interesting findings since anxiety and perfectionism are the most prominent premorbid personality characteristics of women who develop eating disorders. There is also considerable evidence that women who exercise extensively, based on assessments of frequency and commitment, have greater body image concerns and symptoms of disordered eating than those who exercise more moderately. Again, this is not a surprising finding, given that excessive exercising is one of the most common clinical features of patients with anorexia nervosa. Estimates indicate that at least 80% of these patients are hyperactive during periods of acute food restriction and weight loss.

In summary, there is a fairly clear pattern of findings indicating that emotionally vulnerable women with highly perfectionistic tendencies are more likely to exercise for appearance-related reasons, to be critical of their bodies even in the absence of objective reasons for dissatisfaction, and to exercise to the extreme. Elsewhere, I have argued that excessive exercising is the harbinger of an eating disorder and does not really exist as a discreet entity outside the spectrum of this condition—at least not in women. However, other professionals have taken a somewhat different approach and suggested that exercising, even at high levels, is a "healthy" strategy for women who are preoccupied with weight because it is associated with so many physiological benefits, and it may substitute for, or buffer against, more drastic methods of weight loss. I maintain, however, that when exercise is used obsessively and excessively for the primary purpose of expending calories and altering body shape, there is a strong likelihood that it is masking some serious psychological distress. Moreover, the highly positive way in which exercising is regarded in our culture also decreases the likelihood that an eating disorder will be identified in those who tend to overuse exercise.

The causal process is difficult to untangle when attempting to understand the relationship between physical activity and body image. On the one hand, it may be that anxiety-prone women tend to evaluate their bodies more negatively and therefore turn to exercise as a strategy for enhancing appearance. Given the media emphasis on fitness for good looks, this is a strong possibility. Conversely, the milieu of many fitness and exercise facilities, with their mirrored walls and scantily clothed participants, may foster, in some women, a sense of dissatisfaction and a hypercritical view of their body because of the implicit emphasis on exercise for the sake of enhancing appearance.

Future studies should move beyond the strictly cross-sectional, multivariate paradigms that have characterized the bulk of research in this area. Longitudinal designs, incorporating both quantitative and qualitative methods of analysis, as well as case study approaches, would afford a better way of examining the dynamic relationship between subjective body perceptions and the environmental contingencies that affect this image.

INFORMATIVE READINGS

Davis, C. (2000). Exercise abuse. *International Journal of Sports Psychology, 31*, 278–289.—A review that draws strong links between exercise abuse and body image concerns and argues that excessive exercising should be viewed as an "addiction" only when it satisfies the criteria for more conventional addictions.

Davis, C., & Scott-Robertson, L. (2000). A psychological comparison of females with anorexia nervosa and competitive male bodybuilders: Body shape ideals in the extreme. *Eating Behaviors, 1*, 33–46.—A study of competitive male bodybuilders who demonstrated many of the same psychopathological characteristics as women with anorexia nervosa with the exception of reporting very positive perceptions of self-worth and very high body esteem.

Davis, C., & Strachan, S. (2001). Elite female athletes with eating disorders: A study of psychopathological characteristics. *Journal of Sport and Exercise Psychology, 23*, 245–253.—A study comparing eating-disordered patients who had been involved in high-level competitive athletics with nonathlete eating-disordered patients and found no significant differences between the groups on any of the measures of psychopathology or eating-related symptoms. This finding suggests that athletes who develop eating disorders have similar psychological profiles to nonathletes with eating disorders.

Hubbard, S. T., Gray, J. J., & Parker, S. (1998). Differences among women who exercise for "food related" and "non-food related" reasons. *European Eating Disorders Review, 6*, 255–265.—A study demonstrating that women who exercised to work off calories consumed greater body dissatisfaction and elevated scores on measures of eating disturbance than women who exercised for other reasons.

Huddy, D. C., & Cash, T. F. (1997). Body-image attitudes among male marathon runners: A controlled comparative study. *International Journal of Sports Psychology, 28*, 227–236.—A study finding that male marathon runners had better body image and were less likely to be dieting than age-matched controls; however, not surprisingly, they had a lower mean body mass index, which contributed to their more positive self-evaluations.

Johnson, C., Powers, P. S., & Dick, R. (1999). Athletes and eating disorders: The National Collegiate Athletic Association Study. *International Journal of Eating Disorders, 26*, 179–188.—An NCAA study to establish prevalence rates of disordered eating among male and female student athletes.

Smolak, L., Murnen, S. K, & Ruble, A. E. (2000). Female athletes and eating disorders: A meta-analysis. *International Journal of Eating Disorders, 27*, 371–380.—A study of female athletes establishing that, under some circumstances, sport participation can increase risk for body dissatisfaction and eating disturbances, while other circumstances may buffer against these problems.

Terry, P. C., Lane, A. M., & Warren, L. (1999). Eating attitudes, body shape perceptions and mood of elite rowers. *Journal of Science and Medicine in Sport, 2,* 67–77.—A study that found body shape concerns were greater for heavyweight than lightweight rowers and for females compared to males.

Tiggemann, M., & Williamson, S. (2000). The effect of exercise on body satisfaction and self-esteem as a function of gender and age. *Sex Roles, 43,*119–127.—A study finding that the amount of exercise and body satisfaction were inversely related in young women but positively related in older women and young and older men.

Ziegler, P. J., Khoo, C. S., Sherr, B., Nelson, J. A., Larson, W. M., & Drewnowski, A. (1998) Body image and dieting behaviors among elite figure skaters. *International Journal of Eating Disorders, 24,* 421–427.—A study reporting that elite female figure skaters tended to have inadequate calorie intake and delayed menarche but were relatively satisfied with their body image.

Body Image and Congenital Conditions with Visible Differences

NICHOLA RUMSEY

This chapter describes congenital anomalies resulting in visible disfigurement and summarizes the effects on body image, self-concept, and social interaction. Macgregor described visible disfigurement as a social disability, implying that problems experienced by disfigured people set them apart from the general population. However, more recent research suggests that the continuum of emotions, thoughts, and behaviors characteristic of people with disfigurements is not pathological but instead is part of the same continuum experienced by those dissatisfied with aspects of their ostensibly "normal" looks. Factors exacerbating or ameliorating body image effects are also reviewed, as are methodological challenges faced by researchers in this field. Because little research exists that specifically explores body image and congenital conditions, personal accounts and the broader literature on body image in nondisfigured populations are also included.

TYPES OF CONGENITAL CONDITIONS

Some types of disfiguring congenital conditions are fully manifested at birth (e.g., cleft lip), whereas others worsen over time (e.g., neurofibromatosis). Head and neck malformations are the most common visible anomaly. A cleft lip and/or palate occurs approximately once in every 800 births, and can manifest on one (unilateral) or both (bilateral) sides of the face. Other less common abnormalities result from the failure of parts of the face to develop fully, as in the absence of an ear, the underdevelopment of cheek- and jaw-

226

bones (as in Treacher–Collins syndrome), or the early fusion of the cranial bones (as in Cruzon's and Apert's syndromes). Certain congenital conditions have a syndrome of physical features (e.g., Down's with its characteristic facial and oral appearance), as well as brain abnormalities associated with learning difficulties; however, most facial anomalies are not associated with deficits in brain function.

Additional malformations can result from the delayed maturation of blood vessels (as in cutaneous haemangiomata), vascular malformations (e.g., birthmarks), or from the failure of part of a limb to develop. Webbing (syndactyly) refers to the failure of fingers or toes to separate fully, whereas in polydactyly, an extra digit is present on the hand or foot.

Inclusive definitions of disfiguring congenital conditions also cite genetic predispositions to abnormalities that manifest later in life (e.g., vitiligo) or the absence of normal development (as in the absence or asymmetry of breasts). Harris proposes that congenital disfigurements are those that manifest "prememory"; that is, the person has no memory of life without the abnormality. He also notes that the individual's subjective perception of his or her appearance is a better predictor of psychological and body image disturbance than the view of a dispassionate observer.

BODY IMAGE CONCERNS AND DISFIGURING CONGENITAL CONDITIONS

The evaluation of body image concerns in people with disfiguring congenital conditions is complicated by the need to consider the many different types and body sites, the variability in severity and visibility, and the numerous personal, social, and situational characteristics affecting body image and adjustment. However, despite the complexity of the variables involved, there is a remarkable consensus in the problems and difficulties reported. The most common concerns relate to negative self-perceptions and difficulties with social interaction. These problems frequently manifest as combinations of negative emotional reactions (e.g., social anxiety, fear of negative social evaluation), behaviors (e.g., social avoidance), and/or thought patterns (e.g., selective interpretation of feedback from others).

Conceptions of the Self

Grogan, Harter, and others have documented the close relationship between appearance and self-concept. The searing personal accounts of self-doubt and low levels of self-esteem (see, e.g., Storry, Williams, Lacy, & Chapple in Lansdown et al.) leave no doubt that people with disfiguring congenital conditions face formidable hurdles to adjustment. There are few studies of adults with disfigurements caused by congenital conditions. However, Robinson (in Lansdown et al.) highlights common themes of lowered self-confidence and negative self-image. Disturbingly, in 1993 Herskind and colleagues reported a doubled suicide rate among Danish adults with clefts. Turner and colleagues found that 73% of their sample of 15- and 20-year-olds felt their self-confidence had been very much affected by their cleft. Millard and Richman reported in 2001 that cleft-affected children are more at risk than their noncleft peers for self-doubt in relation to interpersonal relationships, for elevated anxiety, and general unhappiness. However, the research findings are not entirely clear-cut. Walters reviewed several studies reporting levels of self-esteem equal to or, in some cases, higher for disfigured children compared with nondisfigured peers. Our work indicates that although 10-year-old children with clefts are less self-confident and socially active than their noncleft peers, 15-year-olds with clefts are more confident and have higher levels of social functioning than a noncleft peer comparison group.

In summary, people with disfigurements of congenital origin appear to be more at risk for body image concerns, low self-esteem, and social interaction problems. Yet whereas many experience difficulties, others find ways of coping effectively. Disfigurement dominates the lives of some, whereas others relegate their visible difference to a minor role in their body image and self-esteem—sometimes even using it to good advantage. In Crank's personal account of living with neurofibromatosis (in Lansdown et al., 1997), he concluded that his appearance had shaped him into someone with "a greater character, compassion, and the vital sense of humor that [he] may not have otherwise developed" (p. 29). However, Williams's description of living with a large facial port-wine stain (in Lansdown et al.) adds a sobering note by concluding that no matter how well a person copes, the feeling will always be there that he or she is "different."

Social Encounters

Visible differences commonly result in strains and distortions in social interaction that can affect, or be affected by, body image. Walters highlighted the frequency of social withdrawal in childhood and the increased likelihood of dependence on significant adults. Turner and her colleagues reported that 100% of their 15- and 20-year-old cleft-affected adolescents reported problems initiating conversations with strangers. Sixty percent reported being teased about their cleft condition, and 25% reporting that this teasing worried them "a lot." Reviewing the problems experienced by adults with congenital and other disfigurements, Robinson and colleagues document difficulties meeting new people, making new friends, and anxieties about developing relationships.

Disfiguring conditions can affect social interaction in many ways. A facial abnormality may lead to unconventional nonverbal and/or verbal communication, resulting from an inability to use particular facial expressions, or from the effects on speech quality (as in the case of a cleft). Anticipation of negative reactions from others can lead to social avoidance or an aggressive, defensive, or reticent interaction style.

Other difficulties can result from the behavior of others. In contrast to the anonymity enjoyed by people with an unremarkable appearance, a person who is visibly different becomes a focus of usually unwanted attention, including staring, comments, and questions. Macgregor describes these behaviors as visual and verbal assaults. Others demonstrate nonverbal and verbal behavior reflecting reactions of aversion, surprise, or discomfort. A key coping difficulty appears to be a disfigured person's lack of control over the amount and type of interactions that occur in the course of everyday life.

FACTORS EXACERBATING OR AMELIORATING BODY IMAGE CONCERNS

Despite these extensive concerns, large individual differences exist in the experiences of people with visible congenital abnormalities. Why do only some become distressed? What physical, social, and/or psychological factors mitigate or magnify distress?

Physical Characteristics of the Disfigurement

A congenital condition may be immediately obvious to others (e.g., extensive disfigurement of the face or hands), apparent only to a few, and/or easily camouflaged. Research and clinical experience clearly demonstrate that the severity and extent of the disfigurement consistently fail to predict distress levels. Lansdown et al. and others have noted that mild disfigurements can cause as much, if not more, anxiety than severe conditions. Less extreme differences may provoke greater variability in the reactions of others, and this unpredictability may raise anxiety levels. Macgregor notes that people with severe disfigurements anticipate negative responses in many situations and are therefore able to develop more consistent ways of coping.

There is a consensus that the location of an abnormality can be an important factor in determining the extent of body image concerns. Facial disfigurements are acknowledged to be particularly distressing, especially if the eyes and mouth are affected. Some conditions are amenable to camouflage; however, a heavy reliance on makeup to conceal a disfigurement may bring its own set of problems. Williams, who uses makeup to conceal her facial port-wine stain, describes how she feels like two different people—her "made-up self" and her "natural self"—and the fear she feels of eventually revealing her disfigurement to others.

Some argue that a congenital disfigurement results in greater body image distress than a disfigurement acquired later in life, whereas others maintain that the ever-present congenital defect offers consistency that allows the affected person to adjust more successfully. Once again, there are no clear answers. The picture is further complicated by the fact that some congenital conditions are progressive (e.g., neurofibromatosis), while others, although very evident at birth (e.g., cleft lip) are amenable to early surgery and become less noticeable over time.

Gender Differences

Although females are thought to value physical appearance more than males, research by Turner and colleagues on the psychosocial needs of cleft-affected children and adolescents found that problems warranting psychological referral were more common in males (69% of their sample) than females (42%). Future research should consider possible gender differences in the coping strategies used to address body image concerns (e.g., males are less likely than females to use makeup to hide a disfigurement).

Coping Style

Adaptive and maladaptive coping styles have been investigated in relation to the body image concerns and adjustment of people with disfigurements, though, once again, the observations are largely anecdotal. A key theme of this research is developing and maintaining a favorable body image and self-esteem, despite stringent social standards of appearance. Until recently, it was assumed that denial or an avoidant coping style was inadvisable because it postponed the development of more effective strategies. More recently, research by Robinson and colleagues suggests that rather than change one or two supposedly maladaptive coping techniques, interventions should focus on broadening the number and variety of skills in the person's repertoire.

Behavioral Strategies

Research summarized in Lansdown and colleagues has demonstrated that people with visible differences who display good levels of social skill (for example, taking the initiative in social interaction) have more self-confidence and are more satisfied with the quality and quantity of their social interactions. Their behavior elicits favorable reactions from others, which further bolsters their positive view of themselves.

BODY IMAGE CONCERNS ACROSS THE LIFESPAN

The initial reaction of parents to the birth of a child with disfigurement includes shock, grief, confusion and guilt. Walters notes that the visibility of the abnormality may interfere with early mother–child bonding. When a facial abnormality affects the infant's expression, caregivers may find it hard to respond appropriately to the baby's needs. Some mothers may hold and stimulate their infant less than mothers of normal babies (see chapters by David Krueger in this volume); however, attachment is by no means always affected, and the longer-term effects on self-concept and body image are unclear.

Each developmental period has associated stressors that may have an impact on body image development. In the first few years of life, many families experience the profound stress associated with initial surgical reconstruction and the changed physical appearance of the child. The parents' attitudes and expectations may influence the child's perception of his or her impairment and the early development of feelings of self-worth.

In early to middle childhood, the child becomes aware that others make evaluative judgments based on appearance; internalization of these social standards also begins during this developmental stage. Many children with disfigurements and their parents report teasing to be a problem. For children affected by a cleft, 7 to 8 years of age is the peak for teasing; yet relevant cognitive and behavioral strategies are poorly developed at this stage.

The physical and psychological changes associated with adolescence are thought to increase the intensity of focus on appearance. Harter reports that teenagers who believed that their appearance determined their self-worth had lower self-esteem and greater depression than adolescents who believed that their self-worth determined their feelings about their appearance. Teenagers who feel uncomfortable about a visible disfigurement may be particularly vulnerable to body image concerns and low self-esteem. Interestingly, however, the 15-year-old cleft-affected patients participating in our research are more socially active and happier with their appearance than a comparative noncleft sample.

Despite the lack of research examining body image concerns in adults with congenital disfigurement, a few observations are noteworthy. Some people with disfigurements report difficulties finding jobs; potential employers may consider a person who is visibly different to be unsuitable as a public representative of a company. One study reported that people with clefts marry less often than a comparative noncleft sample. However, personal accounts of those with congenital disfigurements suggest that most enjoy satisfying permanent partnerships. The issue of whether or not to have children is problematic for those who worry that their offspring might manifest the same abnormality or carry the genetic predisposition on to future generations.

For nondisfigured people, middle and later adulthood may bring stability to body image and self-esteem, together with a reduced reliance on physical appearance and the opinions of others. These processes may also apply to people with visible differences; however, evidence is lacking. Some personal accounts reveal anxieties that the aging process will make an abnormality more noticeable to others.

Transitional Periods

Transitional periods in life, including changing schools, jobs, and neighborhoods, can be inordinately stressful for those who are visibly different. Considerable effort is required to leave familiar support systems, to develop strategies for dealing with the reactions of unfamiliar others, and to progress beyond initial encounters to form new relationships.

FUTURE RESEARCH QUESTIONS

Research in this area is fraught with methodological challenges, not least of which is the wide variation in conditions and the small number of people affected by any one type. The majority of research focuses on young people who agree to participate in studies when in the hospital for treatment. Little is known about the concerns of adults, about those who do not seek treatment, or about the needs of people from minority cultures. In addition, almost all the available research is cross-sectional and correlational. The challenges associated with measuring body image variables across conditions, developmental stages, and cultures remain.

A recent qualitative study by our research group highlights (1) the importance of positive thinking, sociability, and a solid network of social support, (2) the advantages of increasing age and maturity, and (3) the nature of the person's relationship with the health-care team in influencing positive adaptation. This study illustrates the multifactorial nature of adjustment and identifies the many interactional effects that remain to be explored.

CONCLUSIONS

A visible difference in physical appearance places a considerable strain on the affected person and his or her family and increases the risk of a wide range of social and psychological difficulties. No simple formula can explain why some people with disfigurements develop and maintain a positive body image and self-esteem, while others suffer from persistent problems. Among the greatest challenges facing current and future researchers is the task of clarifying the multiplicity of factors influencing adjustment. A greater challenge for those striving to cope successfully with disfigurement is to avoid an overreliance on society's punishing standards of physical appearance as a major component of body image and self-esteem.

INFORMATIVE READINGS

DeBeaufort, I., Hilhorst, M., & Holm, S. (1997). *In the eye of the beholder: Ethics and medical change of appearance*. Copenhagen: Scandinavian University Press.—A collection of papers written from medical, psychological, historical, ethical, and philosophical perspectives.

Grogan, S. (1999). *Body image: Understanding body dissatisfaction in men, women and children*. London: Routledge.—Offers data from interviews with men, women, and children to explore the cultural influences on body image and the findings of previous research.

Harris, D. (1997). Types, causes and physical treatment of visible differences. In R. Lansdown, N. Rumsey, E. Bradbury, T. Carr, & J. Partridge (Eds.), *Visible difference: Coping with disfigurement* (pp. 79–91). Oxford: Butterworth-Heinemann.—A discussion of the definitions and causes of visible differences, together with a summary of surgical, prosthetic, and camouflage approaches to intervention.

Harter, S. (1999). *The construction of the self: A developmental perspective*. New York: Guilford Press.—A synthesis of theory and research, with examples of constructions of the self across the lifespan.

Hughes, M. J. (1998). *The social consequences of facial disfigurement*. Aldershot, England: Ashgate Publishing.—Review of research and report of an empirical enquiry into the social consequences of surgery for facial cancer.

Lansdown, R., Rumsey, N., Bradbury, E., Carr, A., & Partridge, J. (Eds.). (1997). *Visibly different: Coping with disfigurement*. Oxford: Butterworth-Heinemann.—A book designed for health-care professionals and people affected by disfigurement; includes personal accounts, a summary of research, and recommendations for the provision of care.

Macgregor, F. C. (1979) *After plastic surgery: Adaptation and adjustment*. New York: J. F. Bergin.—A follow-up study of patients who underwent surgery to treat disfigurement.

Millard, T., & Richman, L. C. (2001). Different cleft conditions, facial appearance and speech relationship to psychological variables. *Cleft Palate-Craniofacial Journal, 38*(1), 68–75.—A paper investigating the psychological adjustment and learning characteristics of 65 patients, 8–17 years old.

Robinson, E., Rumsey, N., & Partridge, J. (1996) An evaluation of the impact of social interaction skills training for facially disfigured people. *British Journal of Plastic Surgery, 49*, 281–289.—A study of the effects of participation in a group workshop for self-referred adults with facial disfigurements

Turner, S. R., Thomas, P., Dowell, T., Rumsey, N., & Sandy, J. (1997). Psychological outcomes amongst cleft patients and their families. *British Journal of Plastic Surgery, 50*, 1–9.—A paper describing an audit of the psychological status of 112 cleft lip and palate patients and 130 parents.

Walters, E. (1997). Problems faced by children and families living with visible differences. In R. Lansdown, N. Rumsey, E. Bradbury, T. Carr, & J. Partridge (Eds.), *Visible difference: Coping with disfigurement* (pp 112–121). Oxford: Butterworth-Heinemann.—A chapter summarizing the developmental, maturational, and psychological issues faced by children and families affected by disfigurement.

African American Body Images

ANGELA A. CELIO
MARION F. ZABINSKI
DENISE E. WILFLEY

The study of body image is not complete without considering the cultural frameworks that influence people, both as group members and as individuals. This chapter provides an overview of the interethnic differences and intraethnic variation among African Americans that may elucidate the link between cultural contexts and the development and experience of body image.

Body image researchers seldom study African Americans exclusively. Most often, African Americans are compared with whites, although a few studies compare African Americans to other non-white groups. Researchers tend to use the broad term "black" to refer to African Americans, African Caribbeans, and those of continental African descent. However, a variety of influences may affect each of these subgroups' attitudes and values differently. Similarly, the body image literature uses the terms "white," "European American," and "Caucasian" interchangeably. We recognize the problem with such broad categories, yet for simplicity and consistency the terms "black" and "white" will be used throughout this chapter.

BODY IMAGE IDEALS IN BLACKS

In general, there appears to be a more flexible standard of attractiveness and a wider range of acceptable weights and shapes among blacks as compared to whites. While the white standard of female attractiveness consists solely of a slender body shape, black females have described their standard as comprising a multitude of body-focused and non-body-focused factors, including personal style, grooming, fit of clothes, hairstyle, skin tone/color, and ethnic pride. Black female adolescents identify attitude and personality as more important than physical appearance in defining a beautiful black woman. Little is known about attractiveness ideals for black boys and men.

The black community has a unique view of ideal weight and body size compared to white mainstream culture. Black women tend to endorse a larger and more moderate ideal body size than the very thin ideal endorsed by whites. Also, in contrast to overweight white women, overweight black women are more likely to view their own bodies as attractive.

There also appears to be less prejudice against overweight persons among blacks than whites. In 1996, Jackson and McGill reported that when black men were asked to relate several descriptors with the term "obese," they were more likely to associate positive characteristics, such as "attractive" and "generous," and less likely to attribute negative attributes, such as "lazy" or "uneducated," compared to the opinions of white men. Similarly, black women were more likely than white women to relate "sexiness" with "obese" in regard to same-race men. This more tolerant, even appreciative, view of overweight and obese body sizes likely contributes to lower rates of body dissatisfaction in blacks and may also contribute to higher self-esteem. Studies have generally shown that black females have higher self-esteem than white females and that self-esteem may not be as dependent upon body image and weight satisfaction in black women as it is in white women. Self-esteem in black men has been shown to be higher than that of white men, but the specific relationship with body image has gone largely unexamined.

BODY IMAGE SATISFACTION IN BLACKS

Women and Girls

The flexible and multidimensional body ideals promoted in the black culture may increase the probability that black women will have greater body image satisfaction, in stark contrast to the mainstream standards that engender high rates of dissatisfaction among whites. Research has supported this notion, frequently demonstrating that black females of all ages are more satisfied with the current shape and weight of their bodies. Some research has also shown that black girls have greater body satisfaction compared to Hispanic and Asian American girls, and black women as compared to Hispanic women. In addition to being more satisfied with their weight and body size, black women report more satisfaction than white women with their overall appearance and with individual body parts, specifically their lower torso, including hips, buttocks, thighs, and legs. A large sample survey by Smith and her colleagues in 1999 further indicates that black women are more cognitively and behaviorally invested in their bodies than white women.

Regardless of their true weight status, black women are less likely to perceive themselves as overweight and seem to have a higher threshold for what they consider "fat" compared to white women. Black females' perceived body size is closer to their ideal body size than is the case for white females. Nonetheless, it is important to realize that body dissatisfaction exists in black women. For instance, a 2000 study by Striegel-Moore and her colleagues indicated that both black and white girls experience increased body dissatisfaction between the ages of 11 and 16, but that black girls have less dissatisfaction than whites and that whites' dissatisfaction increases more steeply over time.

Men and Boys

In general, much less is known about body dissatisfaction in men and in black men, in particular. As a whole, men tend to have more positive body images than women. However, men are not immune to dissatisfaction with their body shape or appearance. As chapters by Olivardia and by Westmoreland Corson and Andersen discuss, men tend to strive for unrealistic muscular images, and perceived discrepancies with their actual shape can lead to lower self-esteem and maladaptive behaviors, such as anabolic steroid use.

A few studies reveal preliminary evidence about attitudinal body image in black men. Similar to other ethnic groups, black men are more satisfied with their body shape than black women. Some studies have also shown that black men are more satisfied with their body and weight compared to white men. Smith and her colleagues also found that black men reported more cognitive-behavioral investment in their physical appearance than white men did.

FACTORS INFLUENCING BLACKS' BODY IMAGES

Different body ideals may explain some of the differences between blacks' and whites' levels of body dissatisfaction. Several other factors also have been examined as possible contributors to cross-cultural differences and to variations in body image satisfaction within the black community. The following factors have been described in the literature as possible contributors to interethnic and intraethnic differences (with a few noted exceptions, most of this research has been done with females):

- Body mass index
- Socioeconomic status
- Other-sex preferences

- Maternal influences
- Peer influences
- Sexual maturation
- Ethnic identity

Body Mass Index (BMI)

There is a higher prevalence of overweight and obesity in the black population, especially females. Studies show that when comparing black and white women with equal BMIs, black women are more satisfied with their current weight and overall size. However, in black women a positive association does exist between obesity and dissatisfaction, such that black women with higher BMIs are generally more dissatisfied than their less overweight counterparts. Interestingly, some evidence suggests that a higher BMI is also associated with greater satisfaction with specific body parts (e.g., buttocks, hips) in black women, a trend that has not been found for white women. The fact that BMI can have both positive and negative effects on body satisfaction highlights the fact that body weight and shape is less central to blacks' perceptions of overall attractiveness than is the case for whites.

Socioeconomic Status (SES)

As reported by Flynn and Fitzgibbon in their 1998 review, research on the relationship between SES and body image in cross-cultural comparisons has yielded varying results. Lower-SES black females tend to be heavier, have a larger ideal body size, and are more satisfied with their body than upper-SES blacks or whites of all SES. When upper-SES black and white females are compared, they appear to have equal levels of body dissatisfaction. Some data on black girls suggest that body dissatisfaction increases with higher family income. However, other studies have found no relationship between SES and body satisfaction. Some of the inconsistencies in the literature may be due to varying operational definitions of SES (e.g., level of education achieved vs. annual income) and differences in categorization (e.g., high and low SES vs. high, middle, and low SES). The greater number of blacks than whites in lower and middle classes may further complicate interpretations. Standardized definitions and large studies that concurrently take into account multiple explanatory factors are needed in order to clarify the relationship between body image and SES.

Influences of Other-Sex Preferences

Black women tend to believe that black men desire larger and shapelier women. For the most part, these perceptions are consistent with studies directly assessing black men's physical appearance preferences in same-race women. Given a choice among figure silhouettes, black men select moderate-sized body shapes, in contrast to the thinner figures selected by white men. In addition, Jackson and McGill's findings on body part preferences revealed that black males felt wide hips and round buttocks were important characteristics of an attractive black woman. These findings may shed light on why black women, even at higher weights, report greater body satisfaction than white women.

Maternal Influences

Maternal influences also play a key role in determining body image satisfaction, particularly in girls. Typical maternal influences set the expectation for young black girls to be strong, self-reliant, and independent. These expectations may serve as a protective factor against body dissatisfaction. Research on mothers' preferences and perceptions of their daughters has shown that there may be a difference in attitudes about obesity in black and white mothers. For example, Brown and her colleagues reported in a 1995 study that black mothers were less critical of their heavy daughters compared to white mothers of 9- and 10-year-old girls. In addition, a 1996 study by Flynn and Fitzgibbon demonstrated that when black mothers were asked to identify current and ideal images for their daughters from silhouette figures, they perceived their daughters to be at an ideal size, regardless of weight. This research suggests that black mothers may be more accepting than white mothers of overweight body sizes in their children.

Peer Influences

Peer relationships also seem to differ among blacks and whites. Research done by Parker and her colleagues in 1995 suggests that black girls generate supportive, positive peer relationships, complimenting each other on their appearance, whereas white girls may be more competitive or envious with each other. Black girls also seem to value creating a unique, individual style rather than attempting to change their look to conform to mainstream ideals, as is more common among white girls. This value is highlighted by black girls' decreased interest in the brand-name fashions and "ready-made looks" that are currently popular.

Sexual Maturation

The weight gain naturally associated with sexual maturation has been linked to body image dissatisfaction in girls. For boys, puberty-related weight gain takes the form of increased muscle mass and therefore is desired. Notably, black girls begin pubertal development earlier than their white peers, resulting in earlier puberty-related weight gain. However, few studies have specifically examined the relationship between puberty and body image in black girls and boys.

In 1999 a cross-cultural study by Siegel and her colleagues linked perceived timing of sexual maturation in peer groups to body image. This study suggested that perceived late maturation in boys, including blacks, negatively affected their body image satisfaction. However, the findings for black girls diverged from those for other ethnicities: Black girls who perceived themselves to be early developers had the highest body image satisfaction, and those who perceived themselves to be late developers had lowest body image satisfaction. This finding differs from white early developers, who were the least satisfied with their bodies. Consistent with the different cultural body ideals, the fuller figure associated with pubertal development may be acceptable and even desirable to young black girls in comparison to white girls.

Ethnic Identity

Ethnic identity refers to the degree to which a person has adopted beliefs, attitudes, and behaviors that are characteristic of that ethnicity. There are mixed findings as to whether the degree of ethnic identity influences body image satisfaction. A few studies have shown that the more strongly a black woman identifies with black culture, the more likely she is to adopt black standards of beauty and to have greater body satisfaction. Conversely, the less she identifies with the black culture, the more likely she is to adopt the mainstream white standard of beauty, which a few studies have found to be associated with decreased body satisfaction. However, an equal number of studies show no relationship between ethnic identity and body image.

Still, some researchers contend that ethnic identity may play a role in body image satisfaction but that other personal characteristics, such as body mass index and social influences, are more significant contributors. Others contend that the lack of consistent findings can be attributed to the use of different operational definitions and measures of ethnic identity. At this point, the exact role of ethnic identity in body image development is unknown.

Other Factors

Factors such as age and weight-related teasing and criticism should also be taken into account when considering body image satisfaction in blacks. Studies have presented conflicting viewpoints as to whether body image satisfaction in black women increases or decreases with age, and prospective research is needed to further explore this issue. Weight-related teasing and criticism experienced by adolescent and college-age black females have been correlated with body dissatisfaction and the drive for thinness, particularly in those with higher BMIs.

IMPLICATIONS FOR RESEARCH AND CLINICAL PRACTICE

Implications for Research

Given the unique, multidimensional nature of body image in blacks, accurate assessment becomes a central issue. It is essential that selected measures are appropriate and psychometrically sound for this ethnic group (e.g., not validated solely on a white sample) and for each gender (e.g., additional measures are needed for men). In addition, researchers need to evaluate a full range of factors that contributes to body image among this group—including body mass index, social influences, and non-body-focused aspects (e.g., perceptions of personal style, hair type, skin tone). Most of the research to date has focused on relatively small samples; future research needs to examine large, representative samples of age-diverse people. International research would also be helpful; most of the current research has focused on comparisons within the United States. While current treatments exist for improving body image, investigations should determine whether these treatments are effective for black individuals or whether more culturally tailored treatments need to be developed and tested.

Implications for Clinical Practice

The overall trend revealed in the research is one in which blacks experience lower levels of body image dissatisfaction than whites. Consistent with this literature, it appears that blacks are at lower risk for anorexia nervosa and bulimia nervosa, eating disorders for which marked weight/shape concerns play a key role. However, they are equally at risk as whites for binge eating disorder, where other factors are likely to be involved in the onset (e.g., stress, negative affect). In addition, obesity is prevalent among black women, and varying degrees of body dissatisfaction may result. Clinicians can address their dissatisfaction by capitalizing on the flexible cultural views of body ideals and their supportive social environments. Steps must be taken to help obese clients increase or maintain positive views of body image while assisting them in their weight loss efforts. (See Foster and Matz's chapter in this volume.)

It is important to recognize the heterogeneity within the black community and the fact that blacks are not immune to eating disorders or body dissatisfaction. Research needs to inform clinical work as we continue to learn about the multiple factors that shape body image in blacks and the cultural expression of related eating symptoms and syndromes.

CONCLUSIONS

Rates of body image dissatisfaction have consistently been shown to be lower in blacks, who appear to endorse different body ideals than whites. We are just beginning to learn about the unique aspects of body image in blacks and how these differences may affect research and clinical practices. Future research should continue to elucidate the cultural frameworks experienced by the black community.

ACKNOWLEDGMENT

We would like to thank Lara Ray for her assistance in the preparation of this chapter.

INFORMATIVE READINGS

Brown, K. M., Schreiber, G. B., McMahon, R. P., Crawford, P., & Ghee, K. L. (1995). Maternal influences on body satisfaction in black and white girls aged 9 and 10: The NHLBI Growth and Health Study (NGHS). *Annals of Behavioral Medicine, 17*, 213–220.—Presents data from a large sample of black and white mothers on their attitudes towards their daughters' body shape, and eating habits.

Davis, N. L., Clance, P. R., & Gailis, A. T. (1999). Treatment approaches for obese and overweight African American women: A consideration of cultural dimensions. *Psychotherapy, 36*, 27–35.—Integrates research evidence regarding black body image and cultural contexts with treatment recommendations for obesity, advocating an "Afrocentric systems approach."

Flynn, K., & Fitzgibbon, M. (1996). Body image ideals of low-income African American mothers and their preadolescent daughters. *Journal of Youth and Adolescence, 25*, 615–630.

Flynn, K. J., & Fitzgibbon, M. (1998). Body images and obesity risk among black females: A review of the literature. *Annals of Behavioral Medicine, 20*, 13–24.—Reviews over 30 articles on body image in black females, highlighting the complexities and inconsistencies found in the literature.

Jackson, L. A., & McGill, O. D. (1996). Body type preferences and body characteristics associated with attractive and unattractive bodies by African Americans and Anglo Americans. *Sex Roles, 35*, 295–307.—Provides comparative data on body shape preferences and body characteristics associated with attractiveness among black and white males and females.

Kumanyika, S., Wilson, J. F., & Guilford-Davenport, M. (1993). Weight-related attitudes and behaviors of black women. *Journal of the American Dietetic Association, 93*, 416–22.—Presents data from a large study of black women on body image satisfaction, motivations for weight loss, eating behaviors, and other factors deemed important for weight control interventions.

Lovejoy, M. (2001). Disturbances in the social body: Differences in body image and eating problems among African American and White women. *Gender and Society, 15*, 239–

261.—Briefly reviews the literature on body image satisfaction in blacks compared with whites and presents black and white feminist perspectives on body image and eating problems.

Ofosu, H. B., Lafreniere, K. D., & Senn, C. Y. (1998). Body image perception among women of African descent: A normative context? *Feminism and Psychology, 8,* 303–323.—Highlights the heterogeneity of the black population and the cultural influences on black body image, obesity, and incidence of eating disorders.

Parker, S., Nichter, M., Nichter, M., Vuckovik, N., Sims, C., & Ritenbaugh, C. (1995). Body image and weight concerns among African-American and White adolescent females: Differences that make a difference. *Human Organization, 54,* 103–114.—Presents qualitative data from focus groups, interviews, and surveys of black and white adolescents' views on standards of beauty and body image.

Pike, K. M., Dohm, F. A., Striegel-Moore, R. H., Wilfley, D. E., & Fairburn, C. G. (2001). A comparison of black and white women with binge eating disorder. *American Journal of Psychiatry, 69,* 383–388.—Presents findings on the unique presentation of this disorder in black as compared to white women.

Siegel, J. M., Yancey, A. K., Aneshensel, C. S., & Schuler, R. (1999). Body image, perceived pubertal timing, and adolescent mental health. *Journal of Adolescent Health, 25,* 155–165.—Presents data on ethnic differences in body image, depression, and self-esteem in adolescents in relation to pubertal status.

Smith, D. E., Thompson, J. K., Raczynski, J. M., & Hilner, J. E. (1999). Body image among men and women in a biracial cohort: The CARDIA study. *International Journal of Eating Disorders, 25,* 71–82.—Report from a large study of black and white adults presenting data on body dissatisfaction and level of investment in appearance by weight status.

Striegel-Moore, R. H., Schreiber, G. B., Lo, A., Crawford, P., Obarzanek, E., & Rodin, J. (2000). Eating disorder symptoms in a cohort of 11- to 16-year-old Black and White girls: The NHLBI Growth and Heart Study. *International Journal of Eating Disorders, 27,* 49–66.—Large longitudinal study assessing the relationship between race, age, SES, BMI, and symptoms of eating disorders, including body image dissatisfaction.

Striegel-Moore, R. H., Wilfey, D. E., Pike, K. M., Dohm, F., & Fairburn, C. G. (2000). Recurrent binge eating in Black American women. *Archives of Family Medicine, 9,* 83–87.—Presents data on the differences in prevalence of recurrent binge eating and eating disorder symptomatology in black women as compared to white women.

Wilfley, D. E., Pike, K. M., & Striegel-Moore, R. H. (1997). Toward an integrated model of risk for binge eating disorder. *Journal of Gender, Culture, and Health, 2*(1), 1–32.—Discusses pathways of risk for black women, who may be at increased risk for binge eating disorder as compared to anorexia nervosa and bulimia nervosa.

28

Asian American Body Images

KATHLEEN Y. KAWAMURA

In describing Asian American experiences, a differentiation is often made between Asians and Asian Americans. The term "Asian" is generally used either as a broad racial descriptor for any person of Asian or Pacific Islander descent or to refer to a person of Asian or Pacific Islander descent who is a resident of an Asian country or one of the Pacific Islands. The term "Asian American" is often used as an ethnic description of a person of Asian or Pacific Islander descent who is a resident of the United States. Although some of the information presented in this chapter may be generalizable to Asians, the focus is on the body image experiences of Asian Americans.

Over 30 different ethnic subgroups make up the Asian American population, including, though not limited to, people of Chinese, Filipino, Japanese, Korean, Vietnamese, Indian, Hawaiian, Thai, Guamanian, and Samoan descent. Asian American subgroups are diverse not only in ethnicity but in cultural traditions, languages, and values. There is tremendous intragroup and intergroup variability among members of Asian American subgroups in terms of degree of acculturation, generation, and immigration experiences. Despite this variability, there also exist similarities in terms of traditional cultural values, physical appearance (which may differ from Western notions of beauty), and status as an ethnic minority group. This chapter discusses salient differences between Asian Americans and Caucasian Americans in those areas that may affect the body image development of Asian Americans. In addition, this chapter delineates ways in which intragroup differences in acculturation and ethnic identity may influence the body image experiences of Asian Americans.

FACTORS INFLUENCING ASIAN AMERICAN BODY IMAGES

Traditional Asian Values

Many Asian Americans, whether third-generation Japanese Americans or more recent Hmong immigrants, continue to be influenced by traditional Asian values. Though values and beliefs often differ between ethnic subgroups, traditional values common to several Asian American subgroups are likely to influence attitudes towards physical appearance. An understanding of these values, such as collectivism, emphasis on modesty, and restraint of strong emotions, can provide insight into the body images of Asian Americans.

Collectivistic Asian cultures emphasize values that promote interpersonal harmony within the family or the community. There is often pressure to act in a manner that does not reflect poorly on the group; therefore, negative attitudes or behaviors are often accompanied by feelings of shame. Asian Americans have the added responsibility of not only representing their families but also the larger Asian American community, especially if they are one of few Asian Americans in their community. In her discussion of the sociocultural influences on the body images of Asian and Asian American women, Hall hypothesizes that this collectivistic pressure may affect an individual's body image in that maintaining a perfect physical appearance begins to take on great importance. Though studies have found higher levels of perfectionism among Asian Americans, it remains unclear whether these perfectionistic tendencies manifest themselves in the area of physical appearance.

To preserve group harmony, many Asian cultures promote modesty and restraint of strong negative emotions. Inheriting this legacy, Asian Americans may be reluctant to boast of personal achievements, because doing so would disturb group relations by making others feel inferior. This modesty is often interpreted as self-effacement by non-Asians in the United States. In relation to body image, it is possible that Asian Americans are merely reluctant to acknowledge publicly any sense of satisfaction with their physical appearance because of the importance of maintaining modesty. Similarly, the emphasis on the restraint of strong negative emotions may inhibit Asian Americans who are experiencing extreme dissatisfaction with their body image from disclosing this information to others, especially to mental health professionals. Therefore, Asian Americans may appear to be "middle of the road" (neither extremely satisfied nor extremely dissatisfied) regarding their appearance—which may not be an accurate representation of their actual body image experiences.

In the only known study on the effect of Asian values on body image, Mukai and his colleagues studied the effect of the need for social approval on eating disturbances in Japanese college students. They found that the need for social approval predicted eating disturbances, even after controlling for the effects of body dissatisfaction and body mass. Future studies might examine how a collectivist orientation, perfectionistic tendencies, self-concealment, and modesty relate to the body image satisfaction of Asian American men and women.

Asian and Asian American Ideals of Beauty

Some Asian cultures, such as those in Korea, China, Japan, and the Philippines, have traditionally viewed obesity as a sign of prosperity, good health, or beauty. Current research and observations indicate that this is no longer the case among young women in modern industrialized Asia. In fact, studies by both Mukai et al. and Lee et al. reported a desire to be thinner among Japanese and Chinese women, respectively. A study by Mintz and Kashubeck revealed that Asian American women also desire a thinner body size. With regard to weight loss behaviors, the above studies indicated that Asian and Asian American women, as compared to Caucasian American women, engage in dieting behaviors less and evidence a lower incidence of clinical and subclinical eating disorders. It is unclear what mediating factors protect Asian and Asian American women from developing eating disorders, despite high levels of body size dissatisfaction. Perhaps there are ethnic differences in rates of metabolism, or cultural differences in nutrition, lifestyle, or emphasis on dieting, or a combination of the two. Fewer studies have been conducted with Asian and Asian American men, though initial findings by Mintz and Kashubeck revealed no differences between Asian American and Caucasian American men in body dissatisfaction levels.

For Asians, especially those from central Asian countries such as Korea, Japan, and China, common physical features often include the epicanthic eye fold, a broad, flat nose, and yellowish skin pigmentation. In some Asian cultures the idealization of the double eyelid, or eyefold, and the sculpted nose can be interpreted as an attempt to achieve Western standards of beauty. In metropolitan areas of Korea, plastic surgery to create a double eyelid is not uncommon. In a study of Asian American women who undergo cosmetic surgery, Kaw found that eyelid surgery and nasal implants or nasal tip refinements to create a narrower and pointier noise were the most requested procedures. Mintz and Kashubeck also found that Asian American women reported being less satisfied than Caucasian American women with their eyes and faces. The researchers hypothesized that an unattainable Western ideal of beauty contributes to dissatisfaction with racial features and low self-esteem among Asian American women. The idealization of white skin is not thought to be solely a reflection of Western ideals in that, for centuries, some Asian cultures have viewed white skin as a sign of femininity, purity, and upper-social-class status. In many areas of modern Asia, white skin continues to be valued—as can be seen in advertisements for skin whiteners and cosmetics that purport to provide a whiter appearance.

Increased exposure to Western cultures has been implicated in the attitudinal shifts regarding both body size and facial features. Though younger Asian and Asian American women are probably aware of traditional Asian ideals that promote weight gain, they seem to be more likely to subscribe to Western ideals of thinness. Similarly, older generations who are less influenced by Western cultures may be less concerned with racial features such as their eyes and noses. As in Western cultures, there appears to be less of an emphasis on physical appearance for men, and therefore less is known about the body image ideals of Asian and Asian American men. To examine the influence of exposure to Western cultures, the body image of men and women living in areas of Asia that have less contact with the West might be investigated. Furthermore, qualitative research that asks Asian American women and men to identify their beauty ideals along with what they perceive to be the traditional ideals of beauty would elucidate individuals' differentiation of traditional and Western notions of beauty.

Experiences with Racism and Negative Stereotypes

Being a physically distinct ethnic minority group, Asian Americans may have a heightened awareness of racial characteristics that separate them from the dominant group. Even third- or fourth-generation Asian Americans are often perceived to be foreigners and are vulnerable to discriminatory practices, in contrast to Caucasian immigrants from Europe, who are far less likely to encounter discrimination based on their physical features. The media perpetuate racism toward Asian Americans in that until recently, portrayals of Asian characters were primarily negative or stereotyped. Asian Americans are also unlikely to be used as beauty ideals in advertisements, television shows, or the movies—unless it is to portray them as exotic characters. Hall describes how Asian American women must struggle with both racism and sexism because the stereotypical physical features that are often "admired" in Asian women, such as their petite, youthful, feminine appearances, are also seen as submissive and sexualized characteristics. Root, in her discussion on the development of eating disorders in women of color, hypothesized that experiences with racism can lead to internalized racism—the self-loathing of one's own racial characteristics—whereas Caucasian characteristics become equated with respect, acceptance, and self-esteem.

Several studies lend support to the theory that exposure to racism contributes to dissatisfaction with racial features. In their 1998 review of studies on the self-concept of Asian Americans, Lee and Zhan found that when compared to other ethnic minority groups, Asian American youth were the most dissatisfied with their physical appearance and were most likely to prefer to be Caucasian if they could choose to do so. Asian American college students also reported feeling less socially accepted because of their racial features. In Kaw's interviews with Asian American women who had undergone eyelid or nasal surgeries, the women expressed their hopes that these physical alterations would not only enhance their beauty but also elevate their social status. A future empirical investigation of the relationship between satisfaction with racial features and perceived racism could evaluate these theories.

Acculturation and Ethnic Identity

Acculturation is the process by which individuals integrate the customs, attitudes, and habits associated with their traditional cultures with those of the dominant culture. Acculturation affects or is affected by ethnic identity, language use, number of generations in the United States, ethnic composition of one's social network, and adherence to traditional versus dominant values and customs. Theorists have hypothesized that acculturation to "American" culture would be accompanied by the adoption of Western body image ideals; however, published studies have reported no relationship between acculturation and body size dissatisfaction among Asian American women. Acculturation is a multidimensional phenomenon whose various components likely have differing degrees of influence over the development of body image in Asian Americans. Future research is needed to identify and measure specific components of acculturation rather than relying on measures that examine acculturation along a single continuum. For example, it seems likely that stage of ethnic identity, ethnic composition of one's social network, and adherence to traditional values would be primary factors of influence in the development of Asian American body images.

Ethnic identity often plays a large role in the development of Asian Americans' sense of self and therefore warrants further discussion. In a 1996 article on ethnic identity development, Phinney described fluid stages of ethnic identity that appear to change across situations and time. An unexamined ethnic identity characterizes young children or recent immigrants who have had little exposure to the dominant culture and have not yet experienced their ethnicity as requiring reflection. Whether individuals feel positively, negatively, or neutrally about their racial characteristics would be based primarily on the attitudes of the family or the community. As exposure to racism increases, some individuals may respond by rejecting their traditional culture and embracing the dominant culture. This rejection might also include denigration of physical characteristics associated with being Asian. The inability to eradicate salient racial characteristics may lead to low self-esteem and negative body image. On the other hand, others may respond to racism by immersing themselves in their traditional culture and feel anger toward the dominant group. For these individuals, ethnic characteristics may be a celebrated source of pride. An "achieved" ethnic identity occurs when there is a realistic appraisal of racism combined with an acceptance of both positive and negative features associated with both traditional and dominant cultures. This stage would likely be associated with the most stable, positive, body image attitudes. Because exploration of one's ethnic identity often begins to occur in adolescence, body image disturbance may also be indicative of a more general struggle to develop a stable and secure self-concept. Future studies should examine the relationship between self-esteem, stage of ethnic identity, and body satisfaction given that a positive sense of self may contribute to both a stable ethnic identity and body satisfaction.

IMPLICATIONS FOR FUTURE RESEARCH AND CLINICAL PRACTICE

This chapter describes ways in which the experiences of Asian Americans can contribute to differences in Asian American and Caucasian American body images. The explanatory models on the development of body image disturbances that have been based on Caucasian American samples do not adequately capture the experiences of Asian Americans. Unfortunately, few empirical investigations have been conducted to expand the understanding of the development of Asian American body images. This lacuna may be due to the fact that Asian Americans are often characterized as the "model minority group" that suffers from few psychological problems. Furthermore, body image research has traditionally focused on the body size dissatisfaction of young women; perhaps the smaller body size of Asian American women has been mistakenly assumed to protect them from body size dissatisfaction. In addition, dissatisfaction with physical features other than body size, such as facial features, has been largely ignored. Future research needs to differentiate the ethnic subgroups of Asians and Asian Americans and interpret with caution measures of body image that have been normed primarily on Caucasian American samples.

Clinicians who work with Asian Americans will find it helpful to familiarize themselves with the various factors discussed throughout this chapter, as they are likely to influence aspects of psychological functioning beyond that of body image. Mental health professionals should include Asian American women in outreach efforts that are focused on body size dissatisfaction. Discussions with Asian Americans should also include inquiry into degree of satisfaction with racial physiognomic features. Mental health professionals should explore the ways in which their Asian American clients' traditional values, Caucasian ideals of beauty, and experiences with racism have contributed to negative self-images. By understanding the familial and societal influences on the development of body image, clients will be able to challenge these notions of beauty and begin to develop their own definitions of what is attractive.

INFORMATIVE READINGS

Bradshaw, C. K. (1994). Asian and Asian American women: Historical and political considerations in psychotherapy. In L. Comas-Díaz, & B. Greene (Eds.), *Women of color: Integrating ethnic and gender identities in psychotherapy* (pp. 72–113). New York: Guilford Press.—Details the effects of immigration, traditional cultural values, and ethnic minority status on the psychology of Asian American women.

Hall, C. C. (1995). Asian eyes: Body image and eating disorders of Asian and Asian American women. *Eating Disorders, 3*, 8–19.—A literature review of psychological and sociological influences on the body images of Asian and Asian American women.

Kaw, E. (1993). Medicalization of racial features: Asian American women and cosmetic surgery. *Medical Anthropology Quarterly, 7*, 74–89.—Ethnographic research exploring cultural and institutional factors that influence the decisions by Asian American women to undergo cosmetic surgery.

Lee, C. L., & Zhan, G. (1998). Psychosocial status of children and youths. In L. C. Lee & N. W. S. Zane (Eds.), *Handbook of Asian American psychology* (pp. 137–163). Thousand Oaks, CA: Sage.—Theoretical discussions and reviews of empirical research related to the psychology of Asian Americans.

Lee, S., Leung, T., Lee, A. M., Yu, H., & Leung, C. M. (1996). Body dissatisfaction among Chinese undergraduates and its implications for eating disorders in Hong Kong. *International Journal of Eating Disorders, 20*, 77–84.—An empirical investigation of gender differences among Chinese in Hong Kong on satisfaction with various physical features.

Mintz, L. B., & Kashubeck, S. (1999). Body image and disordered eating among Asian American and Caucasian American college students. *Psychology of Women Quarterly, 23*, 781–796.—An examination of gender differences within race and racial differences within gender on measures of body image attitudes and eating-disordered behaviors.

Mok, T. A. (1998). Getting the message: Media images and stereotypes and their effect on Asian Americans. *Cultural Diversity and Mental Health, 4*, 185–202.—A review of media images of Asians and Asian Americans and autobiographical information from Asian American literature.

Mukai, T., Kambara, A., & Sasaki, Y. (1998). Body dissatisfaction, need for social approval, and eating disturbances among Japanese and American college women. *Sex Roles, 39*, 751–763.—A study on the effects of a Japanese cultural value on eating disturbances and a review of the influence of Western culture on body image disturbances in Japan.

Phinney, J. S. (1996). Understanding ethnic diversity: The role of ethnic identity. *American Behavioral Scientist, 40*, 143–152.—Description of a model of ethnic identity development along with ways in which the model can be used to help students explore their own ethnicity.

Root, M. P. (1990). Disordered eating in women of color. *Sex Roles, 22*, 525–536.—A discussion of social, familial, and individual factors that may contribute to the development of eating disorders in women of color.

Uba, L. (1994). *Asian Americans: Personality patterns, identity, and mental health.* New York: Guilford Press.—A comprehensive book on the major issues related to Asian American personality and mental health.

29

Hispanic Body Images

MADELINE ALTABE
KEISHA-GAYE N. O'GARO

In this brief chapter we discuss ideas and evidence regarding Hispanic body images, a fast-growing area of research. Weight-related Hispanic body image has been studied more extensively because of its relationship to eating disorders. However, general appearance body image has been studied to some extent, as has the construct of acculturation in relation to body image. We present a working framework for understanding the issues and research that will emerge over the next decade.

THE CULTURAL CONTEXT

In the United States, the term "Hispanic" is used to refer to groups with backgrounds ranging from South America to the Caribbean. Although there may be some generalities about Hispanic culture, each national group is unique. Indeed, the term "Hispanic" is not universally accepted; many prefer the term "Latino" or "Latina" (for females). The primary comparison group for studies in the United States is referred to as white, Caucasian, European American, or Anglo. We use all these terms in this chapter, depending on the language that authors used in describing their study populations.

The concepts and research presented in this chapter are largely based on U.S. literature and are intended to be helpful in understanding Hispanic American body image. Most research compares Hispanic Americans to European Americans. One could describe Hispanic body image as a construct on its own terms. For a more detailed review of body image in Latin American countries, the interested reader may want to consult the Spanish language psychological literature.

Hispanic Cultural Commonalities and Diversity

Many authors have described the role of the family and its relationship to food and body image in Latino culture. In 1999 Jane, Hunter, and Lozzi observed that young Latina women tend to live with their families longer than their European American counterparts. What a Latino family sees as beautiful is less likely to be a narrowly defined physical ideal like that presented in the U.S. media. Strong family identification can be a protective factor for any group. As Hahn-Smith and Smith found in their 2001 study, maternal identification was associated with better body image and self-esteem for both Hispanic and Anglo girls.

However, two factors may interact to render the thin ideal of the majority culture somewhat more threatening for Latina women than for their European American counterparts: gender role and cultural fatalism. Latino families tend to promote more traditional values. According to Avila and Avila in 1995, the role of the female is characterized by submissiveness, self-sacrifice, and restraint. A more traditional feminine role orientation is associated with more body image and eating disturbances.

Various authors, including Kempa and Thomas in 2000, have described the cultural fatalism of Latinos, a value that stems, in part, from the Catholic belief system that life is hard and that people ought to accept their fate gracefully and await their reward in heaven. *Simpatia*, the value of group harmony, tends to suppress interpersonal conflict and defiance from the group. Taken together with a thinness ideal, Hispanics are left vulnerable because they are less likely than European Americans to question the values of their own culture.

Acculturation

Hispanic groups in the United States have had the experience of adapting to U.S. culture, a process known as acculturation. This process is usually defined as the modification and incorporation of the traditional (ethnic) and the alternate (dominant) cultures' encompassing customs, language, lifestyle, and value orientations. Acculturation can occur in varying degrees. Given two individuals from similar backgrounds, one may find a subculture within the U.S. and retain more customs of the native culture, whereas the other may leave the ethnic neighborhood and become more "acculturated." Acculturation may result in identity confusion due to differences between the traditional and alternate culture. Level of acculturation is best assessed on an individual basis; it is usually measured by self-report of the predominant language spoken at home or by questionnaire regarding food, music, attitudes, and dating practices.

As a cultural group, Hispanics are heavily exposed to mainstream U.S. culture both here and in their native countries. In addition, they are less physically distinctive from Caucasians than other ethnic groups. Thus we expect that many will undergo acculturation. In 1995 Lopez, Blix, and Blix found that age of immigration (marking the beginning of acculturation) significantly affected tendencies toward eating pathology. Immigration to the United States prior to puberty was identified as a risk factor. During adolescence identity is already challenged. Thus, individuals who undergo acculturation in early adolescence may be more likely to develop eating disturbances than those who experience this event earlier or later in life (as Gowen and others discovered).

The findings of these studies about puberty and acculturative stress are consistent, but when level of acculturation is assessed as an individual difference variable, the results are inconclusive. In some studies, level of acculturation and ethnicity are both related to body image. Individuals acculturated to the United States report similar body image attitudes to those of Caucasians. In other studies, ethnic groups vary in their body image, regardless of level of acculturation. Given the variety of acculturation measures and study populations with varying degrees of acculturation, disparities may be explained as methodological. However, other explanations could bear out in time.

One hypothesis is that Latino culture itself is changing with regard to body image. U.S. culture (movies, TV, other products) is heavily exported to Latin American countries. Over time these images influence the culture. Support for the idea that Latino culture has adopted a thin ideal comes from facts such as the increased incidence of eating disorders in Latin American countries. In a Brazilian sample, Darnall and colleagues found that girls in private school have adopted Western body image ideals. The drive to be attractive and thin has led to an increase of laxative and diuretic abuse. Thus it could be the case that an acculturated Hispanic American woman could have a better feeling about her weight than a young woman arriving from Argentina or Brazil today.

Stereotypes of Hispanic women exist within the United States. In the article "Disordered Eating in Women of Color," Root points out that Hispanic women are perceived to be fat, powerless, obedient, and quiet. By striving to be thin, Hispanic American women may be distancing themselves from a negative stereotype of their native culture.

WEIGHT-RELATED BODY IMAGE ISSUES

Recent research is mixed regarding differences between Hispanic and Caucasian women with regard to weight attitudes. Some studies of immigrant and first-generation Latin American women show that their weight satisfaction is higher than that of European American women. For example, Franko and Herrara investigated the body image attitudes of Guatamalan American women who were members of an ethnic student organization. These women were more satisfied with their current weight and less focused on dieting than a comparison group of European American women. Interestingly, there was no difference in investment in physical appearance, even though there were differences in weight satisfaction In addition, the more acculturated Guatamalan American women had lower satisfaction with weight.

Acculturation may account for the similar levels of weight satisfaction reported in some studies of Latina and European American women. For example, in 1997 French and colleagues studied public schoolchildren in Minnesota, where the Hispanic population is about 1%. Not surprisingly, there were few differences between the Latino and European American youths.

Darnall reviewed studies indicating that Brazilian adolescent girls reported greater body dissatisfaction than U.S. adolescent girls. Moreover, in Robinson's 1996 study in a California school that was 28% Latino, the Latina children had greater weight dissatisfaction than European Americans, even after related factors (such as actual degree of overweight) were ruled out. Robinson and colleagues also observed that among the leanest girls in their sample, the Hispanic girls had the greatest body weight dissatisfaction. Perception of mother's body size was also associated with body dissatisfaction.

The first two types of results are consistent with previous our understanding of weight ideals and culture: U.S. culture promotes the thinness ideal; other groups suffer less weight dissatisfaction. As individuals become more acculturated, they accept the U.S. value of thinness and experience more weight dissatisfaction. In a recent comparison of Spanish and American college students in 2000, Gleaves and others found that both groups of women demonstrated similar thin ideals for body weight. By way of explanation, the authors described how Spanish culture has come to value thinness. As evinced by media portrayals, one in four advertisements refers to weight loss. Notably, Spanish men held a thinner ideal for themselves than their American counterparts. According to the authors, the focus on thinness in Spain is a fairly recent phenomenon that coincides with the "Americanization" of Spain.

In 2001 Rieger and colleagues discussed reasons thinness may be valued other than the American beauty ideal. These include religious values of self-sacrifice and denial of the body in order to achieve closeness with the spiritual realm. For example, Saint Catherine was said to have fasted frequently and is depicted in works of art of the time as quite thin. She was trying to be spiritual, not beautiful. Darnall suggested that beauty ideals become even more important in poorer areas of Latin America, as a woman's financial security is more related to attracting men than it would be in the United States. Thus the meaning of the thin ideal in Hispanic culture warrants further study.

BEYOND WEIGHT-RELATED BODY IMAGE

In theory, cultures vary in their views on weight and other physical appearance ideals. In a qualitative analysis of ideal traits, Altabe found that Caucasian and Hispanic college students (men and women) both valued being tall and tan. The Caucasians idealized blond hair, whereas Hispanic individuals identified brown hair as the ideal. Hispanic men also idealized brown eyes. Thus typical Hispanic physical traits (brown hair and eyes, darker skin) were viewed positively by this sample.

Additional body image issues under investigation include sexual body image and appearance investment. For example, Altabe found that Hispanic women were more likely to desire larger breasts; Spencer and colleagues (1999) found that Hispanic women with breast cancer had higher concerns regarding their sexuality than did other ethnic groups. Similarly, when Sommer and colleagues asked American women for their feelings about menopause, Hispanic American women anticipated the most regret at the loss of their menstrual cycle. Unlike Caucasian and African American women, Hispanic women did not associate menopause with freedom or independence. The authors suggest that Hispanic women see their value as more connected with their female role.

Appearance investment modifies the effects of body dissatisfaction. For example, of two people with similar levels of body dissatisfaction, the one with greater appearance investment will suffer more. Franko and Herarra found that appearance investment of Guatamalan American women was similar to that of Caucasian American women. Miller's 2000 study of Hispanic and Caucasian American college students replicated this finding. However, some studies have found that Hispanic Americans have higher appearance investment than other groups. Thus Hispanics investment in appearance leaves them vulnerable to the U.S. ideal of thinness.

PUTTING THE PIECES TOGETHER

Although the Hispanic culture is different from the dominant culture in the United States in its values, the two cultures influence each other here and in Latin America. This process of cultural exchange may be seen in the shift toward thin weight ideals in Latin culture. However, we must consider the possibility that the thin ideal means something different in Hispanic culture. In the dominant U.S. culture, thinness is associated with self-control; what it might mean for Hispanic groups is not yet clear.

The ideal of thinness in Hispanic culture is relatively new and may not represent the cultural experience of all Hispanic Americans. Acculturative stress is likely to occur in some individuals. When this stress coincides with the identity issues of adolescence, the individual may become particularly vulnerable to eating disorders. Conforming to the U.S. standards of weight may appear to be a concrete means of resolving the identity issues. Familial influences, particularly identification with mothers, may provide some protection against weight dissatisfaction for Hispanic girls.

General appearance issues have not been investigated in depth, nor has investment in ideal Hispanic physical traits. Some findings suggest different attitudes toward sexual body image in Hispanic women, who may be more concerned about the physical aspects of their femininity than Caucasian or African American women. They appear to have a more difficult time with menopause and women's medical issues.

As clinicians and researchers, what do we do with this information? The interrelationship between body image, self-esteem, and values is an established dynamic in mainstream U.S. literature. We would argue that the same relations hold true for Hispanics, except that an ideal of thinness is not universally accepted, and the value and meaning of thinness is not yet clear. Female role is likely to be part of the answer. The challenge for the clinician is to explore these ideas while conducting an interview that is mindful of the individual's cultural experience, possible acculturative stress, and body image. For the researcher, important questions remain about the prevalence of the thinness ideal and its meaning in Hispanic culture. The relationship of gender role to body image is also worthy of exploration. Overall we need to keep in mind that cultures are influencing each other at a fast pace. It is useful to understand the form body image ideals take when brought into the values of other cultures.

INFORMATIVE READINGS

Altabe, M. (1996). Ethnicity and body image: Quantitative and qualitative analysis. *International Journal of Eating Disorders, 23*, 153–159.—Discusses general appearance issues in relation to ethnicity.

Avila, D. L., & Avila, A. L. (1995). Mexican-Americans. In N. A. Vacc & S. B. DeVaney (Eds.), *Experiencing and counseling multicultural and diverse populations* (3rd ed.). Philadelphia: Accelerated Development.—Role of female in Latin culture.

Darnall, B. D., Smith, J. E., Craighead, L. W., & Lamounier, J. A. (1999). Modification of the cognitive model for bulimia via path analysis on a Brazilian adolescent sample. *Addictive Behaviors, 24*(1), 47–57.—Examines body image issues in Latin America.

Franko, D. L., & Herrara, I. (1997). Body image differences in Guatamalan-American and White college women. *Eating Disorders: The Journal of Prevention, 5*, 119–127.—Examines weight satisfaction and acculturation in Hispanic women.

French, S. A., Story, M., Neumark-Sztainer, D., Downes, B., Resnick, M., & Blum, R. (1997). Ethnic differences in psychosocial and health behavior correlates of dieting, purging, and binge eating in a population-based sample of adolescent females. *International Journal of Eating Disorders, 22*(3), 315–322.—Lack of ethnic differences in eating symptoms and related factors.

Gleaves, D. H., Cepeda-Benito, A., Williams, T. L., Cororve, M. B., Fernandez, M. D. C., & Vila, J. (2000). Body image preferences of self and others: A comparison of Spanish and American male and female college students. *Eating Disorders: The Journal of Treat-*

ment and Prevention, 8(4), 269–282.—Few differences in Spanish and American women's body ideal and satisfaction.

Gowen, L. K., Hayward, C., Killen, J. D., Robinson, T. N., & Taylor, C. B. (1999). Acculturation and eating disorder symptoms in adolescent girls. *Journal of Research on Adolescence, 9,* 67–83.—Explores relationships among puberty, acculturative stress, and body image.

Guinn, B., Semper, T., & Jorgenson, L. (1997). Mexican American female adolescent self-esteem: The effect of body image, exercise behavior, and body fatness. *Hispanic Journal of Behavioral Sciences, 19*(4), 517–526.—Investigates self-esteem and body image in Mexican Americans.

Hahn-Smith, A. M., & Smith, J. E. (2001). The positive influence of maternal identification on body image, eating attitudes, and self-esteem of Hispanic and Anglo girls. *International Journal of Eating Disorders, 29,* 429–440.—Studies the links between family identification, self-esteem, and body image ideals.

Jane, D. M., Hunter, G. C., & Lozzi, B. M. (1999). Do Cuban American women suffer from eating disorders? Effects of media exposure and acculturation. *Hispanic Journal of Behavioral Sciences, 21*(2), 212–218.—Examines the dual roles of Cuban community and family of origin.

Kempa, M. L., & Thomas, A. J. (2000). Culturally sensitive assessment and treatment of eating disorders. *Eating Disorders: The Journal of Treatment and Prevention, 8*(1), 17–30.—Specific treatment and assessment recommendations for eating disorders in several ethnic groups, including Hispanic Americans.

Lopez, E., Blix, G., & Blix, A. (1995). Body image of Latinas compared to body image of non-Latina White women. *Health Values, 19*(6), 3–10.—Relationship of ethnicity (Latinas), time in the United States, and age of immigration on body image ideals.

Miller, K. J., Gleaves, D. H., Hirsch, T. G., Green, B. A., Snow, A. C., & Corbett, C. C. (2000). Comparisons of body image dimensions by race/ethnicity and gender in a university population. *International Journal of Eating Disorders, 27,* 310–316.—Comparison of several key weight and non-weight dimensions of body image.

Rieger, E., Touyz, S. W., Swain, T., & Beumont, P. J. V. (2001).Cross-cultural research on anorexia nervosa: Assumptions regarding the role of body weight. *International Journal of Eating Disorders, 29*(2), 205–215.—A review of reasons for eating disorders, other than the contemporary U.S. thin beauty ideal.

Robinson, T. N., Killen, J. D., Litt, I. F., Hammer, L. D., Wilson, D. M., Haydel, K. F., Hayward, C., & Taylor, C. B. (1996). Ethnicity and body dissatisfaction: Are Hispanic and Asian girls at increase risk for eating disorders? *Journal of Adolescent Health, 19,* 384–393.—Hispanics showed more weight dissatisfaction.

Root, M. P. (1990). Disordered eating in women of color. *Sex Roles, 22*(7/8), 525–536.—Negative stereotypes of heavy Hispanic women in U.S. media.

Sommer, B., Avis, N., Meyer, P., Ory, M., Madden, T., Kagawa-Singer, M., Mouton, C., O'Neill Rasor, N., & Adler, S. (1999). Attitudes toward menopause and aging across ethnic/racial groups. *Psychosomatic Medicine, 61,* 868–875.—A study of Hispanic women and their negative attitudes toward menopause.

Spencer, S. M., Lehman, J. M., Wynings, C., Arena, P., Carver, C. S., Antoni, M. H., Derhagopian, R. P., Ironson, G., & Love, N. (1999). Concerns about breast cancer and relations to psychological well-being in a multiethnic sample of early-stage patients. *Health Psychology, 18*(2), 159–168.—Hispanic women and their body-related attitudes toward breast cancer.

30

Gay and Lesbian Body Images

ESTHER D. ROTHBLUM

Discontentment with one's body is so common in women in the United States and other Western nations that this phenomenon has been called a "normative discontent." Yet it was not until the late 1980s that the first articles appeared about lesbians and body image. Sari Dworkin postulated that women in Western societies, regardless of sexual orientation, are told how to look and thus are preoccupied with weight and appearance. Laura Brown, on the other hand, drew a parallel between oppression of lesbians and oppression of fat women, arguing that lesbian communities are more accepting of body weight.

The impetus for studies of body image among gay men came from clinical observations in the United States and Europe that gay men were overrepresented among eating-disordered patients. Thus this literature has often focused on clinical samples. For example, although few patients in eating disorders clinics are male, one study found 30% of those few men were self-identified as gay. More recently, there has been discussion of how gay male communities accentuate appearance. For example, Lahti describes how gay male media and erotica highlight and exaggerate gay men's physical proportions, especially muscles and genitals. As a result, gay men are likely to be more dissatisfied with their bodies than heterosexual men.

Another way about thinking of sexual orientation in relation to body image is to include conceptions of both gender and sexual orientation. For example, it has been hypothesized that people sexually involved with men (heterosexual women and gay men) are more focused on appearance than are people sexually involved with women (heterosexual men and lesbians). The result is an interaction of gender and sexual orientation on body image concerns.

As of this writing, data on bisexuals' body image are lacking. This is an important area for future study. It is possible that bisexuals fall somewhere in the middle on the continuum of body image concerns facing gay men, heterosexual women, lesbians, and heterosexual men. On the other hand, as bisexuals increasingly form their own communities and organizations, this group may develop unique body image issues. Because bisexuals are sexually attracted to, and may be involved with, both male and female partners (either simultaneously or sequentially), they could facilitate our study of how body and appearance issues differ for the same person when the sexual partner is male versus female. Taub's qualitative study of bisexual women indicated that bisexual women feel more pressure to conform to heterosexual beauty norms (e.g., dieting, shaving body hair, looking more feminine) when involved with men than with women.

ATTITUDES HELD BY THE GENERAL PUBLIC

Twenty years before the first studies appeared on lesbians, gay men, and body image, social psychologists were studying attitudes about the appearance of lesbians and gay men held by society at large. Studies in the 1970s and 1980s found that college students rated lesbians as less attractive than heterosexual women. Lesbians described as "masculine" were rated as more unappealing, hostile, and disagreeable than were lesbians described as "feminine" or "neutral." College students liked descriptions of heterosexual feminine women the most, although even masculine heterosexual women were liked. Lesbians were liked most when their physical appearance conformed to heterosexual standards for women. Female students who were less tolerant of lesbians selected more unattractive photographs of women as lesbians. Male students, regardless of their tolerance for lesbians, chose unattractive women as lesbians. Female students selected the less attractive photos of men for people they thought to be gay. The general public often views gay men as effeminate and nonmasculine, in contrast to the "gay macho" look in vogue in many gay male communities.

Most lesbians and gay men grew up in households and attended colleges with people who held such attitudes. As a result, lesbians and gay men may internalize these negative attitudes about themselves. They may delay "coming out" to their families and friends or joining lesbian and gay communities in order to avoid negative stereotypes. Their own body image may be affected by these cultural views of the appearance of lesbians and gay men.

SEXUAL ORIENTATION AND WEIGHT

Do lesbians actually weigh more than heterosexual women? Certainly weight is related to body image, given the extreme pressure to be thin in Western nations. Several studies have found lesbians to weigh significantly more than heterosexual women. However, most of these studies recruited lesbians and gay men from community organizations and heterosexual students from colleges. One of the problems with this recruitment method is that noncollege group members tend to be older, and weight is correlated with age, particularly for women. This may explain why lesbians in these studies weighed more than heterosexual women. A recent study I conducted with lesbians and their heterosexual sisters as a control group still found lesbians to weigh significantly more than their sisters. By focusing on sisters, this study controlled for race, ethnicity, and economic factors, as well as for age cohort.

Why do lesbians weigh more than heterosexual women, including their sisters? One possibility is greater comfort with body appearance in the lesbian communities—that is, first a woman becomes a lesbian and, as a result, is more content with and less focused on her weight. We must also consider the opposite: that women who are heavier may become lesbians. For example, is it possible that heavier adolescent girls are less attractive to boys and thus postpone marriage and seek an education? Prior research has shown that girls who weigh more in adolescence are less likely to be married 10 years later. Longitudinal research is necessary to examine the direction of causality between weight and sexual orientation for both women and men.

What about the weight of gay men? In one of the few studies to report such data, gay men weighed less than heterosexual men, and lesbians weighed more than heterosexual women. In this study by Gettelman and Thompson, lesbians and gay men were recruited from college gay and lesbian student associations and friendship networks of these students, and heterosexuals were recruited from college courses.

RESEARCH ON SEXUAL ORIENTATION AND BODY IMAGE

Lesbians

In the 1990s a few studies investigated lesbian body image, with nearly every author citing the two theoretical positions by Dworkin mentioned earlier (lesbians do not differ from heterosexual women on body image) and by Brown (lesbians are more accepting of their bodies than are heterosexual women) as possible alternative outcomes.

In one of the earliest studies, Striegel-Moore, Tucker, and Hsu compared 30 lesbian college students recruited from lesbian/gay social gatherings and a lesbian support group, 25 heterosexual college women recruited from the women's studies department (presumed to be feminist), and 27 heterosexual college women from the psychology research subject pool. There were no differences among the three groups on body image satisfaction or disordered eating, but lesbians had higher self-esteem. Similarly, a qualitative study of 26 lesbian college students found them to place a high value on thinness as ideals for themselves and their partners.

Herzog and his colleagues studied 45 lesbians recruited via gay/lesbian organizations, bars, and advertisements in periodicals, and 64 heterosexual female college students. Lesbians were significantly heavier than heterosexual women, yet lesbians were less concerned with their appearance, were less driven by the thinness ideal, had higher ideal weights, and selected larger figures of women that they thought potential partners would find attractive. In Heffernan's study of 203 lesbians, body esteem was related to self-esteem but not to reported sexual attractiveness, physical condition, or weight concerns. Heavier lesbians were more dissatisfied with their weight and had poorer body esteem.

Gay Men

There have been a few studies of gay men recruited from nonclinical samples. In one study by Herzog and his colleagues, 43 gay men were recruited from gay organizations, bars, and gay periodicals; 32 heterosexual men and 64 heterosexual women were recruited via friends of the authors and periodicals. Gay men were more likely to have an ideal weight below that on the life insurance charts for their height, whereas heterosexual men chose ideal weights above those on the charts.

In a larger study at Yale University by Lisa Silberstein and her colleagues, 71 heterosexual men reported more satisfaction with their upper-body strength and physical condition than did 71 gay men. In addition, the gay men showed a wider gap between actual and ideal bodies than did heterosexual men. Physical appearance was more important to the gay men's sense of self, whereas being physically active was of greater value to the heterosexual men. Similarly, gay men stated that they exercised to improve physical attractiveness, whereas heterosexual men exercised to improve fitness, health, and for enjoyment. There were no differences between groups on body size satisfaction, eating disorders, or self-esteem. Gay men who wanted to be thinner were more likely to diet; heterosexual men who wanted to be heavier had lower self-esteem.

Comparing Lesbians and Gay Men

Susan Beren and her colleagues compared 58 male and 58 female heterosexual college students and 69 lesbians and 58 gay men recruited from gay organizations. Gay men expressed more body dissatisfaction, greater discrepancy between actual and ideal figures, more social pressure to diet, and more public self-consciousness than did the heterosexual men. Lesbians and heterosexual women did not differ on these measures.

In an age-controlled study I conducted with two colleagues, Pamela Brand and Laura Solomon, we compared lesbians at a lesbian music festival, gay men at a gay/lesbian conference, and heterosexual college students. Women were more likely than men to perceive themselves as overweight, as heavier than their ideal weights, which were further, in a heavier direction, than the men's ideal estimates from life insurance recommendations. Women were also more likely than men to have dieted to lose weight. Men were more likely to state that another person's weight would affect their attraction to the person. This study found an interaction between gender and sexual orientation on one variable: Lesbians reported ideal weights that were closer to those on the life insurance charts than did heterosexual women, and gay men reported ideal weights that were lower and closer to the charts than did heterosexual men.

Gettelman and Thompson recruited 32 lesbians and 32 gay men from student organizations and friendship networks, plus 32 heterosexual women and 32 heterosexual men from undergraduate courses. Gay men and heterosexual women were more concerned with appearance, weight, dieting, and body image than were lesbians and heterosexual men. Similarly, Michael Siever conducted a study with 53 lesbians, 59 gay men, 62 heterosexual women, and 63 heterosexual men. He recruited all groups from the same university—a major methodological improvement over other studies. Relative to the other three groups, lesbians were less likely to feel that they or potential partners placed importance on various aspects of their own bodies. Lesbians also placed less importance on a partner's physical attractiveness than did heterosexual women.

In Siever's study, heterosexual men had the highest levels of body satisfaction and the lowest levels of body dissatisfaction and concerns about body shape. Heterosexual women had the highest levels of body dissatisfaction and concerns with body shape, and gay men had the lowest levels of body esteem. On measures of dieting, bulimia, and food preoccupation, heterosexual men scored the lowest and heterosexual women, the highest. This study is notable for finding a strong interaction between gender and sexual orientation on most measures. However, Siever mentions that the lesbian group had a significantly higher body mass index than the other groups, yet he did not control statistically for this difference. In short, lesbians were quite satisfied with their bodies despite weighing more than the other groups.

FACTORS MODERATING BODY IMAGES

Recent research has focused on investigating factors that might buffer lesbians from the weight concerns that so preoccupy heterosexual women. Jeanine Cogan recruited 181 women at a summer gay pride fair; 88% self-identified as lesbian and 12% as bisexual. The women reported that as they "came out" as lesbian or bisexual, they changed aspects of their appearance—for example, wearing more masculine clothing, wearing more comfortable clothing, cutting hair short, giving up beauty rituals, and dressing for oneself rather than for others. Other researchers have found that lesbians who were more involved in lesbian communities were less preoccupied with weight than lesbians who were more isolated. Nevertheless, there seems to be a discrepancy between what lesbians feel they are *supposed* to believe about body image acceptance and what they do feel. For example, Heffernan found lesbians to be more critical of traditional attitudes toward women than were heterosexual women, but this difference was not found for attitudes toward weight and appearance. Lesbians in this study viewed dieting as oppressive, yet about half the lesbians reported having dieted in the past 3 months, were dissatisfied with their weight, and had low body esteem. In the only study that included gay men as well as lesbians, Susan Beren and her colleagues found that affiliation with the gay community increased body dissatisfaction in men but was unrelated to lesbians' body satisfaction.

Interestingly, evidence that feminism serves as a buffer against negative body image has been mixed—lesbians who identify as feminist were found to be more satisfied with their bodies in one study but not in another. Another moderating variable for lesbians has been thought to be the emphasis on fitness. Bergeron and Senn found that physical condition and weight concerns were related to self-esteem in lesbians, whereas only weight concerns were related to self-esteem in heterosexual women. Jeanine Cogan found that the women in her sample reported exercising to maintain health and improve fitness rather than for weight control or to attract others.

MASCULINITY, FEMININITY, AND BODY IMAGE

In the 1950s, lesbian communities divided women into "butches" and "femmes," complete with specific-gender roles. During the women's movement of the 1970s, wearing androgynous, comfortable clothing, having short hair, and using no makeup constituted standard appearance for lesbians. Now there is a reemergence of butch and femme roles among lesbians, though with more fluidity and flexibility than previously. Thus, lesbians of different age cohorts may have different norms about appropriate and desirable ways to look like a lesbian.

Ludwig and Brownell recruited 188 lesbian and bisexual women via the Internet. Women who were feminine in their appearance reported lower body satisfaction than women who were masculine or androgynous; feminine women also rated their friends as more accepting of them and reported a greater likelihood of using their body to attract others. Additionally, women whose friends shared their sexual orientation had greater body satisfaction than those whose friends had a different sexual orientation. This study suggests that lesbians and bisexual women who are feminine in appearance may be subject to similar pressures as heterosexual women.

More recently, Devendra Singh and her colleagues recruited 100 lesbians and 58 heterosexual women via social networks. Lesbians identifying as butch reported more gender-atypical childhood behaviors than did lesbians identifying as femme, with heterosexual women having the least gender-atypical childhood behaviors. Even when the researchers controlled for differences in age and body mass index, lesbians identifying as butch had a higher masculine waist-to-hip ratio than did femmes or heterosexual women. Much more research is needed to examine the relationship between the butch and femme roles and lesbian body image.

METHODOLOGICAL ISSUES AND UNANSWERED QUESTIONS

It should be apparent that a major problem in most research on lesbian and gay male body image is the inconsistency in recruiting gay/lesbian versus heterosexual samples. Rarely are heterosexual and nonheterosexual samples recruited from the same sources. Even when both groups are recruited from the same college, students who join gay and lesbian groups may differ demographically from those who are part of the psychology subject pool, for example. Furthermore, sample sizes are often small, especially given the large numbers of dependent measures. I would urge researchers to use heterosexual brothers and sisters of gay men and lesbians, respectively, as comparison groups, in order to control for race/ethnicity, age, and parental socioeconomic status.

The lesbian and gay male communities have always had norms for physical appearance, and these norms have changed over time. Unlike members of other oppressed groups (e.g., Jews, African Americans) who may first become acculturated within their own group and only later are socialized (e.g., by schools, the media) into the dominant culture, lesbians and gay men are first socialized by the dominant culture and then need to find their communities. Physical appearance has been a major vehicle by which lesbians and gay men have identified "like others," and it continues to provide a sense of group cohesion and identity. In the case of the gay male communities, group identity may also be associated with body dissatisfaction and unrealistic standards of appearance.

This experience of biculturality may also explain the lack of consistent differences in body image satisfaction between lesbians and heterosexual women. The lesbian communities, at least in theory, frown on traditional standards of feminine beauty. Yet when it comes to thinness, lesbians are torn between their beliefs and their interactions with mainstream media, families of origin, and the work setting. More research on moderating factors in the lesbian communities is necessary to determine why some studies find lesbians more satisfied with their bodies and others do not. More focus on women who are in the process of coming out and affiliating with lesbian communities may help us understand the precise mechanisms that facilitate body acceptance versus those that do not differ from the heterosexual macrosociety. Finally, better measures that are normed on lesbian and gay samples may help us understand body image issues that are unique to sexual minority communities.

INFORMATIVE READINGS

Beren, S. E., Hayden, H. A., Wilfley, D. E., & Grilo, C. M. (1996). The influence of sexual orientation on body dissatisfaction in adult men and women. *International Journal of Eating Disorders, 20,* 135–141.—Gay men had more body dissatisfaction than heterosexual men, whereas lesbians did not differ from heterosexual women; affiliation with the gay community was associated with increased body dissatisfaction in gay men but was unrelated to body satisfaction in lesbians.

Bergeron, S. M., & Senn, C. Y. (1998). Body image and sociocultural norms: A comparison of heterosexual and lesbian women. *Psychology of Women Quarterly, 22,* 385–401.— Examined whether lesbian identity buffered women from societal pressures to be thin. Lesbians had more positive attitudes toward their bodies, felt more fit, and had less internalized sociocultural norms about weight than did heterosexual women.

Brand, P. A., Rothblum, E. D., & Solomon, L. J. (1992). A comparison of lesbians, gay men, and heterosexuals on weight and restrained eating. *International Journal of Eating Disorders, 11,* 253–259.—Women, regardless of sexual orientation, were more likely to diet and see themselves as overweight than were men.

Brown, L. S. (1987). Lesbians, weight, and eating: New analyses and perspectives. In Boston Lesbian Psychologies Collective (Eds.), *Lesbian psychologies: Explorations and challenges* (pp. 294–309). Urbana, IL: University of Illinois Press.—Argues that lesbians are less likely to have eating disorders because of fat activism and awareness of oppression in lesbian communities.

Cogan, J. C. (1999). Lesbians walk the tightrope of beauty: Thin is in but femme is out. *Journal of Lesbian Studies, 3,* 77–89.—Asked 181 lesbians and bisexual women about reasons for exercise, body image and satisfaction with weight, feminist identification, and change in appearance after coming out.

Dworkin, S. H. (1988). Not in man's image: Lesbians and cultural oppression of body image. *Women & Therapy, 8,* 27–39.—Speculates that lesbians face the same pressures as heterosexual women to be thin and appearance conscious, due to socialization as women.

Gettelman, T. E., & Thompson, J. K. (1993). Actual differences and stereotypical perceptions in body image and eating disturbance: A comparison of male and female heterosexual and homosexual samples. *Sex Roles, 29,* 545–562.—Compared lesbians, gay men, and heterosexuals on body image, weight, and dieting, and also asked them about "typical" lesbians, gay men, and heterosexuals on these variables.

Heffernan, K. (1999). Lesbians and the internalization of societal standards of weight and appearance. *Journal of Lesbian Studies, 3,* 121–127.—Compared lesbians and heterosexual women on body image, dieting, and self-esteem; involvement in lesbian, but not feminist, activities was a buffer for low body esteem for lesbians.

Herzog, D. B., Newman, K. L., & Warshaw, M. (1991). Body image dissatisfaction in homosexual and heterosexual males. *Journal of Nervous and Mental Disease, 179,* 356–

359.—Heterosexual men weighed more and desired a higher weight than did gay men.

Herzog, D. B., Newman, K. L., Yeh, C. J., & Warshaw, M. (1992). Body image satisfaction in homosexual and heterosexual women. *International Journal of Eating Disorders, 11,* 391–396.—Compared with heterosexual women, lesbians weighed more and were less concerned with weight and appearance.

Lahti, M. (1998). Dressing up in power: Tom of Finland and gay male body politics. *Journal of Homosexuality, 35,* 185–203.—Describes the role of Tom of Finland in contributing to the current-day "gay macho look" of the muscular male body build in gay male communities.

Ludwig, M. R., & Brownell, K. D. (1999). Lesbians, bisexual women, and body image: An investigation of gender roles and social group affiliation. *International Journal of Eating Disorders, 25,* 89–97.—Lesbians and bisexual women who viewed themselves as feminine had less body satisfaction than those who viewed themselves as masculine or androgynous.

Rothblum, E. D. (1994). Lesbians and physical appearance: Which model applies? In B. Greene & G. M. Herek (Eds.), *Psychological perspectives on lesbian and gay issues* (Vol. 1, pp. 84–97). Thousand Oaks, CA: Sage.—This review focuses on ways lesbians are viewed by the general public, the need for lesbians to adapt their appearance in order to be recognized by other lesbians, and how lesbians are affected by the appearance norms faced by heterosexual women.

Siever, M. D. (1994). Sexual orientation and gender as factors in socioculturally acquired vulnerability to body dissatisfaction and eating disorders. *Journal of Consulting and Clinical Psychology, 62,* 252–260.—Compared lesbian, gay, and heterosexual college students on measures of importance of physical attractiveness, body satisfaction, and eating disorders; heterosexual women scored highest and heterosexual men, the lowest.

Silberstein, L. R., Mishkind, M. E., Striegel-Moore, R. H., Timko, C., & Rodin, J. (1989). Men and their bodies: A comparison of homosexual and heterosexual men. *Psychosomatic Medicine, 51,* 337–346.—Gay men were more likely to exercise for physical attractiveness, consider appearance important, and show more body dissatisfaction than were heterosexual men.

Singh, D., Vidaurri, M., Zambarano, R. J., & Dabbs, Jr., J. M. (1999). Lesbian erotic role identification: Behavioral, morphological, and hormonal correlates. *Journal of Personality and Social Psychology, 76,* 1035–1049.—Compares lesbians identifying as butch versus femme to heterosexual women and finds butch lesbians higher on gender-atypical childhood behaviors, waist-to-hip ratio, saliva testosterone levels, and lower on desire to give birth.

Striegel-Moore, R. H., Tucker, N., & Hsu, J. (1990). Body image dissatisfaction and disordered eating in lesbian college students. *International Journal of Eating Disorders, 9,* 493–500.—Found few differences between lesbian and female heterosexual college students on disordered eating and self-esteem.

Taub, J. (1999). Bisexual women and beauty norms: A qualitative examination. *Journal of Lesbian Studies, 3,* 27–36.—Interviewed 74 bisexual women about how coming out as bisexual affected their behavior, thoughts, and feelings about beauty and appearance norms.

V

Body Image Dysfunctions and Disorders

31

A "Negative Body Image"
Evaluating Epidemiological Evidence

THOMAS F. CASH

DISSATISFACTION WITH SPECIFIC PHYSICAL CHARACTERISTICS

The answer to a common question posed by popular media and researchers alike—"How prevalent is a negative body image?"—presupposes an established definition of "negative body image." Unfortunately, there is no clear consensus on the meaning of this term. Typically it has been equated with "body (or body image) dissatisfaction." Accordingly, we refer to the percentage of people in some surveyed population who report dissatisfaction with certain physical characteristics (e.g., weight, shape, facial features, etc.). Thus, in this context, a negative body image means discontent with some aspect of one's physical appearance. An individual might convey on a questionnaire that she or he has some degree of dissatisfaction with one physical feature, even while indicating satisfaction with other physical attributes. In other words, there is *some* aspect of one's appearance that is negatively evaluated.

This type of data has several shortcomings as a representation of valid epidemiological information about negative body image. Nevertheless, Table 31.1 summarizes the prevalence rates cited most often. The data come from a series of large-sample surveys conducted in *Psychology Today* magazine—the first in 1972 by Berscheid and her colleagues, the second in 1985 that my colleagues and I conducted, and the third in 1996 by Garner. In each case, the magazine published a summary report the following year. Beyond offering descriptive information about discontent with specific physical fea-

269

TABLE 31.1. The Results of Three U.S. Surveys on Body Image:
Percentage of Respondents Dissatisfied with Specific Physical Characteristics

Disliked physical attributes	1972 survey		1985 survey		1996 survey	
	Men	Women	Men	Women	Men	Women
Mid-torso	36%	50%	50%	57%	63%	71%
Lower torso	12%	49%	21%	50%	29%	61%
Upper torso	18%	27%	28%	32%	38%	34%
Weight	35%	48%	41%	55%	52%	66%
Muscle tone	25%	30%	32%	45%	45%	57%
Height	13%	13%	20%	17%	16%	16%
Face	8%	11%	20%	20%	NA	NA
Overall appearance	15%	23%	34%	38%	43%	56%

Note. Based on data from Berscheid, Walster, and Bohrnstedt (1973); Cash, Winstead, and Janda (1986); and Garner (1997).

tures, these data are often cited as evidence of gender differences in body satisfaction and as documentation that a negative body image has become increasingly prevalent for both sexes over the past 25 years.

We should exercise caution in believing in the accuracy of the percentages in these surveys and in drawing conclusions from cross-survey comparisons for several reasons. First, samples were self-selected, consisting of those readers of *Psychology Today* motivated to complete and return by mail a lengthy survey. In addition, the preamble to each survey differed. For example, the 1985 survey explicitly encouraged readers to participate regardless of whether "you love your body or hate it." In contrast, the 1996 survey began by discussing the normative aspect of women's body dissatisfaction and related problems (e.g., eating disorders). Whereas the first two surveys analyzed data from a stratified sample selected to match the U.S. census on various demographics, the third survey did not; it was based on the first 4,000 surveys returned. Finally, item wording and scaling formats varied across the surveys. For example, in the 1985 survey body areas were evaluated on a six-point balanced scale, with three levels of satisfaction and three levels of dissatisfaction. The 1996 survey used an unbalanced five-point scale, with three levels of dissatisfaction and only two levels of satisfaction.

Cash and Henry published a more scientifically sound survey of women's body images in 1995. The study utilized representative U.S. population sampling and was conducted by experienced field research personnel. The 803 respondents were compensated for their anonymous completion of the consumer products survey, within which we embedded the validated Multidimensional Body Self-Relations Questionnaire (MBSRQ). The percentages of women reporting any degree of dissatisfaction with various body areas/attributes were: mid-torso—51%, lower torso—47%, upper torso—25%, weight—46%, muscle tone—37%, height—13%, and face—12%. Comparing these data with those in Table 31.1 reveals lower rates of discontent reported in this survey than in those in the 1996 and 1985 *Psychology Today* surveys.

DISSATISFACTION WITH OVERALL APPEARANCE

Focusing on specific physical features in defining negative body image does not capture the body image gestalt. Discontent with a part of the body does not necessarily mean wholesale body image dissatisfaction. Some people might dislike their lower torso or their nose yet retain overall feelings of attractiveness or physical acceptability. Other individuals might experience a single perceived flaw as undermining their overall appearance.

A second approach to defining negative body image assesses an evaluative gestalt based on either a single item of satisfaction–dissatisfaction with one's overall appearance or a composite scale with multiple, globally evaluative items. Although this approach seems to be more valid than the feature-focused method, it too has its limitations. The bottom row of Table 31.1 presents rates of overall appearance dissatisfaction derived from the three *Psychology Today* surveys.

Two extensive surveys in *Glamour* magazine, in 1984 and 1998, are sometimes cited in describing women's body image experiences. The results generated some interesting and quotable findings—for example, 44% of the respondents in 1998 (42% in 1984) said that losing weight would bring them more happiness than would getting a promotion, having a romantic evening, or hearing from an old friend. Of course, readers of this beauty magazine are hardly a representative sample. Moreover, the 1998 survey title included the exclamation "Your Chance to Vent!," certainly conveying a bias. The findings on overall evaluative body image revealed that whereas 41% of respondents reported being moderately or very unhappy with their bodies in 1984, the percentage had increased to 52% 14 years later. These percentages are comparable to the *Psychology Today* rates of women's overall appearance dissatisfaction for the years 1985 and 1996, respectively.

In Cash and Henry's (1995) survey of American women, overall body image was assessed by the Appearance Evaluation subscale of the MBSRQ. Overall body image dissatisfaction was reported by 48% of the sample— somewhat lower than the 1996 *Psychology Today* results, albeit using a different scale.

Smith and her colleagues also used the MBSRQ in a population-based biracial cohort as a part of an epidemiological investigation of 1,837 young men and 1,895 young women. Data were collected during 1992 and 1993. The researchers provided no percentage breakdowns with respect to favorable and unfavorable body images. However, the mean and standard deviation on Appearance Evaluation for the White women indicates that, assuming a normal distribution, approximately 39% of these women would score below the neutral point on the five-point scale, evincing a negative overall body image. These data again give us cause to question the accuracy of the magazine survey findings.

Finally, there is a growing literature comparing various demographic subpopulations on both overall and feature-focused body image. Other chapters in this volume discuss these findings in relation to African Americans, Asian Americans, Hispanic Americans, gay males and lesbians, and older persons.

HAVE BODY IMAGES WORSENED OVER TIME?

Despite the methodological concerns raised above, the three *Psychology Today* surveys are often cited as evidence that negative body images are increasing in both women and men. However, there are other sources of data that address this question. To date, most of these are cross-sectional studies.

In 1998 Feingold and Mazzella published an impressive cross-sectional meta-analysis of body image research, conducted from the pre-1970s to 1995, in which they examined gender differences on a range of evaluative body image measures as a function of when the data were collected. There were 222 coded studies; it should be noted that the *Psychology Today* surveys were excluded due to possible self-selection bias. Analyses confirmed that the effect sizes for gender grew significantly over time; that is, women and men became increasingly divergent in how they evaluated their appearance. The methodology of this meta-analysis precluded a separate evaluation of the sexes over time. However, analyses indicated that women became increasingly overrepresented among people with a poor body image. The authors concluded that, ruling out improvements in male body image over time, the results suggest either that women's but not men's body image has worsened or that both sexes' body images have worsened, with women's discontent increasing more steeply.

Heatherton and his colleagues surveyed 1,200 Radcliffe undergraduates in 1982 and 1992. Although the researchers' primary goal was to compare the two cohorts on weight, dieting, and eating-disordered symptoms, they included an assessment of participants' perceptions of their weight. Not only did results reflect a decline in a variety of eating-disordered symptoms over the decade, the women in 1992 were less likely than those in 1982 to consider themselves overweight (i.e., 31% vs. 42%, respectively), despite the fact that 1992 cohort was significantly heavier (5 pounds). Male cohorts showed few differences between 1982 and 1992.

In 1997 Heatherton and colleagues also published the 10-year longitudinal data from the 1982 cohort. They were able to retest 82% of the women and 76% of the men. Although the responding women had gained an average of 4 pounds over the decade, they reported a reduced drive to be thin and were much less likely to see themselves as overweight, to be dieting, or to desire to lose weight. Bulimic behaviors declined as well. Among the men, who had gained an average of 12 pounds over the decade, the opposite prospective findings occurred. The authors concluded that "body image dissatisfaction remains a problem for a substantial segment of the population" (p. 117).

April Perry and I recently conducted an unpublished cross-sectional investigation using over 15 years of archived MBSRQ data collected at the same university. Drawing from 21 studies that met specific inclusionary and exclusionary criteria, we constructed a sample of 2,192 male and female students who were 18–30 years old. We compared three race- and age-matched cohorts based on when data were collected: 1983–1990, 1991–1994, and 1996–1998. We examined four MBSRQ subscales: Appearance Evaluation, Body Areas Satisfaction, Overweight Preoccupation, and Appearance Orientation (i.e., cognitive-behavioral investment in appearance). Women's appearance evaluation, body satisfaction, and overweight preoccupation worsened significantly from the 1980s to the early 1990s but then improved significantly in the late 1990s. Furthermore, women became progressively less invested in appearance over the 15-year period. Men had a more positive body image and less appearance investment than did women at each time period, and men's body images remained relatively stable over the three periods. The only change was that men's overweight preoccupation declined subsequent to the 1980s. Obviously, we cannot be certain that our results are generalizable beyond this particular university population. Nevertheless, these findings and those from Heatherton's Radcliffe studies provoke interest in whether young women's body images actually might be improving.

TOWARD BETTER CONCEPTIONS OF NEGATIVE BODY IMAGE

Most research that quantifies negative body image using either definitional approach (i.e., dissatisfaction with body attributes or dissatisfaction with overall appearance) ignores the psychological significance and consequences of these negative body image evaluations. For example, were you to ask me how satisfied I am with my waist, I would admit to slight dissatisfaction—the result of an added inch in recent years that has rendered some of my older jeans a bit tighter than I prefer. However, my discontent has no effect on my emotional well-being, my functioning in social situations, or my ability to write this chapter. My waist size (so far) isn't particularly relevant to my sense of self. Of course, someone else might react differently to the same added inch. He or she might "feel fat," wear waist-concealing clothing, forgo or be less comfortable at beach parties, initiate a diet, or ruminate about other erosions of his or her physical appeal. Most attempts to quantify the prevalence of a negative body image neglect to assess (1) the psychological importance that people place in their evaluations of their appearance, and (2) the related impact of the evaluations vis-à-vis personal distress and adaptive functioning.

To address this consideration, Szymanski and I developed the Body Image Ideals Questionnaire (BIQ), guided by Higgins's self-discrepancy theory. In addition to asking respondents to evaluate how discrepant they are from their personal physical ideals (on height, weight, bodily proportions, overall appearance, etc.), the BIQ asks that they rate how important each of these ideals is to them. The latter ratings serve as mathematical weighting factors in calculating body image scores. In other words, among individuals with identical self–ideal discrepancy ratings, those who report greater investment in the attainment of their ideals would have more negative composite dissatisfaction scores. Our data indicate that these ratings enhance the BIQ's validity. Thus, in defining a negative body image continuum, it seems meaningful to ascertain the subjective importance individuals experience regarding the attainment of their physical ideals.

Although the BIQ's approach considers the psychological salience of one's body image satisfaction or dissatisfaction, it does not directly assess the impact of these evaluations on one's life. Impact can be considered in terms of cross-situational personal distress and maladaptation or dysfunctionality. Indeed, in 1992 Kevin Thompson proposed the following definition of what he termed "body image disorder": "A persistent report of dissatisfaction, concern, and distress that is related to an aspect of appearance. Some degree of impairment in social relations, social activities, or occupational functioning must be present" (see Thompson et al.'s *Exacting Beauty*, 1999, p. 11). He further proposed that severity be subcoded from mild to severe, that the physical focus of the concern be indicated, and that the "objectiveness" of the body image complaints be specified (i.e., from valid to delusional).

Three validated body image assessment measures take impairment (i.e., personal distress and psychosocial consequences) into account. First, in the Situational Inventory of Body-Image Dysphoria (SIBID), respondents rate how often they experience negative body image emotions in each of 48 situations (20 situations in the SIBID short form), including those pertaining to eating, exercising, grooming, intimacy, social comparisons, physical self-focus or body exposure, and changes in appearance. Thus SIBID scores reflect a continuum of personal body image distress frequency. (For more information, see my chapter on assessment of body image states.)

A second pertinent body image assessment is James Rosen's Body Dysmorphic Disorder Examination (BDDE), available in both interview and self-administered formats. Respondents complete the BDDE with reference to their most disliked physical characteristic. They use a series of six-point items to rate the importance of this attribute and associated experiences of emotional distress, avoidance, camouflaging, etc. As Phillips discusses in her chapter in this volume, the BDDE can be used in the criteria-based diagnosis of body dysmorphic disorder. Moreover, because it quantifies the continuum of body image dysfunction, the BDDE is valuable in taking us beyond a simple body dissatisfaction conception of negative body image.

Finally, Emily Fleming and I recently developed the Body Image Quality of Life Inventory (BIQLI) (Cash & Fleming, 2002) in order to incorporate the consideration of maladaptation. This instrument, which is also discussed in my subsequent chapter with Tom Pruzinsky, measures the extent of positive and negative consequences of one's body image on 19 facets of psychosocial functioning and well-being (e.g., self-concept, sexuality, social interactions, mood, life satisfaction, etc.). Although data with additional, more diverse samples are essential, our initial findings on the BIQLI with a sample of college women suggest that the percentage who report a negative impact of body image on the quality of life is considerably smaller than typical rates of "body dissatisfaction." For example, we found that 20% of these women reported that body image adversely affected satisfaction with life in general; 35% reported a negative impact on ability to control weight; and only 7% indicated negative effects on relationships with friends.

In sum, as is true of everything in science, the answers we obtain depend on how we ask the questions. I believe that cognitive questions about satisfaction or dissatisfaction with physical characteristics will produce a picture that inflates the prevalence rates of negative body image. Alternatively, assessments that ascertain affect-laden body image experiences and quantify the psychosocial consequences of these experiences provide a more accurate and clinically relevant picture. Unfortunately, we lack large-scale representative studies that provide such data on men, women, adolescents, and children. Greatly needed is a national, demographically diverse survey that administers standardized, reliable, and valid measures of multiple facets of body image and its impact on the quality of life. Of course, the scientific ideal would prescribe the continued, prospective collection of data on this sample.

INFORMATIVE READINGS

Berscheid, E., Walster, E., & Bohrnstedt, G. (1973, November). The happy American body: A survey report. *Psychology Today, 7,* 119–131.—Reports the results of this first in a series of three magazine-based surveys of body image.

Cash, T. F. (2001). *Body image assessment manuals and questionnaires.*—Available from the author's website at *www.body-images.com;* most of the author's body image assessments mentioned in this chapter are available here.

Cash, T. F., & Fleming, E. C. (2002). The impact of body-image experiences: Development of the Body Image Quality of Life Inventory. *International Journal of Eating Disorders, 31,* 455–460—Presents psychometric information on this tool for the assessment of the psychosocial impact of body image experiences.

Cash, T. F., & Henry, P. E. (1995). Women's body images: The results of a national survey in the U.S.A. *Sex Roles, 33,* 19–28.—Provides data from a 1993 representative survey of American women's body images.

Cash, T. F., Winstead, B. A., & Janda, L. H. (1986, April). The great American shape-up: Body image survey report. *Psychology Today, 20,* 30–37.—Reports the results of this second in a series of three magazine-based surveys of body image.

Feingold, A., & Mazzella, R. (1998). Gender differences in body image are increasing. *Psychological Science, 9,* 190–195.—Gives the results of an extensive meta-analysis of gender differences in body image evaluation over time.

Garner, D. M. (1997, January/February). The 1997 body image survey results. *Psychology Today, 30,* 30–44, 75–80, 84.—Reports the results of this third in a series of three magazine-based surveys of body image.

Heatherton, T. F., Mahamedi, F., Striepe, M., Field, A. E., & Keel, P. (1997). A 10-year longitudinal study of body weight, dieting, and eating disorder symptoms. *Journal of Abnormal Psychology, 106,* 117–125.—A prospective comparison of Radcliffe students in 1982 and 1992 that suggests favorable changes in weight-related body image and rates of eating disturbance for women but not for men.

Heatherton, T. F., Nichols, P., Mahamedi, F., & Keel, P. (1995). Body weight, dieting, and eating disorder symptoms among college students, 1982 to 1992. *American Journal of Psychiatry, 152,* 1623–1629.—A cross-sectional comparison of two Radcliffe College surveys that suggests favorable changes in weight-related body image and rates of eating disturbance over the decade.

Rosen, J. C., & Reiter, J. (1996). Development of the Body Dysmorphic Disorder Examination. *Behavior Research and Therapy, 34,* 755–766.—Presents evidence of the reliability and validity of this body image assessment, which is available from the author in structured interview and self-report versions.

Smith, D. E., Thompson, J. K., Raczinsky, J. M., & Hilner, J. E. (1999). Body image among men and women in a biracial cohort: The CARDIA study. *International Journal of Eating Disorders, 25,* 71–82.—An informative body image survey of nearly 4,000 black and white women and men.

Szymanski, M. L., & Cash, T. F. (1995). Body-image disturbances and self-discrepancy theory: Expansion of the Body-Image Ideals Questionnaire. *Journal of Social and Clinical Psychology, 14,* 134–146.—Presents evidence of the reliability and validity of this body image assessment, which is available from *www.body-images.com.*

Body Image and Social Relations

THOMAS F. CASH
EMILY C. FLEMING

Among its many functions, the human body is a "social object." Physical appearance distinctively identifies a person within his or her social world, conveying such basic information as gender, race, approximate age, and perhaps even socioeconomic or occupational information. Throughout history and across cultures, human beings have altered and adorned their outer appearance for purposes of social communication. As Jackson articulated earlier in this volume, physical appearance influences social perceptions and behaviors, often in accordance with social stereotypes. Whether due to cultural socialization (see Jackson's chapter) or to bioevolutionary processes (see Nancy Etcoff's *Survival of the Prettiest*), an individual's degree of physical attractiveness can shape personal and interpersonal experiences over the lifespan.

In this chapter we address the question of how the self-perception of physical appearance, or body image, influences one's social experiences and functioning. Body image is not isomorphic with physical attractiveness—we do not see ourselves as others see us. Physically attractive people are not necessarily satisfied with their appearance, nor are less comely people inevitably unhappy with their looks. Regardless of people's actual physical characteristics, their own perceptions, beliefs, and feelings about their appearance might determine how they *believe* others view them. If so, a positive body image would facilitate social confidence and comfort, whereas a negative body image would lead to social inhibition and anxiety.

"LOOKING-GLASS" REFLECTIONS

Symbolic interaction theorists, such as Charles Horton Cooley and George Herbert Mead, proposed that our self-concept emerges through our appraisals of how other people interact with us. Social interactions are the "looking glass" by which we come to form attitudes and beliefs, or images, about ourselves. Thus body image develops through an internalization of socially reflected appraisals. As discussed in several other chapters of this volume, appearance-related feedback that we receive from peers, family members, and others affects our body image experiences. Such feedback may be explicit—for instance, being teased about some physical characteristic—or implicit—such as receiving fewer compliments about appearance than a sibling receives, or having a parent who overvalues appearance or regularly frets about body image concerns.

The social feedback that contributes to body image creation is not a "one-way street" whereby we passively internalize others' reflected appraisals. Rather, the social influences on body image formation are more reciprocal and interactive. That is, while social feedback undoubtedly shapes individuals' own view of their appearance, these individuals' beliefs and behaviors can influence the nature of the social feedback they receive. For example, the phenomenon of attributive projection, by which individuals infer that others see them as they see themselves, can dramatically influence social cognition and behavior. A woman of average weight who is convinced that she is fat may automatically and habitually assume that others also see what she sees and that they privately agree that she needs to lose weight. This cognitive process will then likely result in certain social behaviors, such as making less eye contact, dressing in a dowdy fashion, or smiling less. In turn, such behaviors may decrease the frequency with which others approach her or compliment her—which she then interprets as "evidence" of her unattractiveness. What is "reflected" back to this individual has been created, at least in part, by her own beliefs and their derivative social behaviors.

Intriguing research conducted by psychologists Kleck and Strenta in 1980 illustrates some of this process. In one condition of their experiment, theatrical makeup was used to construct the appearance of a facial scar on female participants prior to their face-to-face interaction with a stranger. Unknown to the women, the "scar" was removed before the interaction began. The stranger, who did not know that the women had been led to think they had a scar, was actually a research confederate trained to act in a uniform way with all participants. Relative to women who did not believe they had this condition, the "scarred" women felt that the stranger saw them as less attractive. More importantly, during the interactions they "observed" that the stranger was socially uncomfortable and that the stranger's eye contact with them was adversely affected. These findings support the proposition that subjective body image affects how we cognitively and emotionally experience our social interactions. (For readers interested in these cognitive–social processes, consult the chapter by Williamson and colleagues on an information-processing perspective, Rumsey's and Pruzinsky's chapters on physical disfigurement, and Chapman's chapter on AIDS.)

BODY IMAGE, SOCIAL ANXIETY, AND SOCIAL SELF-ESTEEM

"Nonclinical" Evidence

What is the empirical evidence concerning relationships between body image and social functioning? Surprisingly, given the scientific and clinical importance of this question, the research literature is sparse. One answer comes from several studies that examine the associations between body image variables and individual differences in social anxiety. Over the years, in developing and validating new assessments of various aspects of body image attitudes, I (Cash) have routinely included established measures of social confidence or anxiety. Results have consistently confirmed moderately strong relationships between body image and social functioning. For example, the Body Image Ideals Questionnaire measures the extent of congruence–discrepancy between self-perceived and idealized physical attributes and the personal importance of these ideals. Cash and Szymanski discovered that college women (*n* = 284) with greater self–ideal discrepancies *and* with greater investment in attaining their physical ideals reported significantly higher levels of public self-consciousness and anxiety about social evaluation. Cash and Labarge found that women with dysfunctional beliefs about, and psychological investment in, their appearance (on the Appearance Schemas Inventory) had poorer social self-esteem, greater public self-consciousness, and higher levels of social anxiety.

Similarly, Cash, Theriault, and Annis observed significantly higher levels of social evaluative anxiety among 102 men and 125 women who reported less positive appearance evaluations, greater body dissatisfaction, and more dysfunctional appearance investment. Moreover, we found positive correlations between social anxiety and body image dysphoria in everyday contexts. Thus this study confirmed moderate associations between body image and social functioning for *both* sexes.

Clinical Evidence

A few investigations have examined body image and social functioning in relation to clinical body image disorders. Notably, in 1993 Striegel-Moore and her colleagues sought to understand the social disturbances in the lives of women with bulimia nervosa. Their review of the literature indicates that these women experience substantial "social anxiety, impoverished relationships, and social isolation . . . disturbances [that] do not seem to relate simply to eating pathology" (p. 297). The researchers first studied a sample of 222 women from combined college and community samples. Correlational evidence confirmed that women who were more dissatisfied with their bodies reported greater social anxiety, public self-consciousness, and a sense of self as a social imposter. Even after controlling for women's actual body weight, the associations between social concerns and body image remained significant. The researchers' second study compared three groups: 34 patients with bulimia nervosa, 33 women with high levels of eating disturbance (measured by the Eating Attitudes Test), and 67 matched controls. Relative to controls, the two eating-disturbed groups were more dissatisfied with their bodies, socially anxious, publicly self-conscious, and had a sense of self as more socially fraudulent. Although the causal connections among these variables cannot be ascertained, the findings are consistent with our view that the interplay of body image and social functioning is clinically important.

As Phillips and Olivardia discuss in their chapters in this volume, body dysmorphic disorder (BDD) reflects an excessive and distressing preoccupation with a minor or imagined defect in one's appearance. Accompanying this severe body image disturbance is considerable impairment in social self-concept and interpersonal functioning. Persons with BDD are intensely self-conscious in, and avoidant of, many social situations. In fact, Rosen has pointed to the phenomenological and behavioral similarities between BDD and social phobia. In her book *The Broken Mirror*, Phillips presents data on the comorbidities of BDD and other psychological disorders. Among those who meet diagnostic criteria for BDD, social phobia is second only to major depression as the most common comorbid condition; specifically, the current and lifetime co-occurrence rates are 26% and 36%, respectively. Noteworthy is the fact that these percentages reflect comorbidity rates with "primary" social phobia; cases in which the social anxiety and/or avoidance were judged to be symptomatic of BDD, per se, were excluded. Otherwise, as Phillips states, "the percentages would be much higher" (p. 336).

BODY IMAGE, SOCIAL INTERACTIONS, AND SOCIAL PERCEPTIONS

Thus far we have seen that body image attitudes are clearly related to individuals' reported comfort and confidence in their social relations. Recently, we developed a novel assessment tool to measure the extent to which people feel that their body image affects their life (including the quality of their social life). We found that evaluative body image was significantly positively related to its reported effects on social experiences. In descending magnitude of effect size, these social experiences included interactions with people of the other sex, meeting new people, interactions with friends and same-sex individuals, and relationships with family members.

Day-to-Day Interactions

Most evidence concerning body image and social functioning is in the form correlations among various trait-level scales answered at a single point in time. An alternative but seldom used approach examines how body image predicts the quality of social interactions over the course of everyday life. In 1999 Nezlek conducted such an investigation, employing the well-established Rochester Interaction Record (RIR), a methodology used previously by Reis and his colleagues to compare the day-to-day social interactions of physically attractive and unattractive people. After assessing evaluative body image among 66 women and 58 men, Nezlek had them use the diary-like RIR continuously for 3 weeks to monitor, code, and rate all their social interactions that lasted for 10 minutes or more. This naturalistic study confirmed that body image predicted the quality of social interactions. In general, individuals with a more positive body image experienced their day-to-day interactions (same- or other-sex) as more intimate. They also had feelings of greater confidence and influence in these interactions, an effect that was stronger for women than for men.

Women's Social Relations

A largely ignored topic of research is how body image influences relationships among women. If beauty is an especially valued commodity by women, which is sought, in part, to attract a mate and acquire other social reinforcers, then beauty becomes a criterion of competition among women. Beautiful women represent an object of upward social comparison and envy, as well as a reminder of one's own physical "shortcomings." Most women are familiar with the common ambivalent reactions to beautiful or thin women: "I hate you. You look so great." It logically follows that women who are highly psychologically invested in their appearance and in the cultural standards of beauty should be particularly ambivalent about attractive "competitors."

Recently, my students and I (Cash, Roy, & Strachan, 1997) developed the Women's Appearance Relations Scale (WARS) to assess women's attitudes toward other females based on physical attractiveness. The WARS measures three attitudes one might hold toward attractive women: antipathy and disparagement, salience and envy, and manipulativeness and competition. In a study of 185 college women, we found that these three attitudes were espoused to a greater extent by women who were more invested in their own appearance, aspired to cultural standards of beauty, were less satisfied with their own bodies, and held a more traditional view of male–

female relations. Thus, body image has important bearing on women's relationships with one another.

Romantic Relations

How does one's body image affect romantic relationships? As Wiederman articulates elsewhere in this volume, evaluative body image clearly influences the quality and quantity of sexual relations. My own recent research (Rieves & Cash, 1999) investigated 93 heterosexual couples in terms of their body images and perceptions of how their partners viewed them. Both sexes underestimated their partners' evaluations of their appearance, typically expecting partners' views to reflect their own body image evaluations. Also, the more they assumed that their partners' views of their appearance were positive, the more they were satisfied with their relationships, in general, and their sexual relationships, in particular. Of course, these data are not causally conclusive, but they do support the notion of attributive projection—the assumption that others, even intimate others, see us as we see ourselves.

BODY IMAGE AND INTERPERSONAL ATTACHMENT

Over 25 years ago, John Bowlby articulated and tested the profound ideas of attachment theory. In 1977 he noted that the attachment system was "the propensity of human beings to make strong affectional bonds to particular others" (p. 201). While early work in this area focused largely on parent–child attachment, recent years reveal a growing interest in the formulation of adult attachment models. Bartholomew and Horowitz, for example, have described four such prototypes:

1. *Secure* individuals have a sense of worthiness and lovability and are comfortable with intimacy and autonomy.
2. *Preoccupied* people lack this sense of worthiness yet seek others' love and acceptance.
3. *Fearful* people lack a sense of lovability and avoid others in anticipation of rejection.
4. *Dismissing* individuals feel worthy of love yet detach from others whom they generally regard as untrustworthy.

One can reasonably propose that attachment styles might have implications for body image experiences. Individuals who are insecure in attachment, whether due to self-perceived inadequacies or expectations of social rejection, may also be insecure about their physical worth and acceptability. Surprisingly little research has examined links between attachment styles and body image. Based on evidence that eating-disordered women display insecure attachments, Sharpe and her colleagues compared securely and insecurely attached preadolescent and adolescent girls with respect to their weight concerns. The results confirmed that, although the two groups judged themselves to be of equivalent size (on figural stimuli), the insecurely attached girls reported significantly more preoccupations about thinness and body shape. The authors suggested that insecure attachment may lead girls and young women to internalize and pursue societal appearance standards to attain a sense of self-worth and social acceptability. Thus insecure attachment may place them at risk for the development of eating disturbances.

In the aforementioned study by Cash, Theriault, and Annis, we examined associations between attachment styles and body image in male and female college students. We used a psychometrically sound assessment of attachment styles vis-à-vis social relationships in general and romantic relationships in particular, as well as measures of several body image dimensions. For both sexes, we found that general attachment security was significantly related to greater body satisfaction and less dysfunctional investment in one's appearance. Among Bartholomew and Horowitz's three styles of insecure attachment (i.e., preoccupied, fearful, and dismissing), only the preoccupied style, for both men and women, was significantly associated with greater body dissatisfaction, more dysfunctional investment in appearance, and more body image dysphoria across a range of situations. With respect to romantic relationships, men and women with a more anxious (preoccupied) attachment style reported more body image dissatisfaction, dysfunction, and dysphoria.

In 2000, Suldo and Sandberg investigated the relationship between these four attachment styles and eating-disordered symptomatology in 169 college women. They too found that only preoccupied attachment was predictive of the drive for thinness and bulimic behavior.

Although, again, we cannot infer causality from the above studies, the findings highlight the potential value of understanding body image experiences in relation to attachment processes. As Krueger discusses in his chapter on psychodynamic perspectives and Kearney-Cooke asserts in her chapter on familial influences, feelings about one's body may mirror one's securities and insecurities in human relationships (and vice versa).

CONCLUSIONS AND IMPLICATIONS FOR RESEARCH AND CLINICAL PRACTICE

The present review reveals that body image and social functioning are intertwined—conceptually, empirically, and experientially. We urge more scientific inquiry into how body image attitudes shape and are shaped by social relations and interpersonal experiences. Such research should include eating-disordered populations as well as other clinical/medical groups. In-

vestigators must consider the experiences of both sexes in a full range of social contexts, including same- and other-sex acquaintanceships, friendships,
and romantic relations. We need more naturalistic research, such as that conducted by Nezlek, to explore the roles of body image evaluation, investment, and emotions in everyday human relationships. We must continue to
elucidate how these specific parameters of body image impact social cognition, as people process information about their social interactions. We especially need studies that include observations of actual social behaviors. Furthermore, the investigation of linkages between body image and attachment
appears to hold promise. Because attachment processes may be fundamental to our understanding of the development of personality and personality
disorders (e.g., Theodore Millon's perspective, among others), we encourage
further research on body image experiences and personality disorders.

The prevention and treatment of body image disorders and discontentment must address the social contexts and consequences of these difficulties.
As Cash and Strachan discuss later in this volume, cognitive-behavioral
therapy (CBT) is an empirically validated treatment for body image disturbances. Clinical trials with CBT have confirmed that positive body image
outcomes following the administration of this approach generalize to improvements in social anxiety and social self-esteem. The issues and evidence
reviewed in the present chapter suggest the merit of turning even greater
therapeutic focus on the interpersonal aspects of body image. In their
interesting *Comprehensive Guide to Interpersonal Therapy* (IPT), Weissman,
Markowitz, and Klerman discuss published and in-progress research on IPT
with people who have eating disorders (e.g., studies by Fairburn and by
Wilfley) and individuals with body dysmorphic disorder. Controlled evaluations of the efficacy of IPT for body image change, per se, are clearly warranted.

Both medical and mental health practitioners encounter patients with
body image problems that vary in severity and impact on the quality of life.
The present chapter attests that, in their assessments and assistance of these
individuals, clinicians must pose a crucial question: "How does your body
image affect your life, particularly your social interactions and relationships
with other people?" The impact of body image on social relations is a potentially fertile topic for research and clinical intervention.

INFORMATIVE READINGS

Bartholomew, K., & Horowitz, L. M. (1991). Attachment styles among young adults: A test
of a four-category model. *Journal of Personality and Social Psychology, 61,* 226–244.—
Provides an informative overview of attachment and examines a specific model of
adult attachment.

Bowlby, J. (1977). The making and breaking of affectional bonds. *British Journal of Psychiatry, 130*, 201–210.—One of the author's many seminal works in the study of human attachment and its implications for psychosocial development.

Cash, T. F. (1997). *The body image workbook: An 8-step program for learning to like your looks.* Oakland, CA: New Harbinger.—Details a body image CBT program that includes specific interventions to improve how body image affects interpersonal relations and experiences.

Cash, T. F., & Fleming, E. C. (2002). The impact of body-image experiences: Development of the Body Image Quality of Life Inventory. *International Journal of Eating Disorders, 31*, 455–460.—Presents information on the psychosocial impact of body image experiences, including effects on social relations.

Cash, T. F., & Labarge, A. S. (1996). Development of the Appearance Schemas Inventory: A new cognitive body-image assessment. *Cognitive Therapy and Research, 20*, 37–50.—Presents evidence of the relationships between body image schemas and social functioning.

Cash, T. F., Roy, R. E., & Strachan, M. D. (1997). *How physical appearance affects relations among women: Implications for women's body images.* Poster presented at the convention of the American Psychological Society, Washington, DC.—Reports initial research using the Women's Appearance Relations Scale.

Cash, T. F., & Szymanski, M. L. (1995). The development and validation of the Body-Image Ideals Questionnaire. *Journal of Personality Assessment, 64*, 466–477.—Presents evidence of the relationships between body image parameters and social functioning.

Cash, T. F., Theriault, J., & Annis, N. M. (in press). Body image in an interpersonal context: Adult attachment, fear of intimacy, and social anxiety. *Journal of Social and Clinical Psychology.*—Confirms significant relationships between various facets of body image, attachment styles, and social anxiety.

Etcoff, N. (1999). *Survival of the prettiest: The science of beauty.* New York: Doubleday.—Presents a provocative, in-depth scientific treatise on sociobiological/evolutionary perspectives on how human appearance shapes lives.

Kleck, R. E., & Strenta, A. (1980). Perceptions of the impact of negatively valued physical characteristics on social interaction. *Journal of Personality and Social Psychology, 39*, 861–873.—A series of studies demonstrating that self-perceived "physical deviance" biases people's perceptions of their social interactions.

Nezlek, J. (1999). Body image and day-to-day social interaction. *Journal of Personality, 67*, 793–817.—Using a social interaction diary, findings indicate that evaluative body image is associated with qualitative aspect of social relations in everyday life.

Phillips, K. A. (1996). *The broken mirror: Recognizing and treating body dysmorphic disorder.* New York: Oxford University Press.—A comprehensive volume on body dysmorphic disorder and its profound effects on social functioning.

Rieves, L. C., & Cash, T. F. (1999). *Do you see what I see?: A study of actual and perceived physical appearance attitudes in romantic relationships.*—An unpublished investigation of the accuracy and impact of self- and partner-perceived body image among 93 couples.

Sharpe, T. M., Killen, J. D., Bryson, S. W., Shisslak, C. M., Estes, L. S., Gray, N., Crago, M., & Taylor, C. B. (1998). Attachment style and weight concerns in preadolescent and adolescent girls. *International Journal of Eating Disorders, 23*, 39–44.—Presents evidence that attachment styles may play a role in weight-related body image.

Striegel-Moore, R. H, Silberstein, L. R., & Rodin, J. (1993). The social self in bulimia nervosa: Public self-consciousness, social anxiety, and perceived fraudulence. *Journal of Abnormal Psychology, 102,* 297–303.—Supports the hypothesized relationship between social-self concerns and body dissatisfaction and bulimia nervosa.

Suldo, S. M., & Sandberg, D. A. (2000). Relationship between attachment styles and eating disorder symptomatology among college women. *Journal of College Student Psychotherapy, 15,* 59–73.—Reveals significant correlations between a preoccupied attachment style and higher scores on drive for thinness and bulimic behavior.

Szymanski, M. L., & Cash, T. F. (1995). Body-image disturbances and self-discrepancy theory: Expansion of the Body-Image Ideals Questionnaire. *Journal of Social and Clinical Psychology, 14,* 134–146.—Presents evidence of the interconnectedness of body image and social relations.

Weissman, M. M., Markowitz, J. C., & Klerman, G. L. (2000). *Comprehensive guide to interpersonal therapy.* New York: Basic Books.—An impressive volume that articulates and applies the basic framework that psychological disorders reflect influential interpersonal contexts.

33

Body Image and Sexual Functioning

MICHAEL W. WIEDERMAN

Sexual functioning involves the complex interplay of thoughts, feelings, physical processes, and behaviors. Accordingly, it seems obvious that body image, which represents the intersection of the physical body with cognitive and emotional activity, would be an important component of sexual functioning. Body image is likely to influence sexual functioning as well as be shaped by sexual experiences. Despite what might seem like an obvious notion, it is surprising how little research has been conducted on the relationship between body image and sexual functioning.

It is important to draw certain distinctions. *Body image* may include self-evaluation of overall physical attractiveness or "sex appeal," as well as specific perceptions and evaluation of one's own genitals. In turn, these possible aspects of body image may be experienced either as a general, enduring disposition or as a more transient effect of a particular sexual situation. For example, one individual may feel self-conscious about his or her overall appearance (or genitals) across sexual situations, whereas another person might experience such self-consciousness only in particular sexual settings or with certain partners.

Sexual functioning is also multiply construed and includes the extent of one's experience as well as how well one functions within any particular episode of sexual activity. To complicate matters, sexual functioning typically entails involvement with a partner. To the extent that there is overlap between one's body image and one's physical attractiveness to others, it may be difficult to determine the degree to which body image, per se, exerts direct effects on sexual functioning. Apparent relationships between body image and sexual functioning may instead be a function of the degree of physical attraction potential partners experience toward a particular individual.

These and other issues are discussed below; for sake of organization, they are discussed separately with regard to sexual experience versus immediate sexual functioning (within a sexual episode).

BODY IMAGE AND SEXUAL EXPERIENCE

Gaining interpersonal sexual experience requires both attracting a partner and being comfortable enough with one's body to bare it (or at least certain parts of it) to a partner. So (assuming that sexual experience with a partner is consensual) both physical attractiveness as well as comfort with one's body may influence sexual experience.

Logically, attractive people may have more sexual experience than unattractive people because of increased opportunity. Indeed, over the years, several researchers have found a generally positive relationship between physical attractiveness and sexual experience. However, physical attractiveness typically has been measured via self-report. So it may be more accurate to say that body image (in this case, self-evaluation of physical attractiveness) is positively related to sexual experience. Why is this an important distinction? Other research has shown that relationships between self-ratings of physical attractiveness and ratings performed by judges are typically small. There are a few obvious possibilities, then, for the generally positive correlation between self-rated attractiveness and sexual experience.

Perhaps viewing oneself as attractive results in greater confidence when interacting with potential partners, thereby leading to greater sexual experience. Conversely, perhaps greater sexual interest shown by potential and actual sexual partners leads individuals to view themselves as physically attractive. Of course, it is also possible that self-rated attractiveness and sexual experience do not have a causal relationship but rather are correlated because of their shared relationship with some third variable, such as social popularity or certain personality characteristics.

Gender is another important variable to consider when attempting to understand relationships between body image and sexual experience. Perhaps particularly in Western cultures, and among heterosexuals, a woman's appeal as a sexual partner appears to be heavily dependent on her role as a visual stimulus for her male partner. Compared to women, men's appeal as sexual partners may be more based on non-appearance-related characteristics such as personality, attentiveness, and sexual skill. The implication is that perhaps physical attractiveness and body image are more relevant to women's than to men's heterosexual experience.

Unfortunately, there has been a paucity of research that would illuminate possible gender differences in the relationships between physical attractiveness, body image, and sexual experience. In this regard, however, it is worth noting that those adolescent boys who mature earlier than their peers tend to be seen as more attractive by peers, have more positive body image, and have increased sexual experience. These relationships can be explained by increased testosterone levels in these boys, which leads to maturity of physical features (which, presumably, are seen as more attractive than immature features and therefore lead to a positive body image) and increased sexual drive. In contrast, adolescent girls who mature earlier than their peers tend to be the objects of male sexual attention and teasing, which often seems to lead to self-consciousness, negative body image, and perhaps disordered eating.

Assuming that physical attractiveness and body image are more important factors in women's sexual experience than in men's, Wiederman and Hurst studied the self-rated attractiveness of 192 female college students in relation to independent assessments of rated on physical attractiveness by a female and a male research assistant to provide an "objective" measure. Similar to previous research, these experimenter ratings of attractiveness were only weakly related to self-rated attractiveness. Finally, the women were privately weighed and their height measured so that an overall index of body size (body mass index) could be calculated.

In considering these aspects of physical attractiveness and body image as related to dating and sexual experience, a clear pattern emerged. Body size and experimenter ratings of attractiveness were consistently related to dating and sexual experience: Those respondents who were relatively thin and seen as attractive by the experimenters were most likely to be involved in a dating relationship and to have experienced a variety of sexual activities. Self-rated physical attractiveness, general body image satisfaction, avoidance of social situations due to body image concerns, and personal investment in one's physical appearance were relatively unimportant in explaining dating and sexual experience. The one notable exception occurred in regard to receiving oral sex. Here women's self-rated bodily attractiveness was one of the most prominent correlates. This finding likely indicates the importance of women's body satisfaction as a prerequisite for exposing the body to the scrutiny of a male partner who is performing oral sex.

We interpreted their findings to mean that, perhaps at least among young college women, physical attractiveness to men was more important in determining women's sexual experience than was women's body image. At this developmental stage, perhaps receiving male romantic or sexual attention is more important in determining dating and sexual experience than is how the young woman feels about her own body. This interpretation received additional support when we considered the respondents' sexual attitudes. Correlations between sexual attitudes and all of the measures of body size, attractiveness, and body image were small and not statistically significant. So it did not appear that larger women, or those rated as relatively unattractive, held comparatively more conservative or more negative sexual attitudes.

We also measured women's sexual self-schema and sexual esteem. Those individuals who scored highest on these measures indicated that they saw themselves as romantic, uninhibited sexually, and overall as "good" sexual partners. In contrast to dating and sexual experience, body size and experimenter ratings of attractiveness were unrelated to sexual self-schema and sexual esteem. However, self-rated attractiveness was positively related to both sexual self-schema and sexual esteem. The important issue was how the women saw themselves, rather than their actual size or attractiveness.

It is important to note that the research discussed thus far involved global evaluations of physical attractiveness and body image satisfaction. Wiederman speculated that such dispositional measures of body image may not be as predictive of sexual experience as a measure of body image self-consciousness during physical intimacy with a partner. It is conceivable that an individual might carry a negative body image, in general, yet when involved in a potentially sexual interaction tend not to focus on the negative body image, thereby making sexual decisions unaffected by body image. Conversely, another individual might carry a relatively positive body image, yet when involved in a potentially sexual interaction tend to focus on perceived deficits in physical appearance, perhaps because of the perceived scrutiny of an intimate partner.

To examine women's experience of body image concerns specifically within the context of physical intimacy with a partner, Wiederman developed a self-report questionnaire on which respondents could indicate the extent to which they felt self-conscious about their body size when physically intimate with a partner. In administering the new measure to two samples of college women, approximately a third of the respondents indicated experiencing body image self-consciousness at least "sometimes," and scores were moderately related to body size and more general body image satisfaction. Interestingly, however, even after statistically controlling for effects related to body size, general body image satisfaction, social avoidance due to body image concerns, and tendencies to feel anxious in sexual situations, scores on the new measure of body image self-consciousness during physical intimacy predicted dating and sexual experience, sexual esteem, sexual avoidance, and sexual assertiveness, each in the expected way. In their unpublished research, Cash and his colleagues have reported similar findings.

Taken as a whole, the pattern of limited research findings indicates that, at least among college women, it is important to make the distinctions between body image satisfaction and more objective physical attractiveness as well as between dispositional body image satisfaction and body image self-consciousness specific to instances of physical intimacy with a partner. One's physical attractiveness to others may contribute more to sexual opportunities and attention than does one's body image. However, how one views one's physical attractiveness may contribute to sexual assertiveness, pursuit of sexual experience, and comfort within interpersonal situations that may develop sexually.

BODY IMAGE AND IMMEDIATE SEXUAL FUNCTIONING

How might body image concerns affect sexual functioning within a specific episode? Sex therapists have long considered the phenomenon that Masters and Johnson termed "spectatoring." Traditionally this phenomenon was applied to men who experienced difficulty achieving or maintaining an erection; for such an individual in a sexual situation, concern over achieving and maintaining an erection would result in cognitive distraction from erotic stimuli, as he monitored the erectile functioning of his penis. Of course this monitoring, or spectatoring, would further reduce sexual functioning by mentally removing the distracted individual from the evocative cues of the sexual situation.

Although the classic notion of spectatoring was applied to men and erectile functioning, certainly it is possible to be cognitively distracted over a variety of issues while engaged in a sexual situation. For women, cognitive distraction is liable to interfere with sexual arousal, thereby inhibiting genital vasocongestion and subsequent vaginal lubrication. Attempted intercourse following such a situation is likely to be uncomfortable or painful for the woman. It is possible that, at least for women in Western cultures, concern over physical attractiveness and bodily appearance serves as the focus of a good deal of spectatoring that inhibits sexual arousal and interferes with sexual satisfaction. With this possibility in mind, Dove and Wiederman administered questionnaires to a sample of college women who were experienced in sexual intercourse. The respondents completed measures of general body image satisfaction, general tendency to engage in self-focus, general sexual attitudes, and sexual desire. We also constructed a self-report measure of the tendency to become cognitively distracted by appearance concerns while involved in a sexual interaction with a partner.

Even after statistically controlling for general body image satisfaction, general tendency to engage in self-focus, general sexual attitudes, and sexual desire, results indicated that the degree to which the respondents reported experiencing cognitive distraction due to appearance concerns was related to decreased sexual esteem, decreased sexual satisfaction and consistency of orgasms, and increased likelihood of pretending or "faking" orgasm with a partner. The measure of appearance concern was general in focus, but it is possible that concern over the appearance, smell, or taste of one's genitals serves as a specific form of cognitive distraction. In other words, one's genital body image satisfaction may be important to consider.

Reinholtz and Muehlenhard may have conducted the only study examining men's and women's perceptions of their own genitals and how such genital body image satisfaction is related to sexual experience. Interestingly, the degree to which respondents (college students) indicated liking their own genitals and worrying about their partners' reactions to their genitals was unrelated to having engaged in various genital sexual experiences. However, as expected, those students who indicated the greatest liking for their own genitals and the least worry associated with their partners' reaction to their genitals, reported the greatest satisfaction with receiving oral sex.

IMPORTANT QUESTIONS FOR FUTURE RESEARCH

As indicated at the outset, the existing research on possible links between body image and sexual functioning is sparse, leaving many questions unanswered. For example, previous research relies virtually exclusively on college respondents, particularly females, who are Caucasian and heterosexual. To what extent do these findings pertain to older respondents, those with more sexual and relationship experience, those with greater diversity of body sizes and types, and those from different ethnic groups and sexual orientations? Other research indicates that African American men seem to be more accepting and desirous of relatively larger women than are American men of European descent, and that lesbian women place less emphasis on physical appearance in sexual attraction than do gay men or heterosexual individuals (see chapters by Altabe and by Rothblum in this volume). To the extent that these characterizations are accurate, body size and body image may be less important in the sexual functioning of heterosexual men and African American and lesbian women than among white women, heterosexual women, and gay men.

One area of research that is entirely lacking would investigate links between sexual functioning and body size and body image within specific contexts. For example, no published research has included the distinction between the first sexual encounter with a new partner versus a sexual encounter with a longstanding and trusted partner. However, in one unpublished study, Yamamiya and Cash found that when having sex with a partner for the first time, women who were sexually self-conscious were more ambivalent/acquiescent sexual decision makers, more emotionally detached during sex, and more regretful and concerned about acceptance after sex. Another area to explore: What about the individual characteristics of specific sexual partners? Particular verbal or behavioral reactions to one's bodily appearance made by one's sexual partner may have an important influence on subsequent body image and sexual functioning, particularly with that partner. When such reactions do not have an effect, why not? Why are people more or less influenced by reactions of sexual partners to their bodily appearance? What effects do sexual experiences have on body image, both globally and specific to body image self-consciousness during sexual activity? With respect to prevention, what can be done to ensure that individuals do not develop body image self-consciousness during physical intimacy with a partner? What can be done clinically, once such self-consciousness interferes with sexual functioning?

CLINICAL IMPLICATIONS

The research on body image and sexual functioning, though limited, has important clinical implications. First, clinicians should be aware that body image concerns during physical intimacy with a partner may be salient for a substantial proportion of women, perhaps especially among those presenting for sex therapy, eating disorders, or relationship counseling. Individuals experiencing such concerns may not express them to a mental health professional, perhaps because they believe that their body is truly unappealing and there would be no point in broaching the issue with someone who could not "fix" their appearance. Clinicians should not assume that a large body size or a negative general body image necessarily leads to body image self-consciousness during physical intimacy with a partner, nor that a thin body or positive general body image ensures feeling uninhibited in sexual interactions. The potential effects of specific partners, particular settings, and certain sexual activities on body image sexual consciousness and sexual functioning should also be assessed.

Addressing body image in sex therapy, clinicians should consider graded exposure or systematic desensitization to the sexual situations or activities that prompt body image discomfort. To the extent that the individual experiencing self-consciousness during physical intimacy with a partner is engaging in "mind reading" by assuming that the partner finds his or her body unappealing, couple's counseling to clarify perceptions and expectations may be beneficial.

INFORMATIVE READINGS

Dove, N., & Wiederman, M. W. (2000). Cognitive distraction and women's sexual functioning. *Journal of Sex and Marital Therapy, 26,* 67–78.—A report of research on college women using a new measure of cognitive distraction about appearance concerns during sexual activity with a partner.

Ellison, C. R. (2000). *Women's sexualities: Generations of women share intimate secrets of sexual self-acceptance.* Oakland, CA: New Harbinger.—Only a small portion of this book addresses body image, but the respondents represent diversity with regard to age and ethnicity.

Regan, P. C. (1996). Sexual outcasts: The perceived impact of body weight and gender on sexuality. *Journal of Applied Social Psychology, 26,* 1803–1815.—Documents the sexual stigmatization of large individuals, particularly females.

Reinholtz, R. K., & Muehlenhard, C. L. (1995). Genital perceptions and sexual activity in a college population. *Journal of Sex Research, 32,* 155–165.—Perhaps the only research report on genital body image satisfaction and its relationship to sexual activities with a partner.

Stuart, R. B., & Jacobson, B. (1987). *Weight, sex, and marriage: A delicate balance.* New York: Norton.—Addresses the multiple levels at which weight and body image may function within intimate relationships.

Werlinger, K., King, T. K., Clark, M. M., Pera, V., & Wincz, J. P. (1997). Perceived changes in sexual functioning and body image following weight loss in an obese female population: A pilot study. *Journal of Sex and Marital Therapy, 23*, 74–78.—One of several studies demonstrating the generally positive change in sexual functioning following weight loss.

Wiederman, M. W. (2000). Women's body image self-consciousness during physical intimacy with a partner. *Journal of Sex Research, 37*, 60–68.—Presents a psychometrically sound self-report measure, albeit developed with two samples of college women.

Wiederman, M. W. (2001). "Don't look now": The role of self-focus in sexual dysfunction. *The Family Journal, 9*, 210–214.—Discusses the role body image self-consciousness may play in sexual dysfunction and how to treat it.

Wiederman, M. W., & Hurst, S. R. (1997). Physical attractiveness, body image, and women's sexual self-schema. *Psychology of Women Quarterly, 21*, 567–580.—Report of research examining the relationships among body image, physical attractiveness, and self-schemas related to sexuality among unmarried college women.

Wiederman, M. W., & Hurst, S. R. (1998). Body size, physical attractiveness, and body image among young adult women: Relationships to sexual experience and sexual esteem. *Journal of Sex Research, 35*, 272–281.—Report of research examining the relationships among body image, body size, and sexuality among unmarried college women.

34

Body Image and Anorexia Nervosa

DAVID M. GARNER

DIAGNOSTIC SIGNIFICANCE AND CLINICAL RELEVANCE

Body image disturbance is one of the most common clinical features attributed to anorexia nervosa. Most contemporary theories consider body dissatisfaction to be the most immediate or proximal antecedent to the development of anorexia nervosa. Empirical studies indeed confirm that a strong concern about physical appearance predates the onset of the disorder. Anorexia nervosa has also been explained in terms of a more fundamental perceptual deficit related to size estimation. This explanation has intuitive appeal because it provides an explanatory construct for the perplexing claim by many of these emaciated patients that they have a morbid fear of gaining weight because they "feel too fat." The importance of the body image construct is reflected in its inclusion in the diagnostic criteria for anorexia nervosa in the fourth edition of the *Diagnostic and Statistical Manual of Mental Disorders* (DSM-IV-TR; American Psychiatric Association, 2000): "an intense fear of gaining weight or becoming fat, even though underweight" and "disturbance in the way in which one's body weight or shape is experienced, undue influence of body weight or shape on self-evaluation, or denial of the seriousness of current low body weight" (p. 589).

This definition reflects the consensus at the time that the body image construct is multidimensional, involving perceptual as well as attitudinal components. Even though there is widespread acceptance that body image is a key contributor to anorexia nervosa, there have been authors who have argued that it is not diagnostically distinctive or that it is a largely culture-bound concept and should not be considered essential for a diagnosis. Nevertheless, there is mounting evidence that body image disturbance, operationalized by various measurement techniques, is a *useful* construct, as Cash and Deagle revealed in an extensive meta-analysis in 1997. Body image disturbance is believed to be an important risk factor for the development of anorexia nervosa. Even after weight restoration, the majority of anorexia nervosa patients continue to worry excessively about body weight and shape. Body image is a major predictor of relapse in anorexia nervosa, and patients who do recover report that it is one of the major impediments to lasting change. Although body dissatisfaction is one of the most relevant and immediately antecedent variables leading to the development of anorexia nervosa, body image therapy it is not included or stressed in many approaches to treatment.

There have been two primary lines of research into the specific nature and measurement of body image disturbance in anorexia nervosa. The first hypothesis proposes a perceptual body size distortion wherein the patient misperceives the actual size of her body. The second proposes a cognitive-evaluative disturbance composed of body dissatisfaction or disparagement. These two forms of body image disturbance have generally been conceptualized as independent processes and operationally defined via quite different methodologies.

PERCEPTUAL BODY SIZE DISTORTION

Clinical Relevance

More than 30 years ago, Hilde Bruch described distorted body size perception as a core feature of anorexia nervosa. The discrepancy between the patient's actual appearance and her mental picture of her body provides compelling clinical evidence for the presence of a perceptual disturbance. Despite an intellectual understanding that they are horribly underweight, many anorexia nervosa patients really do appear to overestimate their body size. This remarkable clinical observation has resulted in decades of research aimed at operationally defining and studying body size misperception in anorexia nervosa.

Whole Body versus Body Part Estimation

Clinical observations of body image disturbance in anorexia nervosa have led to at least two different operational measures of size misperception: (1) body part size estimation procedures that involve estimation of the width or depth of specific regions of the body (i.e., face, chest, hips, etc.), and (2) whole body techniques that involve the estimation of the whole body size, using a distorted image of the subject's own body. Cash and Deagle's meta-analysis revealed that whole body methodologies produced larger clinical control effect size differences than body part methods. According to this analysis, the average eating-disordered patient distorts her size to a greater extent than about 73% of controls. The explanation for the modest advantage of the whole body techniques is not clear but may relate to the fact that these methods involve direct exposure to one's self-image rather than the more indirect estimation the width of a particular body region. This focus may heighten the negative emotional experience related to body size and magnify the size distortion. In addition, according to this meta-analysis, perceptual distortion differences between eating-disordered and control subjects do not seem to reflect a generalized sensory-perceptual deficit because eating-disordered patients and controls do not differ in appraisals of object size.

Size Overestimation Is Common but Not Universal

The overall findings from the meta-analysis indicate that the body size overestimation tends to be "relatively weak, unstable, or nonpathognomic" (p. 177) among eating-disordered patients. The observation that size misperception is not unique to anorexia nervosa has led some to conclude that body size misperception should not be considered of any diagnostic significance. However, it has been argued by other researchers that it may be premature to abandon size misperception entirely in anorexia nervosa, because it has been shown to predict higher levels of psychopathology, including external loss of control, low ego strength, higher levels of depression, introversion, anxiety, physical anhedonia, atypical thinking, eating problems, prior treatment failure, lack of clinical progress, and poor clinical outcomes. Body size misperception is unstable in anorexia nervosa and can be triggered by negative mood states, viewing thin images of women in the media, and perceived overeating. Goals of future research include the search for better operational measures of body size misperception and understanding possible underlying psychological and neurobiological mechanisms of action.

Explanatory Constructs

Smeets and her colleagues have proposed two possible explanations of observed size overestimation in anorexia nervosa. The first is that size overestimation reflects pure visual misperception. In this case, the patient retrieves a fatter image of herself from visual memory, and her size estimations reflect this image. The second explanation attributes size misperception to the reconstruction of visual representations based on particular thoughts and feelings. In this case, distorting the size of the visual body image is a function of memory rather than perception. The inability of anorexic patients to "perceive" themselves accurately may be related to impaired hemispheric symmetry in storing visual representations of the body or impaired interhemispheric interaction, with reduced updating of body image in the right hemisphere by the left hemisphere, where it is maintained. The third explanation is based on the fact that overestimation may simply be an artifact related to absolute size being smaller. According to this notion, women with smaller bodies may be more prone to overestimation regardless of their level of eating pathology. This may be due to the fact that smaller sizes are inherently harder to estimate accurately (e.g., it may be harder to estimate the width of a pencil than a desk) because of the limited range for the distribution of estimation errors. These is some evidence that body size overestimation may be understood as a form of information-processing bias that reflects a cognitive judgment rather than a perceptual event. In this case, rather than having a fixed and distorted body image, anorexia nervosa patients may have a loose, unstable, or weak mental representation of their body, biased by reactivity to cultural ideals for beauty as well as cognitive and affective variables. There is some evidence for each of these explanatory constructs.

BODY DISSATISFACTION: COGNITIVE-EVALUATIVE FEATURES

Cultural, developmental, familial, and personality factors have been described as determinants of body dissatisfaction in anorexia nervosa. Both feminist and cognitive-behavioral perspectives on anorexia nervosa emphasize the cultural context in the formation of beliefs and feelings about appearance. Given the current cultural pressures for thinness, it is not hard to understand how women, particularly those with persistent self-doubts, could arrive at the conclusion that personal failings are related to weight, to some degree, or that the attainment of slenderness would measurably improve self-esteem. Moreover, anorexia nervosa is more common among women and in adolescence, at a time when conspicuous changes in body fat converge with increasing challenges from social and family environments. However, cultural pressures and body dissatisfaction clearly lead to the expression of eating disorders in only a small fraction of the population. Thus it is assumed that cognitive vulnerability to anorexia nervosa has its origins in certain personality and temperamental traits, such as obsessionality, perfectionism, rigidity, and harm avoidance, as well as variations in neuronal systems that influence cognitive style and information processing.

Nevertheless, one of the most striking features of anorexia nervosa is the supreme importance given to physical appearance and its connection to self-evaluation. The disorder most often develops out of the person's conviction of a perceived physical defect that can be corrected by restrictive dieting, exercise, and weight loss. Prospective studies have found that body dissatisfaction and dieting are significantly associated with the emergence of eating-disordered symptomatology as well as full-blown eating disorders. Body dissatisfaction translates into dysfunctional beliefs about weight and shape, such as, "Being thin is a sign of self-control and self-discipline" and "My self-worth is measured by how thin I am." It has been postulated that once these beliefs are kindled, basic reasoning and information-processing errors, such as selective attention, confirmatory bias, and cognitive rigidity, perpetuate them. (See the chapter by Williamson and colleagues in this volume.) The result is that certain idiosyncratic beliefs become inexorably tied to the positive and negative reinforcement contingencies associated with success or failure at weight controlling behaviors. Once weight loss is achieved, the process is further maintained by attitudinal, emotional, and physiological "starvation symptoms" that tend to sustain idiosyncratic beliefs and weight control behavior.

Body Dissatisfaction and Body Weight

According to studies of young women with and without eating disorders, one of the strongest predictors of body dissatisfaction is actual body weight. Nevertheless, the meaning of body dissatisfaction is more complicated in anorexia nervosa, because at the worst stage of their disorder, many patients are quite satisfied with, or even proud of, their emaciated shape. Body dissatisfaction may have been the impetus for weight loss, but once diagnostic criteria for anorexia nervosa are met, the average patient has a body dissatisfaction score on the Eating Disorders Inventory that is very similar to the average female college student. Clearly, body dissatisfaction must be interpreted within the context of actual body weight, since the same level of body dissatisfaction may have very different clinical implications for patients at different body weights. Body dissatisfaction may be a positive sign in anorexia nervosa if it reflects a desire to gain weight; however, if it indicates a wish to lose even more weight, it may denote even greater emotional disturbance.

Attitudinal versus Perceptual Measures

As Cash and Deagle point out, there have been fewer studies of body dissatisfaction than of perceptual distortion, perhaps reflecting researchers' belief that size overestimation is the central feature of eating disorders. Their meta-analytic results indicate that measures of attitudinal dissatisfaction yielded substantially larger effects (almost twofold) than those of body size distortion in overall eating clinical control comparisons. However, this effect is largely attributable to the bulimia nervosa patients. The magnitude of anorexia control effect size differences in body dissatisfaction is about one-half of that observed for bulimia nervosa.

Body Dissatisfaction Is Culture-Bound in Anorexia Nervosa

Although body dissatisfaction is clearly common among patients with anorexia nervosa, some scholars have mounted a compelling argument questioning the central and defining role of body dissatisfaction in the disorder. Although body dissatisfaction is one of the most common modes of entry into anorexia nervosa, early case descriptions and evidence from non-Western cultures indicate that some patients voluntarily reach an emaciated weight for a variety of psychological reasons but do not show the characteristic body dissatisfaction. Some of the earliest clinical descriptions of anorexia nervosa, dating back to the 19th century, do not even mention body dissatisfaction as a feature of the disorder. Cases of apparent anorexia nervosa in China and India lack indication of the "fear of becoming fat" or the body dissatisfaction so prominent in Western cases. Even in Western culture, research studies as well as clinical experience indicate that there is a small minority of patients who present with a very low weight but who deny body dissatisfaction at any point the development of their disorder. Some of these patients began restricting their food intake because of "spiritual" concerns, fears of choking, aversion to the texture of certain foods, food allergies, or a brief phase of physical illness. These cases have been typically classified as "atypical" or "eating disorder not otherwise specified"; however, these designations may be too restrictive. Robert Palmer has suggested changing the diagnostic criteria for the main eating disorders to emphasize persistent dietary restraint rather than body image disturbance. This alteration would broaden the diagnostic criteria for eating disorders to include many of the cases described in different cultures and at different points in time.

TREATMENT APPROACHES TO BODY IMAGE IN ANOREXIA NERVOSA

Treatment approaches to addressing body image disturbance in cases of anorexia nervosa can be divided into those aimed at perceptual distortion and those aimed at cognitive or attitudinal disturbances.

Distorted Body Size Perception

Various methods have been used in attempts to correct distorted body size perception in anorexia nervosa patients. One method has been to provide corrective feedback with the aim of improving accuracy over time. This approach can be executed in several ways. One strategy involves providing feedback on standardized measures of size estimation. Another involves directing patients to study their body in a mirror and try to develop a more objective or realistic view of their weight or shape. Some studies have shown that this exercise may have value in helping patients overcome denial of the severity of their disorder. However, most clinicians agree that directly changing body size perceptions plays a very limited role in the treatment of anorexia nervosa. It is not surprising that confronting patients with their own distorted self-perception has little therapeutic impact, since most patients have a long history of receiving feedback from friends, family, and therapists that they are too thin and must gain weight.

I prefer a cognitive approach aimed at reinterpreting the meaning of body size overestimation rather than trying to change it directly. I explain body size overestimation to patients as a perceptual anomaly that is similar to other situations where people are encouraged to *not* rely on a particular perceptual state but rather defer to a higher-order judgment regarding the perception—for instance, a person trying to decide whether or not to drive a car after drinking alcohol. Accordingly, patients are encouraged to view their body size misperception as an unfortunate perceptual disability, like that experienced by a color-blind person trying to coordinate her wardrobe. Thus it is preferable to rely on objective data or a trustworthy person rather than on self-perception to reach conclusions about actual body size. Body image usually does not improve early in the process of recovery from anorexia nervosa. In fact, it often becomes worse during weight gain. If body image does improve, it is often not until the later stages of recovery.

Body Dissatisfaction, Dysfunctional Attitudes, and Behavioral Disturbances

There has been remarkable advancement in recent years in the strategies and techniques created for treating body dissatisfaction in those at risk for eating disorders and in obese individuals. The application of these approaches to anorexia nervosa has been less fully developed. As mentioned earlier, those with anorexia nervosa are often more satisfied specifically because they have achieved a low weight. Treatment requires increasing weight and inadvertently but predictably increasing body dissatisfaction in the short term. The cognitive view of anorexia nervosa emphasizes the array of cognitive, emotional, and interpersonal adaptive functions that dietary restraint, weight loss, and other eating-disordered symptoms can serve. Accordingly, cognitive restructuring first focuses on identifying the idiosyncratic meaning that "being thin" and "weight control" has for the patient. Then the aim is to find more elegant personal and interpersonal solutions that do not require the lifelong physical, psychological, and interpersonal disadvantages of maintaining anorexia nervosa.

We have found that group therapy focused on the "appearance assumptions" from Cash's *Body Image Workbook* can be particularly useful as part of a cognitive-behavioral approach to therapy that has been adapted to include family therapy and interpersonal relationship themes. (See Cash and Strachan's chapter on cognitive-behavioral body image therapy.) Moreover, developing a more positive body image often involves avoiding certain self-defeating practices (e.g., weighing, looking in the mirror, wearing revealing clothing, and compulsive exercise) that provide short-term relief but become rituals that only accentuate anxiety, discontentment, and dysphoria. These can be replaced by body image enhancement activities (yoga, movement, pleasure walks, listening to music, massage by trusted friend) that emphasize the body as a source of pleasure rather than a vehicle for control, mastery, and self-definition.

INFORMATIVE READINGS

Cash, T. F. (1997). *The body image workbook*. Oakland, CA: New Harbinger.—A practical resource of assessment tools and detailed body image interventions based on a cognitive-behavioral approach.

Cash, T. F., & Deagle, E. A. (1997). The nature and extent of body-image disturbance in anorexia nervosa and bulimia nervosa: A meta-analysis. *International Journal of Eating Disorders, 22*, 107–125.—A key reference representing a quantitative distillation of more than 20 years of empirical literature on perceptual and attitudinal body image disturbance in eating disorders.

Cooper, M. (1997). Cognitive theory in anorexia nervosa and bulimia nervosa. *Behavioral and Cognitive Psychotherapy, 25*, 113–145.—A review of cognitive theory as applied to anorexia nervosa; existing models and the knowledge needed to understand the mechanisms that may influence body image and self-schemas are highlighted.

Garner, D. M., Vitousek, K., & Pike, K. (1997). Cognitive-behavioral therapy for anorexia nervosa. In D. M. Garner & P. E. Garfinkel (Eds), *Handbook of treatment for eating disorders* (2nd ed., pp. 94–144). New York: Guilford Press.—Provides the rationale for patients' enduring negative body image while they address the multiple personal and interpersonal functions that weight and shape can serve in maintaining the disorder.

Hermans, D., Pieters, G., & Edlen, P. (1998). Implicit and explicit memory for shape, weight, and food-related words in patients with anorexia nervosa and nondieting controls. *Journal of Abnormal Psychology, 107*, 193–202.—A comprehensive review of the literature and a promising experimental paradigm based on information-processing theory that indicates a strong explicit memory bias in anorexia nervosa.

Palmer, R. L. (1993). Weight concern should not be a necessary criterion for the eating disorders: A polemic. *International Journal of Eating Disorders, 14*, 459–465.—A controversial but pivotal theoretical treatise raising the major dilemmas in considering body dissatisfaction and concern about weight and shape as essential components in defining the two main eating disorders.

Rosen, J. C. (1997). Cognitive-behavioral body image therapy. In D. M. Garner & P. E. Garfinkel (Eds.), *Handbook of treatment for eating disorders* (2nd ed., pp. 188–201). New York: Guilford Press.—A well-organized and concise scholarly review of perceptual, cognitive, affective, and behavioral elements of body image therapy for eating disorders.

Sweets, M. A. M., Ingleby, J. D., Hoek, H. W., & Panhuysen, G. E. M. (1999). Body size perception in anorexia nervosa: A signal detection approach. *Journal of Psychosomatic Research, 46,* 465–477.—A scholarly analysis and experimental study aimed at clarifying the visual and cognitive mechanisms that are responsible for size overestimation in anorexia nervosa.

Thompson, J. K. (1996). *Eating disorders, obesity, and body image: An integrative guide to assessment and treatment.* Washington, DC: American Psychological Association.—A comprehensive text that provides an introduction to the body image area as well as scholarly reviews by leading authors in the field.

Thompson, J. K., & Smolak, L. (2001). *Body image, eating disorders, and obesity in youth: Assessment, prevention, and treatment.* Washington, DC: American Psychological Association.—Leading authors review a broad range of topics on current research, assessment techniques, and suggestions for treatment and prevention of body image disturbance in children and adolescents.

35

Body Image and Bulimia Nervosa

ERIC STICE

Bulimia nervosa is a prevalent and chronic psychiatric disorder associated with marked comorbid psychopathology. In addition, bulimic pathology increases the risk for subsequent onset of obesity, substance abuse, and major depression. Accordingly, it is important to elucidate the processes that result in the onset and maintenance of this serious psychiatric disturbance so that optimally effective preventive and treatment interventions can be developed.

Body image disturbances have emerged as one of the most potent risk factors for the development and maintenance of bulimia nervosa. The broad construct of body image disturbances refers to (1) internalization of the socioculturally prescribed body image ideal (thin-ideal internalization), (2) negative subjective evaluations of one's physical appearance (body dissatisfaction), and (3) distorted perceptions of body image (body image distortions). Body image disturbances should be distinguished from the overemphasis placed on weight and shape in determining self-worth, which is a symptom of bulimia nervosa. The importance of understanding the adverse effects of body image disturbances is underscored by the fact the majority of women in Western cultures report at least moderate body dissatisfaction. This chapter describes the theoretical accounts of the origins and consequences of body image disturbances, summarizes extant empirical findings, notes conceptual and methodological limitations of this literature, discusses clinical implications of these findings, and suggests potentially profitable directions for future research.

THEORETICAL ACCOUNTS

Body image disturbances are thought to arise primarily in response to sociocultural pressures to be thin and from physical deviation from the current cultural thin-ideal. Pressure to be thin emanates from a variety of sources, including the mass media, families, and peers. These pressures take numerous forms, such as glorification of ultraslender fashion models, direct messages that one should lose weight (e.g., weight-related teasing), and indirect influences to conform to the ideal (e.g., a friend's persistent obsessions about weight and appearance). The results may include an internalization of the current thin-ideal, elevated investment in appearance, and a generalized belief that attainment of thinness will result in a plethora of social and interpersonal benefits (e.g., greater personal acceptance and enhanced career success). Pressures to be thin and their internalization are thought to promote body dissatisfaction because this ideal is virtually unattainable for most individuals. Moreover, elevated adiposity is theorized to contribute to body dissatisfaction because of its disparity from an ultrathin figure. As Williamson and his colleagues discuss in this volume, heightened internalization of the thin-ideal is thought to foster information-processing biases that result in body image distortions.

Body image disturbances, in turn, increase the risk for bulimic pathology through two hypothesized mechanisms. The most widely accepted account is that body image dissatisfaction and distortion result in elevated dieting because of the common belief that this is an effective weight control technique. Dieting, in turn, increases risk for onset and maintenance of bulimic pathology because individuals may binge eat to directly counteract the effects of caloric deprivation. Dieting might also promote binge eating because violating strict dietary rules can result in overeating (i.e., the abstinence-violation effect). Moreover, dieting requires a shift from relying on physiological cues to enforcing a cognitive-driven control over eating behaviors; this shift leaves individuals vulnerable to overeating when these cognitive processes are disrupted, possibly due to intense emotions.

In addition to the putative dietary pathway that progresses from body image disturbances to bulimic pathology, theorists have suggested a negative affect regulation pathway. Specifically, body image dissatisfaction distortions are thought to contribute to negative affect because appearance is a central evaluative dimension for females in Western culture. Elevated negative affect, in turn, is thought to increase the risk of binge eating for those individuals who binge in an effort to provide comfort and distraction from adverse emotions. Individuals might also use radical compensatory behaviors, such as vomiting, to reduce anxiety about weight gain consequent to overeating or because they believe that purging serves as an emotional catharsis.

EMPIRICAL FINDINGS

Accumulating empirical findings support the assertion that sociocultural pressures foster internalization of the thin-ideal, body dissatisfaction, and body image distortions. First, perceived pressure to be thin correlates positively with thin-ideal internalization, body dissatisfaction, and body image distortions. Second, several prospective studies confirm that perceived pressure to be thin predicts increased body dissatisfaction. Third, randomized experiments indicate that exposure to media-portrayed thin-ideal images and interpersonal pressure to be thin result in increased body dissatisfaction. Finally, experimental evidence confirms that an intervention that decreases internalization and endorsement of the thin-ideal significantly reduces body dissatisfaction.

There is also support for the proposition that elevated adiposity contributes to body image disturbances. First, body mass correlates positively with body dissatisfaction. Second, elevated body mass prospectively predicts increases in body dissatisfaction. Finally, controlled randomized trials indicate that successful weight loss interventions result in improved body satisfaction.

There is mounting evidence that body image disturbances, in turn, are related to increased bulimic pathology. Cross-sectional studies have documented that individuals with bulimia nervosa from clinical and community samples report elevated thin-ideal internalization, investment in appearance, body dissatisfaction, and body image distortions relative to non-eating-disordered individuals. Although bulimic individuals typically overestimate their body size, a sensory deficit does not appear to be the cause. Rather, the overestimation seems to be due to attitudinal disturbances rooted in an internalization of the thin-ideal. Furthermore, differences between individuals with bulimia nervosa and those without eating disorders are much stronger for body dissatisfaction than for body image distortion. Prospective studies have also documented that initial elevations in body dissatisfaction increase the risk for subsequent onset and increases in bulimic pathology. In a recent meta-analytic summary, Stice found that the average prospective effect for body dissatisfaction in the prediction of bulimic pathology was a correlation of .19, making it the second most potent predictor of increases in bulimic pathology (second only to dieting). Finally, interventions that reduce body dissatisfaction result in decreases in bulimic pathology. Thus there is consistent prospective and experimental support for the assertion that body image disturbances increase the risk for bulimic pathology.

Research supports the contention that body image disturbances give rise to dieting—which, in turn, increases the risk for bulimic pathology. First, cross-sectional studies reveal significant correlations among the variables of body dissatisfaction, body image distortions, dieting, and bulimic pathology. Second, initial elevations in body dissatisfaction predict subsequent increased dieting. Third, dieting predicts the onset of, and subsequent increases in, bulimic pathology. In support of the assertion that dieting mediates the relation between body dissatisfaction and bulimic pathology, Stice found that a prospective relation from body dissatisfaction to increases in bulimic symptoms became nonsignificant when the effects of change in dieting were controlled.

The suggestion that negative affect may mediate the relation between body image disturbances and bulimic pathology also has support. First, body dissatisfaction, body image distortions, negative affect, and bulimic symptoms are positively correlated. Second, prospective studies have found that initial elevations in body dissatisfaction predict increases in negative affect and onset of depression. Third, negative affect predicts increases in bulimic pathology, although this relation has not been observed in some longitudinal studies. My meta-analysis indicates that the average effect of negative affect on bulimic pathology is weaker than that for dieting ($r = .14$ vs. $r = .21$, respectively), which may partially explain why this effect is less consistently observed. Still, as Cash and Strachan review in this volume, interventions that reduce body dissatisfaction result in decreased negative affect. In direct support of the negative affect mediational hypothesis, Stice found that a significant relation between initial body dissatisfaction and subsequent increases in bulimic symptoms became nonsignificant when the effects of change in negative affect were statistically controlled.

Although numerous studies have tested whether body image disturbances increase risk of bulimic pathology, few investigations tested whether these factors predict maintenance of bulimic symptoms. A distinction between risk and maintenance factors is important. The former are germane to the design of prevention programs, whereas the latter are relevant to the design of optimally effective treatments.

Wilson and colleagues have found that initial elevations in body dissatisfaction attenuate the effects of cognitive-behavioral therapy for bulimia nervosa—the current treatment of choice for this disorder. However, this relation has not been replicated in other investigations. Nevertheless, testing whether elevations in a factor impede the effects of a treatment program is not isomorphic with testing whether elevations in this factor predict persistence of pathology in a community sample of eating-disordered individuals. There is evidence that most individuals with bulimia nervosa do not seek treatment and those who do evince greater psychiatric disturbances. Thus, findings from treatment studies concerning the factors that predict persistence of bulimic pathology may not generalize to the larger population of individuals with bulimia nervosa.

Two studies examined the predictors of bulimic symptom persistence using data from nonclinical samples. Stice and Agras found that initial elevations in body dissatisfaction predicted persistence, versus remission, of bulimic symptoms over time. Although a study by Fairburn and colleagues did not directly assess body dissatisfaction, they did find that weight and shape concerns predicted an increased risk for the persistence of bulimic symptoms in individuals who met criteria for bulimia nervosa at baseline. These data provide preliminary support for the assertion that body dissatisfaction may play an important role in the maintenance of bulimic pathology.

CONCEPTUAL AND METHODOLOGICAL LIMITATIONS

Perhaps the most serious conceptual limitation of this body of research is that few theorists have considered the possibility that some third variable may explain the relation of body image disturbances to dieting, negative affect, and bulimic pathology. Because most pertinent studies were correlational or prospective, they cannot rule out the possibility that some other variable accounts for the observed findings. For example, a tendency toward caloric overconsumption may result in elevated adiposity, social pressure to be thin, body dissatisfaction, dieting, and eventual onset of bulimic pathology. Alternatively, the observed relation between body dissatisfaction and eating pathology may arise solely from the fact that attitudinal internalization of the thin-ideal produces both of these outcomes—that is, there may be no causal relation between body image and eating disturbances. Accordingly, it would be useful if more careful theoretical consideration were given to the possibility that some third variable could explain the relation of body image disturbances to these putative precursors and sequelae.

A second conceptual shortcoming is that few researchers have considered the possibility that body dissatisfaction is reciprocally related to dieting, negative affect, and bulimic pathology. For example, episodes of binge eating might lead an individual to feel more negatively about his or her body. Similarly, negative affect might be associated with a negative information-processing bias that results in body image distortions.

A third conceptual limitation is the paucity of theoretical work concerning factors that may potentiate or mitigate the relation of body image disturbances to dieting, negative affect, and bulimic pathology. For instance, elevated self-esteem in a domain that is independent of appearance, such as academic or artistic pursuits, may render individuals more resilient to the adverse effects of the sociocultural pressure to be thin. One exception to this trend is the evidence that the adverse effects of exposure to media-portrayed thin-ideal images are stronger for individuals with initial elevations in thin-ideal internalization and body dissatisfaction. Tiggemann's chapter in this volume addresses this topic.

Among the methodological limitations of this literature is the under-utilization of prospective designs. Because it is not possible to use cross-sectional data to differentiate a precursor from a consequence of body dissatisfaction, such studies do not permit inferences regarding the nature of observed effects and therefore do little to advance our understanding of these relations. Prospective studies permit greater inferential confidence regarding the putative direction of effects between variables.

A second methodological limitation is the rarity of randomized experiments. Even prospective studies do not rule out third-variable explanations. Accordingly, greater use should be made of experiments that manipulate suspected causes of body image disturbances. Similarly, experiments that manipulate body image disturbances should be used to establish the consequences of these disturbances. Various laboratory-based experiments have successfully manipulated the variable of social pressure for thinness and documented adverse consequences on body dissatisfaction. It is also possible to use randomized prevention trial methodology to determine the effects of reducing body image disturbances on putative consequences.

Third, many studies have used unrepresentative samples, such as college students or patients from clinical settings, which limits the generalizability of findings. Greater use should be made of community-recruited samples.

Finally, some researchers have used measures with questionable reliability or validity. For example, the Restraint Scale has been found to be *uncorrelated* with actual caloric intake and to predict *increases* in weight over time and thus does not appear to tap dietary restraint, as implied by the scale's name.

CLINICAL IMPLICATIONS

This body of literature has several implications for prevention efforts. First, interventions that reduce sociocultural pressure to be thin or that render individuals more resilient to these pressures may prove useful in reducing body image disturbances. For example, Posavac and colleagues found that brief interventions that helped women become more critical consumers of media buffered them from adverse effects of exposure to thin-ideal images. Second, interventions promoting healthy weight management skills (e.g., regular moderate exercise and reduced fat consumption) might decrease body dissatisfaction by lowering obesity. Indeed, in one preliminary experiment by our research group, a healthy lifestyle intervention produced increased body satisfaction. Third, eating disorder prevention programs might be strengthened by inclusion of a module to decrease thin-ideal internalization, body dissatisfaction, and body image distortions. Fortunately, cognitive-behavioral interventions exist that effectively achieve these aims, as this volume's chapters by Cash and Strachan and by Winzelberg and his colleagues attest. Modules in eating disorder prevention interventions that reduce unhealthy dietary restriction and negative affect—factors that appear to increase the risk for subsequent onset of bulimic pathology—might prove useful.

Because so few studies have tested whether body dissatisfaction predicts maintenance of bulimic pathology, treatment implications from this review are tentative. Nonetheless, available data suggest that treatment interventions for bulimia nervosa might be improved by a more explicit focus on reducing body image disturbances. Although cognitive-behavioral therapy for bulimia nervosa focuses on reducing overvaluation of shape and weight in determining self-worth, directly targeting body dissatisfaction, thin-ideal internalization, and body image distortions may further improve treatment outcome. Cash and Strachan discuss this issue in their chapter in this volume. In addition, it is important to assess the specific facets of body image disturbances for each patient to facilitate treatment planning so that the areas of greatest disturbance can be targeted.

DIRECTIONS FOR FUTURE RESEARCH

In sum, greater use should be made of prospective and experimental studies when investigating the precursors and consequences of body image disturbances because this would permit far greater inferential confidence. Randomized prevention trials that target one specific factor may offer a powerful way of experimentally investigating the hypothesized relations. More research should be directed toward elucidating factors that promote body image disturbances and those that mitigate or potentiate the predictors and consequences of body image disturbances. In a related vein, research should consider the possibility there are qualitatively different routes from body image disturbances to bulimic pathology (e.g., a dieting pathway versus an affect regulation pathway). Exploratory data analytic techniques, such as classification tree analysis, may prove useful for addressing these questions. Finally, more research should examine the maintenance role of body image disturbances in bulimic pathology. Although impressive advances have been made in understanding the precursors and consequences of body image disturbances, many questions remain unanswered.

INFORMATIVE READINGS

Cash, T. F., & Deagle, E. A. (1997). The nature and extent of body-image disturbances in anorexia nervosa and bulimia nervosa: A meta-analysis. *International Journal of Eating Disorders, 22,* 107–125.—A comprehensive review of body image disturbances among eating-disordered individuals.

Cash, T. F., & Strachan, M. D. (1999). Body images, eating disorders, and beyond. In R. Lemberg (Ed.), *Eating disorders: A reference sourcebook* (pp. 27–36). Phoenix, AZ: Oryx

Press.—An overview of evidence for the effectiveness of cognitive-behavioral body image therapy for body dissatisfaction, including the implications of its use in treating eating disorders.

Cattarin, J. A., & Thompson, J. K. (1994). A three-year longitudinal study of body image, eating disturbance, and general psychological functioning in adolescent females. *Eating Disorders: Journal of Treatment and Prevention, 2,* 114–125.—One of only a few prospective examinations of the risk factors for body image disturbances.

Cooley, E., & Toray, T. (2001). Body image and personality predictors of eating disorder symptoms during the college years. *International Journal of Eating Disorders, 30,* 28–36.—A prospective study documenting body image disturbance as a risk factor for eating pathology.

Fairburn, C. F., Stice, E., Cooper, Z., Doll, H. A., Norman, P. A., & O'Connor, M. E. (in press). Understanding persistence of bulimia nervosa: A five-year naturalistic study. *Journal of Consulting and Clinical Pschology.*—A community-based investigation of the maintenance factors that predict persistence of bulimia nervosa.

Field, A. E., Camargo, C. A., Taylor, C. B., Berkey, C. S., Roberts, S. B., & Colditz, G. A. (2001). Peer, parent, and media influences on the development of weight concerns and frequent dieting among preadolescent and adolescent girls and boys. *Pediatrics, 107,* 54–60.—An epidemiological investigation of the risk factors for body image disturbances.

Irving, L. M., DuPen, J., & Berel, S. (1998). A media literacy program for high school females. *Eating Disorders, 6,* 119–131.—Description and evaluation of a media literacy intervention designed to increase adolescent girls' resilience to sociocultural pressures.

Killen, J. D., Taylor, C. B., Hayward, C., Haydel, K. F., Wilson, D. M., Hammer, L., Kraemer, H., Blair-Greiner, A., & Strachowski, D. (1996). Weight concerns influence the development of eating disorders: A 4-year prospective study. *Journal of Consulting and Clinical Psychology, 64,* 936–940.—One of the most rigorous investigations of risk factors for bulimic pathology.

Posavac, H. D., Posavac, S. S., & Weigel, R. G. (2001). Reducing the impact of media images on women at risk for body image disturbance: Three targeted interventions. *Journal of Social and Clinical Psychology, 20,* 324–340.—An evaluation of preventive interventions designed to make women more resilient to the adverse effects of exposure to thin-ideal media.

Stice, E. (2001). A prospective test of the dual pathway model of bulimic pathology: Mediating effects of dieting and negative affect. *Journal of Abnormal Psychology, 110,* 124–135.—A prospective evaluation of an etiological model of bulimia nervosa that centers on body image disturbances.

Stice, E., & Agras, W. S. (1998). Predicting onset and cessation of bulimic behaviors during adolescence: A longitudinal grouping analysis. *Behavior Therapy, 29,* 257–276.—A prospective investigation of the risk factors that predict onset of bulimic pathology.

Wilson, G. T., Loeb, K. L., Walsh, B. T., Labouvie, E., Petkova, E., Liu, X., & Waternaux, C. (1999). Psychological versus pharmacological treatments of bulimia nervosa: Predictors and processes of change. *Journal of Consulting and Clinical Psychology, 67,* 451–459.—One of the most comprehensive investigations of the predictors of response to bulimia nervosa treatment.

Body Image and Body Dysmorphic Disorder

KATHARINE A. PHILLIPS

Body dysmorphic disorder (BDD), also known as dysmorphophobia, is a fascinating disorder of body image that has been described around the world for more than a century. BDD appears to be relatively common in the general population and in psychiatric, dermatological, and cosmetic surgery settings. Still, it is underrecognized in many clinical settings and has received relatively little scientific study.

According to criteria in the *Diagnostic and Statistical Manual of Mental Disorders*, fourth edition (DSM-IV), BDD entails a preoccupation with an imagined defect in appearance; if a slight physical anomaly is present, the person's concern is markedly excessive. This preoccupation must cause clinically significant distress or impairment in social, occupational, or other important areas of functioning, and it cannot be better accounted for by another mental disorder, such as anorexia nervosa. In DSM-IV, BDD is classified as a somatoform disorder. Its delusional variant is classified as a psychotic disorder—a type of delusional disorder, somatic type. A patient with delusional BDD would receive diagnoses of both BDD and delusional disorder.

CLINICAL FEATURES

Appearance Preoccupations

Individuals with BDD are preoccupied with the idea that some aspect of their appearance is unattractive, deformed, or "not right" in some way, when in reality the perceived flaw is minimal or nonexistent. Preoccupations commonly involve aspects or features of the face or head, most often the skin, hair, or nose (e.g., acne, scarring, thinning hair, or a large or crooked nose). However, any part of the body can be the focus of concern. "Muscle dysmorphia" is a type of BDD in which individuals (usually men) worry that their body build is small and puny, when in reality they are typically large and muscular.

BDD preoccupations are distressing, time consuming, and typically difficult to resist or control. Clinical observations and research findings suggest that the preoccupations are usually associated with low self-esteem, shame, embarrassment, unworthiness, and fear of rejection. Most patients either have poor insight or are delusional, not recognizing that the flaw they perceive is actually minimal or nonexistent. A majority has ideas or delusions of reference, thinking that others take special notice of the supposed defect, staring at it, talking about it, or mocking it.

Repetitive Behaviors

Nearly all individuals with BDD perform repetitive, often time-consuming, and compulsive behaviors, the usual intent of which is to inspect, hide, obtain reassurance about, or fix the perceived defect. Among these behaviors are excessively checking the perceived flaw in mirrors, other reflecting surfaces, or directly; excessive grooming; camouflaging the perceived deformity (e.g., with hair, makeup, body position, or clothing); seeking reassurance; comparing with others; and skin picking (i.e., picking at minor blemishes in an attempt to improve their skin's appearance). Although the goal of such behaviors is to diminish the anxiety provoked by the body image concerns, these behaviors often increase and maintain the anxiety.

Complications

BDD often causes severe distress and markedly impaired social and occupational/academic functioning. In a study by Phillips and Diaz of 188 patients with BDD, more than a quarter of them had been completely housebound for at least one week, more than half had been psychiatrically hospitalized, and nearly 30% had attempted suicide. A 1997 study by Cotterill and Cunliffe of dermatology patients who committed suicide found that most had acne or BDD. Quality of life is notably poor for these individuals; in the only study of this topic, patients with BDD had poorer mental health-related quality of life than reported for patients with type II diabetes, a recent myocardial infarction, or depression.

Demographic Features, Comorbidity, and Course of Illness

Some clinical series of patients with BDD contain more men than women, whereas others contain more women than men. In the largest published series (Phillips & Diaz), 51% were men. BDD affects people of all ages, usually beginning during adolescence and occurring even in childhood. Little has been published on race/ethnicity and BDD, although it is known that the disorder, reported around the world, may affect individuals of any race. In most studies, a majority of patients have never been married.

Most BDD patients seen in psychiatric settings have other mental disorders, most commonly major depression, a substance use disorder, social phobia, or obsessive–compulsive disorder. A majority of patients has a personality disorder, most often avoidant personality disorder.

BDD appears to usually be chronic, although the course is more favorable when patients receive appropriate treatment. Prospective studies are needed to better elucidate the disorder's course over time.

Prevalence

BDD appears to be relatively common but underdiagnosed in psychiatric settings. BDD is particularly common in patients with atypical depression, social phobia, and obsessive–compulsive disorder. In cosmetic surgery settings, BDD rates of 6%, 7%, and 15% have been reported. In 2000, Phillips and colleagues found that among patients seeking dermatological treatment, 11.9% of them screened positive for BDD.

CASE EXAMPLE

Ms. A, a 26-year-old single white female, presented with the chief complaint: "I look ugly and deformed." She was obsessed with many aspects of her appearance, including her "crooked" nose, "ugly" eyes, "pimply" skin, "bushy" facial hair, and "fat" thighs. She estimated that she thought about her perceived appearance flaws for 10 hours a day and checked them in mirrors for 5 hours a day. She repeatedly sought reassurance about how she looked from family members but could not accept reassurance that she looked normal. She also compulsively compared herself with other people, applied makeup for hours a day, picked her skin with pins, covered her face with her hand, and tweezed her facial hair. As a result of her appearance concerns, she had dropped out of high school. After getting her GED, she enrolled in college classes but could not take a full course load because her obsessions distracted her from studying and because she felt too self-conscious and ugly to go to class. Ms. A avoided friends, dating, and most other social interactions. She was chronically suicidal and had attempted suicide because, as she said, "I'm ugly and I look like a freak."

BODY IMAGE DISTURBANCE IN BDD

Despite the fact that body image dysphoria is a central feature of this disorder, little is known about body image disturbance in BDD. In a 1982 study by Hardy, compared to normal controls, patients with BDD were less satisfied with their body image and more likely to feel that their body was unacceptable. In a recent study, when rating the attractiveness of photos, including their own, patients with BDD overestimated the attractiveness of beautiful faces and underestimated their own attractiveness. And in a Stroop study, patients with BDD selectively attended to words like "beauty," indicating a preoccupation with their beauty ideal.

Regarding body image distortion, it is not known whether patients' views of their appearance have a basis in abnormal sensory (perceptual) processing or in attitudinal/cognitive-evaluative dissatisfaction. Clinical observations suggest that at least some individuals with BDD have abnormal sensory processing, perhaps experiencing a visual illusion or hallucination. However, preliminary empirical reports do not support the presence of a primary sensory-processing deficit. To the contrary, persons with BDD may have even better discriminatory ability than normal controls. In a 1995 study by Thomas and Goldberg, BDD patients' assessments of facial proportions were more accurate than those of normal controls or cosmetic surgery patients. Another pilot study, by Jerome in 1991, similarly suggested that BDD patients may have a more accurate perception of nose size and shape than normal controls.

Individuals with BDD have been found to have deficits in verbal and nonverbal memory, compared to normal controls. The deficits seem to be due to organizational (i.e., executive) dysfunction that entails overfocusing on minor or irrelevant stimuli. This finding raises the question of whether appearance-related beliefs in BDD arise from hyperattentiveness to minor, isolated details rather than attention to overall appearance.

ASSESSING BDD

Reasons for the underrecognition and underdiagnosis of BDD include the disorder's past omission from the DSM, patients' tendency to seek nonpsychiatric treatment (e.g., cosmetic surgery), and, perhaps most importantly, patients' reluctance to reveal their appearance concerns because of embarrassment and shame. Several studies that investigated BDD's prevalence in clinical populations found that the patient's clinician missed the diagnosis of BDD in all cases in which it was present. The best approach to diagnosing BDD is to specifically ask every patient the questions listed below, which follow the diagnostic criteria for BDD, and to be alert to the clues listed below. Unless BDD is specifically asked about, the diagnosis is likely to be missed.

BDD can be diagnosed with the following questions:

- Are you very worried about your appearance in any way? *If yes*: What is your concern?
- Does this concern preoccupy you? Do you think about it a lot and wish you could worry about it less? If you added up all the time you spend thinking about your appearance each day, how much time do you think it would be?
- What effect has this preoccupation with your appearance had on your life? Has it interfered with your job (or schoolwork), your relationships or social life, other activities, or other aspects of your life? *If yes*: How has it interfered?
- Have your appearance concerns caused you a lot of distress? *If yes*: How much?
- Have your appearance concerns affected your family or friends? *If yes*: How?

BDD is diagnosed if the person is preoccupied with minimal or nonexistent appearance flaws. A useful guideline is whether the person thinks about the perceived flaw for at least an hour a day. Clinically significant distress or impairment in functioning must be present for the diagnosis to be made. Clues to the diagnosis include mirror checking or avoidance, comparing one's appearance with that of others, seeking reassurance about the perceived flaw(s), excessive grooming (e.g., hair combing or shaving), skin picking, camouflaging, frequent clothes changing, frequent body measuring, excessive exercising or weightlifting, seeking unnecessary dermatological treatment or surgery, and anabolic steroid use. Additional clues include ideas or delusions of reference, being housebound, and symptoms of depression, anxiety, panic attacks, social anxiety, and/or self-consciousness.

Several instruments are available for diagnosing BDD. I have included some of these in my 1996 book, *The Broken Mirror*. The Body Dysmorphic Disorder Diagnostic Module is a reliable semistructured clinical interview with a format similar to that of the Structured Clinical Interview for DSM-IV (SCID-P). This instrument has the advantages of brevity and strict adherence to DSM-IV criteria. The Body Dysmorphic Disorder Questionnaire (BDDQ) is a brief self-report version of this scale that has good sensitivity and specificity for the BDD diagnosis. The Yale–Brown Obsessive–Compulsive Scale modified for BDD (BDD-YBOCS) is a 12-item measure of current BDD severity that is reliable, valid, and sensitive to change. Advantages include its brevity, suitability for assessing BDD symptoms of any degree of severity, and the fact that ratings do not depend on the specific content of BDD symptoms. Instead it uses constructs such as time spent preoccupied or performing compulsive behaviors. This last advantage, however, may also be a disadvantage, in that it does not assess the specific content of appearance concerns and associated behaviors. The Body Dysmorphic Disorder Examination (BDDE), developed by James Rosen, is a semistructured clinical interview that both diagnoses and assesses the severity of BDD. It has good reliability, validity, and sensitivity to change. Advantages include its assessment of both the presence and severity of BDD and its evaluation of multiple content domains (e.g., negative evaluation of appearance, excessive importance given to appearance in self-evaluation, checking behaviors, and avoidance of activities). Disadvantages of the BDDE include its omission of certain features of the disorder (e.g., skin picking), the fact that it is relatively time-consuming to administer, and its suitability only for patients with milder BDD.

PATHOPHYSIOLOGY AND ETIOLOGY

BDD's pathoetiology has received little investigation and is currently unknown. Family history data, while limited, indicate that BDD occurs in 6–10% of first-degree family members, which is almost certainly higher than in the general population, suggesting that BDD is familial. Neuropsychological studies indicate that BDD's pathogenesis may involve executive dysfunction, implicating frontal–striatal pathology. Available treatment data, while offering only indirect evidence about etiology, suggest a role for serotonin. In several case reports, BDD symptoms were worsened by serotonin antagonism. Perceptual abnormalities may be present, the neuroanatomical and neurochemical bases of which require elucidation.

BDD's pathoetiology is likely multifactorial, with neurobiological, evolutionary, sociocultural, and psychological factors playing a role. A study by Phillips and colleagues conducted in 1996 found that BDD patients reported receiving poorer parental care than normal controls. It seems plausible that frequent criticism of, or teasing about, one's appearance would be a risk factor for BDD, but potential risk factors such as this have not been studied.

TREATMENT

Pharmacotherapy

Case reports, case series, open-label studies, and several controlled studies indicate that serotonin reuptake inhibitors, also referred to as SRIs or SSRIs, are often effective for BDD and more effective than other psychotropic medications. SRIs currently marketed in the United States are fluvoxamine (Luvox), fluoxetine (Prozac), paroxetine (Paxil), citalopram (Celexa), sertraline (Zoloft), and clomipramine (Anafranil). In two open-label studies of the SRI fluvoxamine, 19 (63%) of 30 subjects and 10 (67%) of 15 subjects responded. A double-blind crossover study of 40 patients (29 of whom were randomized) found that clomipramine was superior to desipramine, a non-SRI antidepressant. In the only placebo-controlled pharmacotherapy study of BDD ($n = 74$), I found that the SSRI fluoxetine was more effective than placebo. It appears that relatively high SSRI doses are often needed to effectively treat BDD.

Although fluvoxamine, clomipramine, and fluoxetine are the best studied SRIs in BDD treatment, clinical experience suggests that all of the SRIs may be effective. Of note, SRIs also appear effective for delusional BDD. Although other psychotropic medications have been less well studied, available evidence suggests that they are generally ineffective for BDD when used as single agents. However, certain medications (e.g., buspirone) may be useful as adjunctive agents in combination with an SRI.

Cognitive-Behavioral Therapy

Cognitive-behavioral therapy (CBT) also appears effective for BDD. Exposure (e.g., to avoided social situations) and response prevention (e.g., not seeking reassurance) as well as cognitive techniques have been used in most published studies. In a 1993 report by Neziroglu and Yaryura-Tobias, four of five patients improved in 90-minute individual sessions conducted 1 day or 5 days per week (with the total number of sessions ranging from 12 to 48). A report of 13 patients published by Wilhelm and colleagues in 1999 found that BDD significantly improved in patients who participated in 12 90-minute group therapy sessions. In a 1995 study by Rosen and colleagues, 8 weekly 2-hour group sessions of CBT were effective for 77% of 27 women, and CBT produced greater improvement than shown by untreated patients on a waiting list. In this study (the only study to my knowledge to assess change in body image in BDD patients with treatment), compared to subjects on the waiting list, those who received CBT also had greater improvement on the Multidimensional Body Self-Relations Questionnaire Appearance Evaluation scale, which assesses feelings of physical attractiveness or unattractiveness and satisfaction or dissatisfaction with one's looks. In Veale and colleagues' 1996 controlled study of 19 patients, individual CBT resulted in significantly greater improvement than no treatment, with seven of nine patients no longer meeting criteria for BDD. In a 1999 case series, published by McKay, 10 patients treated individually in an intensive behavioral therapy program, which included a 6-month maintenance program, maintained their improvement after 2 years.

Other Treatments

The efficacy of other types of therapy for BDD has not been well studied, although limited data suggest that supportive psychotherapy and insight-oriented psychotherapy are generally ineffective for BDD, when used alone. Clinical experience suggests, however, that these treatments may have a useful adjunctive role in combination with an SRI and/or CBT.

A majority of BDD patients seen in a psychiatric setting have sought and received nonpsychiatric treatment, most commonly dermatological treatment and cosmetic surgery. Although the efficacy of these treatments has not been studied prospectively, available data suggest that they are usually ineffective and may even worsen appearance concerns.

FUTURE RESEARCH

Although research on BDD is rapidly increasing, it is still limited and at an early stage. Investigation of virtually all aspects of this disorder is imperative. Greatly needed are placebo-controlled pharmacotherapy studies, psychotherapy studies using an attention-control group or an alternative treatment, and studies of the combination of psychotherapy and pharmacotherapy. Nearly all treatment studies have been short term; continuation and maintenance studies are essential to elucidate longer-term outcomes.

Because body image disturbance is likely central to BDD's pathophysiology and maintenance, it is a key area for future inquiry. Neuroimaging studies are needed, as are other approaches to investigating the temporal and occipital lobes, which process facial images and (along with the parietal lobes) are involved in neurological disorders involving disturbed body image. Psychological and sociocultural contributors to BDD must be investigated, as knowledge of this disorder's pathogenesis may ultimately guide much-needed treatment and prevention strategies.

ACKNOWLEDGMENTS

This chapter was adapted in part from K. A. Phillips (2002). Body image and body dysmorphic disorder. In C. G. Fairburn & K. D. Brownell (Eds.), *Eating disorders and obesity: A comprehensive handbook* (2nd ed., pp. 113–117). New York: Guilford Press. Copyright 2002 by The Guilford Press. Adapted by permission.

INFORMATIVE READINGS

Cotterill, J. A., & Cunliffe, W. J. (1997). Suicide in dermatological patients. *British Journal of Dermatology, 137*, 246–250.—An important clinical report on a series of patients who committed suicide and were in treatment with a dermatologist.

Hardy, G. E. (1982). Body image disturbance in dysmorphophobia. *British Journal of Psychiatry, 141*, 181–185.—An early study of body image disturbance in BDD.

Hollander, E., Allen, A., Kwon, J., Aronowitz, B., Schmeidler, J., Wong, C., & Simeon, D. (1999). Clomipramine vs. desipramine crossover trial in body dysmorphic disorder: Selective efficacy of a serotonin reuptake inhibitor in imagined ugliness. *Archives of General Psychiatry, 56*, 1033–1039.—The first controlled pharmacotherapy study of body dysmorphic disorder.

Jerome, L. (1991). Body size estimation in characterizing dysmorphic symptoms in patients with body dysmorphic disorder (letter). *American Journal of Psychiatry, 36*, 620.—An unpublished study of perception of nose size and shape in BDD patients.

McKay, D. (1999). Two-year follow-up of behavioral treatments and maintenance for body dysmorphic disorder. *Behavior Modification, 23*, 620–629.—The only report, to my knowledge, on maintenance treatment for BDD and longer-term outcomes of treated patients.

Neziroglu, F. A., & Yaryura-Tobias, J. A. (1993). Exposure, response prevention, and cognitive therapy in the treatment of body dysmorphic disorder. *Behavior Therapy, 24*, 431–438.—One of the first reports of CBT for patients with BDD, a strength of which is its relatively detailed description of the patients and treatment provided.

Phillips, K. A. (1991). Body dysmorphic disorder: The distress of imagined ugliness. *American Journal of Psychiatry, 148*, 1138–1149.—The first comprehensive review of body dysmorphic disorder.

Phillips, K. A. (1996). *The broken mirror: Recognizing and treating body dysmorphic disorder.* New York: Oxford University Press.—The most comprehensive source of information on body dysmorphic disorder for both professionals and lay audiences; it includes assessment instruments.

Phillips, K. A. (2000). Quality of life for patients with body dysmorphic disorder. *Journal of Nervous and Mental Disease, 188*, 170–175.—The only paper on quality of life in patients with body dysmorphic disorder.

Phillips, K. A., & Diaz, S. (1997). Gender differences in body dysmorphic disorder. *Journal of Nervous and Mental Disease, 185*, 570–577.—An investigation of gender similarities and differences in the largest published series of patients with DSM-IV BDD.

Phillips, K. A., Dufresne, Jr., R. G., Wilkel, C., & Vittorio, C. (2000). Rate of body dysmorphic disorder in dermatology patients. *Journal of the American Academy of Dermatology, 42*, 436–441.—To my knowledge, this is the only published report on the rate of BDD in patients seeking dermatological treatment.

Phillips, K. A., McElroy, S. L., Keck, Jr., P. E., Pope, Jr., H. G., & Hudson, J. I. (1993). Body dysmorphic disorder: 30 cases of imagined ugliness. *American Journal of Psychiatry, 150*, 302–308.—The first descriptive series of body dysmorphic disorder using modern assessment methods.

Phillips, K. A., Steketee, G., & Shapiro, L. (1996). Parental bonding in OCD and body dysmorphic disorder. *New Research Program and Abstracts.* New York: American Psychiatric Association 149th annual meeting, p. 261.—An unpublished study of parental bonding, using the Parental Bonding Instrument, in patients with BDD.

Pope, H. G., Phillips, K. A., & Olivardia, R. (2000). *The Adonis complex: The secret crisis of male body obsession.* New York: Free Press.—An overview of body dysmorphic disorder, muscle dysmorphia, and eating disorders in men for professionals and lay readers.

Rosen, J. C., & Reiter, J. (1996). Development of the body dysmorphic disorder examination. *Behaviour Research and Therapy, 34,* 755–766.—A report on the development and psychometric properties of one of the few instruments developed to assess BDD.

Rosen, J. C., Reiter, J., & Orosan, P. (1995). Cognitive-behavioral body image therapy for body dysmorphic disorder. *Journal of Consulting and Clinical Psychology, 63,* 263– 269.—One of the two controlled psychotherapy studies of body dysmorphic disorder.

Thomas, C. S., & Goldberg, D. P. (1995). Appearance, body image and distress in facial dysmorphophobia. *Acta Psychiatrica Scandinavica, 92,* 231–236.—One of the few studies on body image distortion in BDD.

Veale, D., Gournay, K., Dryden, W., Boocock, A., Shah, F., Willson, R., & Walburn, J. (1996). Body dysmorphic disorder: A cognitive behavioural model and pilot randomized controlled trial. *Behaviour Research and Therapy, 34,* 717–729.—One of the two controlled psychotherapy studies of body dysmorphic disorder.

Wilhelm, S., Otto, M. W., Lohr, B., & Deckersbach, T. (1999). Cognitive behavior group therapy for body dysmorphic disorder: A case series. *Behaviour Research and Therapy, 37,* 71–75.—A report of group therapy for BDD, which is a useful addition to the growing literature on CBT for BDD.

Body Image Disturbances in Psychotic Disorders

THOMAS PRUZINSKY

This chapter describes body image disturbances in psychotic disorders, including schizophrenia, somatic delusions, and the psychotic variant of body dysmorphic disorder (BDD). Many challenges exist in reviewing psychotic forms of body experience. The admonition of the *Diagnostic and Statistical Manual of Mental Disorders–IV—Text Revision* (DSM-IV-TR) that the term psychotic "has historically received a number of different definitions, none of which has achieved universal acceptance" (p. 827) addresses a central challenge. Relatively little is known about psychotic aspects of body image. This lacuna is partially due to the lack of body image measures developed specifically for psychotic populations and infrequent use of available measures to assess these individuals.

BODY IMAGE AND SCHIZOPHRENIA

Historically, body image distortion often has been viewed as a central feature of schizophrenia. Psychodynamic theorists, in particular, have presented clinical observations and theories propounding the central role of body image in schizophrenic etiology and phenomenology. Guimón comprehensively reviews the body image disturbances described in schizophrenia, including experiences of body deterioration, depersonalization, body boundary disintegration, and transmuted feelings of masculinity and femininity. He describes a range of body image perceptions and beliefs pertaining to missing or misshapen body parts, perceptions of the body as unusually weak or strong, changes in body size or consistency (e.g., turning into stone), denial of the existence of body parts, reports of body parts being re- placed with those of another person, failure to recognize oneself in mirror reflections, and modifications of internal organs. Autoscopic symptoms are also reported, in which patients believe they see a replica of their body pro- jected in front of them.

These observations are clinically fascinating and worthy of consider- ation for the expanded view of body image they provide. However, Fisher's extensive review of body image and schizophrenia concluded that

> there is no solid evidence that adult schizophrenics experience their bodies in any unique fashion or that they suffer from some extraordinary "body image deficit." Why empirical studies fail to verify the flamboyant body image dramas that abound in so many clinical vignettes about schizo- phrenics remains a mystery. (p. 299)

Priebe and Röhricht decried the lack of systematic investigation of body-focused symptoms in schizophrenia and the inconsistent findings in extant research. For example, some studies document perceptions of in- creased body size while others document decreases. These authors also de- scribe common methodological problems, including poor specification of body image pathology, lack of diagnostic homogeneity, and use of non- standardized measures.

Interestingly, Chapman and colleagues used one standardized measure, the Body Image Aberration Scale, and documented that body image distor- tions were one component of a "broader conceptual aberration." Similarly, Priebe and Röhricht used standardized measures and found that individu- als with schizophrenia had consistent body size perceptual disturbances, which the authors speculated could be indicative of a "sensory information processing" dysfunction.

The conclusions of these two studies highlight the central question re- garding body image and schizophrenia: Are the body image distortions the result of either conceptual aberrations or sensory dysfunction that results in myriad distorted perceptions, including perceptions of the self, others, the world, as well as the body? If the answer is yes, then there is nothing distinc- tive about body image distortion in schizophrenia—it is just one of many perceptual distortions. Unfortunately, there is no definitive answer to this question.

SOMATIC DELUSIONS

Munro points out that although somatic delusions are the most extensively researched of all delusional disorders, there has been little explicit focus on body image functioning in these patients. Nonetheless, a brief review of somatic delusions provides insight into how perceptions and conceptions of body appearance and functioning can be psychotically disturbed.

According to DSM-IV-TR, the diagnosis of delusional disorder, somatic type (DDST), "applies when the central theme of the delusion involves bodily functions or sensations" (p. 325). Such individuals present with nonbizarre delusions that cannot be accounted for by another psychiatric disorder. Munro notes that while the severity of somatic delusions fluctuates considerably over time for any particular individual, the disorder tends to be chronic and causes the person to persistently seek inappropriate treatments. In addition to delusions of body odor and psychotic forms of BDD (addressed later), two common manifestations of DDST are delusional infestation and hypochondriacal delusions.

Delusional Infestation

The individual with delusional infestation is convinced that he or she is infested with parasites, despite the absence of any objective evidence of such infestation. These individuals almost invariably seek the services of dermatologists, infectious disease physicians, or even entomologists rather than mental health professionals. As described in Baker and colleagues' 1995 review, delusional infestation appears to derive from tactile hallucinations. These patients differ from individuals with schizophrenia in that they evince no decline in social or occupational functioning. Similar to many individuals with somatic delusion, they often function reasonably well outside the context of their delusional focus.

Hypochondriacal Delusions

Kingdon and colleagues, reviewing the literature on psychotic disorders with hypochondriacal features, describe the many forms that hypochondriacal beliefs can take. They use the term developed by Munro, "monosymptomatic hypochondriacal psychosis," to describe the symptoms of an individual with a single, long-term hypochondriacal belief that is of delusional intensity.

There is little empirical documentation of the nature of delusional experience or body image functioning in hypochondria. However, there is much clinical evidence that levels of patient conviction in hypochondriacal beliefs vary widely; some hypochondriacal patients are delusional, and some are not. Determining the difference between the delusional and nondelusional forms is clinically and empirically challenging. Côté and colleagues document the decision-making process for defining DSM-IV diagnostic criteria for hypochondria. They note the challenges in differentiating somatic delusions, in which patients never recognize the irrationality of their beliefs, from an "unshakable conviction" that can vary in intensity over time for many patients.

One key diagnostic distinction in determining the severity of hypochondriacal beliefs is whether patients have insight into their illness. Clinicians need to assess a patient's degree of insight into the hypochondriacal beliefs, as noted by the inclusion of the diagnostic specifier "With Poor Insight" in the DSM-IV (and DSM-IV-TR). Poor insight is evident "if, for most of the time during the current episode, the person does not recognize that the concern about having a serious illness is excessive or unreasonable" (DSM-IV-TR, p. 507). Similar issues regarding assessing delusionally held beliefs and degree of patients' insight into their illness are central to understanding the psychotic features of BDD.

PSYCHOTIC FEATURES OF BODY DYSMORPHIC DISORDER

Katharine Phillips describes BDD in this volume as "a preoccupation with an imagined defect in appearance." In their chapter, Allen and Hollander note that two forms of body image disturbances in BDD include body dissatisfaction and the less common and more "dramatic" perceptual distortions that have a greater likelihood of being delusional in nature.

The history of BDD is replete with references to its psychotic variants. Phillips and Hollander note that BDD often has been considered a precursor to, or a variation of, schizophrenia. Current evidence, however, reveals little, if any, genetic connection between BDD and schizophrenia.

In contrast, there is convincing evidence of psychotic features in a significant percentage of BDD patients. Phillips (in this volume) notes that the "majority" of BDD patients "have ideas or delusions of reference" and that many BDD patients are delusional in terms of their perception of their "deformities."

DSM-IV-TR's categorical approach to classification requires that patients with delusional forms of BDD receive a BDD diagnosis *and* a diagnosis of DDST. This dual diagnostic approach raises the question of whether delusional and nondelusional forms of BDD are two different disorders or whether they are the same disorder that varies in severity along a dimension of insight/delusionality. Phillips and Hollander report that this issue was debated during the drafting of DSM-IV's diagnostic criteria for BDD. Current evidence supports the conclusion that there is "a single disorder with widely varying levels of insight"(Allen & Hollander, 2000, p. 620), with some patients exhibiting delusional forms of the disorder at some time.

Phillip's 2000 review of BDD indicates many similarities between its delusional and nondelusional forms in terms of phenomenology, course, associated features and comorbities, and the fact that both forms respond to selective serotonin reuptake inhibitors (SSRIs) but not to antipsychotic medications given alone. The primary difference between the two forms is in the severity; delusional patients experience greater impairment in social and work/academic functioning, more frequent reports of suicidality, histories of being housebound or hospitalized due to BDD, and overall lower quality of life.

Therefore, despite the DSM-IV's categorical approach, it appears from extant data that a dimensional approach to describing the functioning of BDD patients is more valid. That is, instead of delusional BDD patients being diagnosed with two separate and distinct disorders (BDD and DDST), it is more accurate to regard BDD as one disorder in which there is a wide range of functioning across patients as well as within patients over time.

Partially reflecting this viewpoint, the description of BDD has been updated in DSM-IV-TR to include the observation that "insight about the perceived defect is often poor, and some individuals are delusional; that is, they are completely convinced that their view of the defect is accurate and undistorted, and they cannot be convinced otherwise" (p. 508). However, unlike the criteria for obsessive–compulsive disorder and hypochondriasis, the specifier "With Poor Insight" has *not* been added to the DSM-IV-TR's diagnostic considerations for BDD. I would recommend adding such a specifier to the future DSM-V. (Widiger and Clark's 2000 review in *Psychological Bulletin* addresses the possibility of combining categorical and dimensional approaches to classification when developing the DSM-V.)

The dimensional viewpoint concerning BDD has not received universal acceptance. Munro, who has conducted seminal research on monosymptomatic hypochondriacal psychosis and has written extensively on the classification and treatment of delusional disorders, believes that there are two distinct forms of the disorder—one that is delusional in nature, and one that is not.

One major area of apparent disagreement between Munro and other researchers pertains to the efficacy of SSRIs and neuroleptics in treating delusional forms of BDD. In the present volume, Allen and Hollander as well as Phillips report that delusional forms of BDD respond to SSRIs but *not* to neuroleptics given as a monotreatment. Munro, however, reports that in his and others' experience, delusional disorders are most commonly chronic illnesses that respond *only* to neuroleptic treatment.

Despite Munro's dissenting view, it is helpful in understanding BDD patients to view insight and delusionality as falling along a continuum. That is, patients with a DSM-IV-TR diagnosis of BDD or the dual BDD–DDST diagnosis fall somewhere along this continuum, in terms of degrees of insight and delusionality, at any one point in time. As illustrated in Phillips and McElroy, some BDD patients exhibit no delusionality and fair to excellent insight into the nature of their symptoms. Other patients have what are best described as "overvalued ideas," which DSM-IV-TR defines as "An unreasonable and sustained belief that is maintained with less than delusional intensity (i.e., the person is able to acknowledge the possibility that the belief may not be true)" (p. 826). Most extreme are those BDD–DDST patients who have no insight into their illness and are blatantly delusional.

In determining where patients fall along this continuum, it is clinically

and empirically essential to assess the nature and extent of delusional beliefs. Eisen and colleagues documented the validity of the Brown Assessment of Beliefs Scale for this purpose. The seven dimensions of this clinician
rating scale are: (1) conviction, (2) perception of others' view of beliefs, (3)
explanation of differing views, (4) fixity of ideas, (5) attempt to disprove beliefs, (6) ideas/delusions of reference, and (7) insight. This measure assesses
the predominant belief present during the previous week and has been used
to evaluate BDD treatment outcomes.

The research of Phillips and colleagues makes it clear that assessing
BDD patients' delusional beliefs must be combined with evaluating severity
of impairment (using a modified version of the Yale–Brown Obsessive–
Compulsive Scale). Such a comprehensive approach to patient evaluation
helps specify treatment outcomes. As Phillips and colleagues have also emphasized, it is not yet clear to what degree patients' insight improves with
specific forms of treatment, or if degree of insight is prognostic of future
functioning or treatment outcome. Phillips has proposed evaluating the efficacy of augmenting SSRI treatment (fluoxetine) with pimozide, the neuroleptic reported by Munro to be effective in treating hypochondriacal and
other somatic delusions. The result could shed light on the optimal treatment of patients with delusional variants of BDD. Given the large number of
patients who experience BDD and the level of suffering that it entails, well-
designed treatment outcome research is imperative.

CONCLUSION

The preeminent body image scholar Seymour Fisher has taught us to appreciate the full range of "unreal" body image perceptions. A comprehensive
understanding of body image functioning requires even greater knowledge
of the psychotic forms of body image disturbance—including the body image experiences of patients with schizophrenia, somatic delusions, and delusional variants of BDD.

Body image delusions sometimes occur in persons with disorders other
than those discussed in this chapter. For example, delusional body image experiences are evident in some self-mutilating patients. Phillips, Kim, and
Hudson have also described examples of delusional perceptions in anorexia
nervosa. Moreover, given substantial correlational evidence that body dissatisfaction is associated with depressive symptomatology, the study of
body image delusions in severe depressive disorders is warranted.

Whatever the exact symptomatic presentation, patients with psychotic
forms of body image disturbances are intensely and unshakably committed
to their beliefs and perceptions as well as to their misguided demands for ineffective treatments. They almost invariably push the limits of a clinician's
ability to be compassionate. Our recognition of the depth of their concerns
can help us continue our efforts to understand and relieve their suffering.

INFORMATIVE READINGS

Allen, A., & Hollander, E. (2000). Body dysmorphic disorder. *Psychiatric Clinics of North America, 23*, 617–628.—A review of diagnostic and treatment issues related to BDD in the context of considering the full range of obsessive–compulsive spectrum disorders.

Baker, P. B., Cook, B. L., & Winokur, G. (1995). Delusional infestation: The interface of delusions and hallucinations. *Psychiatric Clinics of North America, 18*, 345–361.—A review of issues related to differential diagnosis, etiology, and treatment of delusional infestation.

Chapman, L. J., Chapman, J. P., & Raulin, M. L. (1978). Body-image aberration in schizophrenia. *Journal of Abnormal Psychology, 87*, 399–407.—This study used the 28-item Body Image Aberration Scale to compare patients with schizophrenia and normal control subjects.

Côté, G., O'Leary, T., Barlow, D. H., Strain, J. J., Salkovskis, P. M., Warwick, H. M. C., Clark. D. M., Rapee, R., & Rasmussen, S. A. (1995). Hypochondriasis. In *DSM-IV sourcebook* (pp. 933–947). Washington, DC: American Psychiatric Press.—A review of the data and decisions that influenced the development of DSM-IV diagnostic criteria for hypochondriasis, including a specific discussion of somatic delusions.

deLeon, J., Bott, A., & Simpson, G. M. (1989). Dysmorphophobia: Body dysmorphic disorder or delusional disorder, somatic type? *Comprehensive Psychiatry, 30*, 457–472.—Offers historical perspective on BDD and related diagnoses.

Eisen, J. L., Phillips, K. A., Baer, L., Beer, D. A., Atala, K. D., & Rasmussen, S. A. (1998). The Brown Assessment of Beliefs Scale: Reliability and validity. *American Journal of Psychiatry, 155*, 102–108.—Reports the psychometric characteristics of this scale that is utilized for assessing the extent of delusionality in patients with many different types of psychiatric conditions, including mood disorders, BDD, and OCD.

Fisher, S. (1986). *Development and structure of the body image (Vols. 1 & 2)*. Hillsdale, NJ: Erlbaum.—Comprehensive scholarly review of body image research.

Guimón, J. (1997). Corporality and psychoses. In J. Guimón (Ed.), *The body in psychotherapy* (pp. 63–72). Basel, Switzerland: Karger.—Describes a broad range of psychotic body image symptoms.

Kingdon, D., Rathod, S., & Turkington, D. (2001). Psychotic disorders with hypochondriacal features: Delusions of the soma. In G. Asmundson, S. Taylor, & B. Cox (Eds.), *Health anxiety: Hypochondriasis-related conditions* (pp. 324–337). New York: Wiley.—Reviews historical, diagnostic, etiological, and treatment issues.

Munro, A. (1999). *Delusional disorder: Paranoia and related illnesses*. New York: Oxford University Press.—Comprehensive review of the history, diagnosis, and treatment of delusional disorders, with extensive coverage of somatic delusions.

Phillips, K. A. (2000). Body dysmorphic disorder: Diagnostic controversies and treatment challenges. *Bulletin of the Menninger Clinic, 64*, 18–35.—A comprehensive, yet relatively concise overview of the research and clinical literature.

Phillips, K. A., & Hollander, E. (1996). Body dysmorphic disorder. In T. A. Widiger, A. J. Frances, H. A. Pincus, R. Ross, M. B. First, & W. W. Davis (Eds.), *DSM-IV sourcebook* (Vol. 2, pp. 949–960). Washington, DC: American Psychiatric Association.—Documents the decision-making process regarding BDD classification for DSM-IV.

Phillips, K. A., Kim, J. M., & Hudson, J. I. (1995). Body image disturbance in body dysmorphic disorder and eating disorders: Obsessions or delusions? *Psychiatric*

Clinics of North America, 18, 317–334.—One of the few articles specifically addressing body image and the psychotic aspects of BDD as well as eating disorders.

Phillips, K. A., & McElroy, S. L. (1993). Insight, overvalued ideation, and delusional thinking in body dysmorphic disorder: Theoretical and treatment implications. *Journal of Nervous and Mental Disease, 181*, 699–702.—Brief article providing helpful descriptions and clinical examples illustrating distinctions among levels of insight and between overvalued ideas and delusional thinking.

Phillips, K. A., McElroy, S. L., Keck, Jr., P. E., Hudson, J. I., & Pope, Jr., H. G. (1994). A comparison of delusional and nondelusional body dysmorphic disorder in 100 cases. *Psychopharmacology Bulletin, 30*, 179–186.—Documents more similarities than differences in psychotic and nonpsychotic forms of BDD, providing support for BDD as existing along a continuum of functioning.

Priebe, S., & Röhricht, F. (2001). Specific body image pathology in acute schizophrenia. *Psychiatry Research, 101*, 289–301.—Uses refined research methodology to document the historically critical issue of significant body image disturbances in schizophrenia.

Widiger, T. A., & Clark, L. A. (2000). Toward DSM-V and the classification of psychopathlogy. *Psychological Bulletin, 126*, 946–963.—A helpful review of issues that can lead to improving the DSM classification system.

VI

Body Image Issues
in Medical Contexts

38

Body Image Issues in Dermatology

JOHN Y. M. KOO
JENSEN YEUNG

GENERAL PSYCHOLOGICAL ISSUES
WITH REGARD TO THE SKIN

A discussion of body image would not be complete without considering its interconnections with the field of dermatology. The importance of the skin for an individual's psychosocial equilibrium can easily be appreciated. First and foremost, the skin represents the "outward packaging" of our being. The cutaneous surface is what society initially perceives; for that reason, having a healthy, unblemished skin enhances one's self-esteem and identity. As discussed in Barnard's book *Touch: The Foundation of Experience*, many psychological studies have attested to the importance of cutaneous, tactile experience that is empathic and stimulatory in the development of healthy body image and psychological differentiation of self from others. Moreover, even in the 21st century, in some societies skin pigmentation unfortunately still determines social rank and status, either explicitly or implicitly. In addition, numerous psychological studies have demonstrated that those who are afflicted with visible, disfiguring disorders are more likely to be stigmatized and ill-treated than those with obvious physical disabilities.

Having a presentable skin surface is usually a prerequisite for maintaining optimal body image. Disfigurement, disease, or a blemish on the skin can lead to embarrassment, humiliation, and other negative body image experiences, which in turn can diminish self-esteem and engender depression and other psychological difficulties. For example, in 1997 Rapp and his colleagues found that as many as 25% of patients with psoriasis have wished that they were dead at some point in their lives because of it, and about 8%

333

of them currently felt that their lives were not worth living because of the condition. Clearly, the psychosocial sequelae of skin disease should not be underestimated.

DETERMINANTS AFFECTING MAGNITUDE OF SKIN DISORDER'S IMPACT ON BODY IMAGE

Although any visible disfigurement of the cutaneous surface can have a negative impact on body image, the intensity with which the individual experiences the negative impact varies depending on variables such as age of onset, gender, anatomical location, the nature of the skin disorder, premorbid personality, and family and social support networks.

Age of Onset

Although there are individual differences, the effect of skin disorders tends to be more intense in adolescents and young adults than in older persons. In fact, there is a roughly inverse relationship between the intensity of the negative psychosocial impact of the skin disorder and the age of the afflicted individual. This is easily conceivable, given that younger patients tend to be less firmly grounded with regard to their personal identity and that they are also challenged by dating and peer acceptance issues where appearance is critically important. By contrast, the elderly population, such as those of retirement age, is least affected, presumably because social pressures related to physical appearance are not as prominent.

Gender

In general, females are more disturbed by hair and skin disorders than males—clearly illustrated by the fact that the majority of consumers of hair and skin products and services are females. However, it should be noted that over the past decade, males have become much more physically and psychologically conscious about their skin condition, thereby narrowing the gender difference in this respect.

Anatomical Location

Any disfigurement or skin disorder involving visible areas such as the face, dorsal hands, or nails has much more negative consequences for the sufferers than those involving areas that can be covered with clothing. One exception to this is the genital area, where any involvement can greatly inhibit the patient's comfort level with intimacy. Furthermore, intense involvement of the hands and feet (psoriasis, eczema, lichen planus, or any other chronic dermatosis) can easily erode the patient's quality of life, even if the rest of the skin is uninvolved.

The Nature of the Skin Disorder

There are at least three major types of skin disorders, each with differing impacts on body image. The first group includes bona fide skin disease, such as eczema or psoriasis. Even though many of these conditions are not contagious, the issue of perceived contagiousness unfortunately plays a role. Because the general public often misunderstands or misdiagnoses skin disease, sexual promiscuity or impropriety can be wrongly presumed in patients afflicted with these common skin disorders, in addition to the fear of contagiousness. Patients suffering from chronic, recurrent dermatosis, such as psoriasis and eczema, frequently feel "contaminated" or "dirty," even though they know intellectually that their condition is not contagious. In addition, these conditions are often associated with physical discomfort and disability, which can further contribute to the negative impact on body image.

The second group of skin or hair conditions, such as vitiligo or alopecia areata, where the disease manifestation is purely appearance-related does not entail physical discomfort or disability. However, as with the previous group, others can still misunderstand these conditions as being contagious. Patients suffering from this class of disorder frequently face enormous struggles with insurance companies, mass media, and the general public, who may have the tendency to trivialize their condition. They often have to prove that their condition, which compromises their body image, is a serious handicap, not just a "cosmetic concern."

The third group of patients comprises those with significant body image dissatisfaction secondary to changes related to aging. In the contemporary American society, undergoing cosmetic procedures has become a mainstream activity. The general perception has shifted from the view that acquiring a cosmetic procedure is a sign of mental imbalance to a less stigmatizing view that such procedures are merely a means of bridging the gap between the age one feels and the age one looks. Nevertheless, there will always be a minority of patients whose desire for cosmetic procedure does signify underlying psychopathology, such as body dysmorphic disorder (see Phillips's discussion of this topic in this volume).

Premorbid Personality

As in other medical or psychiatric conditions, the individual's premorbid adjustment plays a large role in determining how he or she is affected by a cutaneous disorder or disfigurement. Certainly, the individual's degree of emotional investment in his or her appearance is an important variable. On one extreme are patients whose cutaneous presentability is at the core of their self-esteem; *any* cutaneous imperfection or disorder can easily devastate patients who are highly psychologically invested in their appearance. On the other extreme are those who are least affected by cutaneous conditions because appearance plays little to no role in sustaining their healthy self-esteem and self-identity.

Family and Social Support Networks

The presence of strong family and social support networks significantly ameliorates the negative impact of skin disorder. This network may include the positive and supportive attitude of intimate contacts as well as the availability of patient-run support groups such as the National Psoriasis Foundation, National Eczema Foundation, and National Alopecia Areata Foundation. These supportive networks help diminish the person's sense of isolation. Moreover, by disseminating information about currently available and possible future treatments, these groups can greatly remedy the patient's sense of hopelessness and helplessness.

THE RELATIONSHIP BETWEEN THE PHYSICAL SEVERITY OF THE SKIN CONDITION AND THE MAGNITUDE OF ITS PSYCHOSOCIAL IMPACT

In dermatology, the quantitative psychometric evaluation of the impact of skin conditions on quality of life is in its infancy. Several tools, however, now exist, such as the Dermatology Life Quality Index and Skindex (dermatology-specific instruments) and the Psoriasis Disability Index (a disease-specific instrument). As discussed above, there is tremendous variability in the way different individuals respond to a similar magnitude of skin disfigurement. To our knowledge, none of these instruments have been able to demonstrate a strong correlation between the physical severity of the dermatological condition and its impact on quality of life, even with large groups of dermatological patients. This finding suggests that physicians should not rely primarily on physical severity of the disease to determine the plan of care for the patient. Doing so runs the risk of undermining the emotional and social impact of the disease. For example, the physician may judge a patient's mild rosacea to be too minor to warrant any aggressive treatment. However, the patient may be bothered by it to the extent that his or her social life is impaired. Therefore, the psychosocial consequences of skin disease should be thoroughly explored with each patient. Quality-of-life measurement instruments are needed for use with dermatological patients in order to tailor clinical management and enhance their psychosocial well-being.

ASSESSMENT OF PSYCHOSOCIAL CONCERNS
BY DERMATOLOGIST

In contemporary dermatological practice in North America, psychological assessment that includes body image concerns is not adequately conducted. There are several reasons for this deficiency. First, the busy pace of dermatological practice, in which a patient is seen within the span of a few minutes, is not conducive to conducting adequate psychological assessment. Second, many dermatologists may feel uncomfortable with psychological concepts and issues due to the fact that the psychological aspect of skin disease is rarely incorporated into dermatology residency programs. Consequently, dermatologists who are trained to be "visually oriented" feel more comfortable undertaking purely visual assessment based on skin morphology and the extent of body surface involvement, thereby neglecting the assessment of the psychosocial and occupational impact of the skin disease.

These realities frequently result in perceptual discrepancies between the dermatologist and the patient. For example, a 50–75% improvement in the skin condition is often considered "therapeutic success" by the dermatologist, especially if the more severe manifestations of the skin disease, such as cracking, bleeding, scaling, and crusting, resolve. However, the patient may continue to experience negative reactions, such as rude stares and avoidance behavior, with this degree of improvement. Thus, overt symptomatic improvements may not be enough for the patient to live a normal lifestyle. This discrepancy illustrates the acute need for the education of dermatologists regarding the impact of skin disorders on patients' psychological, social, and occupational functioning and how to incorporate this understanding into the process of deciding how aggressively to treat a given skin condition. For example, consider a patient with moderate to severe acne who is found to have a severely negative body image as a result. The clinician may decide to treat him or her with Accutane, a much more powerful acne medication than tetracycline or other less effective but also less risky oral agents. Similarly, consider a fashion model with a case of resistant psoriasis on her face or other visible area that could ruin her career. She might be a candidate for serious oral medications such as cyclosporine or methotrexate, whereas similar lesions on a less appearance-concerned elderly man might only be treated partially with topical agents.

As mentioned previously, instruments that capture the psychosocial aspects of skin disease are still at the early stage of development. (See also Pruzinsky and Cash's chapter on the assessment of body image quality of life in this volume.) In 1996 Chren and her colleagues devised a dermatology-specific tool, Skindex, which is a quality-of-life measure for patients with skin disease. It allows the comparison of quality of life measurements among different dermatological diseases. However, it was found to be not sensitive and specific enough for comparisons within the same skin disorder. For example, flushing, which is a common finding in rosacea, is not included in Skindex. A few disease-specific instruments have been constructed subsequently, with many more underway. As these instruments are still relatively novel, they are not widely used, and much work is needed in the field to gain more global acceptance.

IMPROVEMENT IN BODY IMAGE PERCEPTION
WITH DERMATOLOGICAL THERAPY

Even though the psychometric instruments available to assess quality of life and body image improvements are relatively limited in the field of dermatology, published studies have shown improved quality of life and body image perception following treatment for dermatological disease. For example, Salek and her colleagues found that cyclosporin greatly improves the quality of life of adults with severe atopic dermatitis. Kurwa and Finlay demonstrated that patients with psoriasis and severe atopic dermatitis showed a significant decrease in impairment of life quality following inpatient treatment. Perhaps one could argue that documenting quality-of-life improvement is obviously easy when the disease is severe and the treatment is aggressive. However, it has been possible to demonstrate quality-of-life improvement even in mild cases of psoriasis, if the instrument used has sufficient sensitivity and disease specificity. Koo has shown this improvement using the Psoriasis Quality of Life Questionnaire with mild to moderate psoriatic patients treated with Tazarotene, a topical retinoid.

MENTAL HEALTH REFERRAL
IN DERMATOLOGICAL PRACTICE

For the majority of dermatological patients who have more chronic, recurrent conditions such as psoriasis, eczema, or alopecia, common issues such as helplessness, hopelessness, and isolation can be effectively addressed through a referral to nationwide patient-organized support groups such as those previously mentioned. However, for those with relatively minor conditions the result can be unexpectedly negative. Upon seeing others with more severe conditions, those with mild to moderate manifestations might actually feel more discouraged about their future. Therefore, if the clinician feels it is advisable to refer a patient to a support group, proper education regarding his or her prognosis is warranted prior to participation in the group.

Referral to a mental health professional is warranted if the patient presents with a diagnosable psychiatric condition such as depression, body dysmorphic disorder, social phobia, or agoraphobia. Referral also can be beneficial for patients whose situational stress is exacerbating their skin disease. It should be noted that not everyone who needs mental health assistance requires the help of a psychiatrist. Mental health professionals of various disciplines can provide effective psychotherapeutic treatments of choice for these psychological disorders. The authors in Part VIII in this volume discuss a range of psychotherapeutic approaches for helping persons with body image disturbances.

Dermatologists in North America need to become comfortable with managing milder psychodermatological diseases and with prescribing psychotropic medications (e.g., antipsychotics for delusions of parasitosis; SSRIs for trichotillomania). Often times, patients with mild psychiatric problems do not believe that they have such problems and are very resistant to the idea of seeking psychiatric help; they may become hostile and lose their trust in the dermatologist if such a referral is even mentioned.

FUTURE RESEARCH DIRECTIONS

Efforts to develop psychometrically reliable and valid body image and quality-of-life instruments for dermatological diseases are underway. Other questions that deserve research attention include the following:

1. What is the best way for the average practicing dermatologist to evaluate body image, quality of life, and other psychological issues in view of the fact that, as a group, practicing dermatologists have very little formal training in psychology or psychiatry?
2. What type of instruments or other tools will allow dermatologists to accomplish the above goal and still be able to maintain a relatively hectic practice style?
3. How can the referral system and the working relationship between dermatologists and other mental health professionals be facilitated in light of the fact that many dermatological patients resist mental health referrals?
4. How can practicing dermatologists systematically incorporate body image and quality-of-life issues into their decision making regarding how aggressively to treat the patient's condition?

SUMMARY

Due to the visible nature of skin disorders, dermatological conditions can have a tremendously negative impact on the patient's body image. To varying degrees, every practicing dermatologist probably recognizes the importance of body image issues. However, at least in North America, practicing dermatologists' lack of training and experience in psychology and mental health make it difficult for them to give these issues appropriate emphasis. We hope that this situation will improve in the future through better education and research.

INFORMATIVE READINGS

Barnard, K. E., & Brazelton, T. N. B. (Eds.). (1990). *Touch, the foundation of experience*. Madison: International Universities Press.—Thorough discussion of the importance of touch in many domains of life.

Ben-Tovin, D. I., & Walker, M. K. (1995). Body image, disfigurement and disability. *Journal of Psychosomatic Research, 39*(3), 283–291.—Studied body image self-perception of women suffering from physical disorders that were disfiguring and/or disabling.

Cash, T. F. (1999). The psychosocial consequences of androgenetic alopecia: A review of the research literature. *British Journal of Dermatology, 141*, 398–405.—A thorough review of body image and quality-of-life issues relevant to androgenetic alopecia.

Chren, M. M., Lasek, R. J., Quinn, L. M., Mostow, E. N., & Zyzanski, S. J. (1996). Skindex, a quality-of-life measure for patients with skin disease: Reliability, validity, and responsiveness. *Journal of Investigative Dermatology, 107*, 707–713.—A newly developed instrument to evaluate the effect of skin disorders on quality of life.

Finlay, A. Y., & Kelly, S. E. (1987). Psoriasis—an index of disability. *Clinical and Experimental Dermatology, 12*, 8–11.—Illustrates the early development of a quality of life measure of psoriasis—Psoriasis Disability Index.

Finlay, A. Y., & Khan, G. K. (1994). Dermatology Life Quality Index (DLQI): A simple practical measure for routine clinical use. *Clinical and Experimental Dermatology, 19*, 210–216.—A general quality-of-life measure in dermatology.

Ginsburg, I. H. (1996). The psychosocial impact of skin disease. *Dermatologic Clinics, 14*(3), 473–483.—An in-depth discussion of quality-of-life issues in dermatology.

Halious, B., Beumont, M. G., & Lunel, F. (2000). Quality of life in dermatology. *International Journal of Dermatology, 39*, 801–806.—Addresses contemporary views of quality of life in the field of dermatology.

Koblenzer, C. (1996). Psychologic aspects of aging and the skin. *Clinics in Dermatology, 14*, 171–177.—A review of aging-related psychological issues in dermatology.

Koo, J. Y. M. (1995). The psychosocial impact of acne: Patient's perceptions. *Journal of the American Academy of Dermatology, 32*, S26–S30.—Focuses on the psychological domain of this common skin disease.

Koo, J. Y. M. (1996). Population-based epidemiological study of psoriasis with emphasis on quality of life assessment. *Dermatologic Clinics, 14*(3), 485–496.—Development of the Psoriasis Quality of Life Questionnaire to quantify the psychosocial impact of psoriasis.

Kurwa, H. A, & Finlay, A. Y. (1995). Dermatology in-patient management greatly improves life quality. *British Journal of Dermatology, 133*, 575–578.—Demonstrates quality-of-life improvement in patients with psoriasis and eczema following inpatient treatment using the Dermatology Life Quality Index questionnaire.

Rapp, S. R., Exum, M. L., Reboussin, D. M., Feldman, S. R., Fleischer, A., & Clark, A. (1997). The physical, psychological and social impact of psoriasis. *Journal of Health Psychology, 2,* 525–537.—Examines how psoriasis can affect the physical and the psychosocial self.

Salek, M. S., Finlay, A. Y., Luscombe, D. K., Allen, B. R., Berth-Jones, J., Camp, R. D. R., Graham-Brown, R. A. C., Khan, G. K., Marks, R., Motley, R. J., Ross, J. S., & Sowden, J. M. (1993). Cyclosporin greatly improves the quality of life of adults with severe atopic dermatitis. A randomized, double-blind, placebo-controlled trial. *British Journal of Dermatology, 129,* 422–430.—An experimental study using the United Kingdom Sickness Impact Profile and the Eczema Disability Index to illustrate the benefit of short-term treatment of cyclosporin on the quality of life of patients with severe atopic dermatitis.

39

Body Image Issues in Dental Medicine

H. ASUMAN KIYAK
MARISA REICHMUTH

This chapter focuses on the development and change of oral–facial body image. Children's development of overall body image, self-concept, and interpersonal skills is affected by the presence of dentofacial features that deviate from the normal range. How facial body image may change as a function of elective procedures, such as conventional and surgical orthodontics and the use of dental implants to replace natural teeth, is explored within this developmental framework.

It is widely recognized that facial attractiveness is a social asset that results in greater acceptance by others, including peers, teachers, and employers. Conversely, unattractive facial features can be a social liability that results in peer rejection, academic difficulties, and (later) employment problems. The concept of "what is beautiful is good" has been widely demonstrated in studies with raters and targets of all ages. Numerous studies have shown that preference for symmetrical facial features and teeth emerges in early childhood. By age 8, children appear to use the same criteria as adults for judging facial attractiveness. Teachers' academic expectations and evaluations of their students have been found to be correlated with their perceptions of each child's attractiveness. Both teachers and classmates rate physically attractive children as friendlier and more intelligent, even with no objective data on these characteristics!

Attractiveness continues to be a social asset in adulthood, for example, when employees who are judged to be more attractive are given better job performance ratings by their supervisors. Similarly, laypersons with no information about an individual beyond a photo rate attractive strangers as friendlier and more socially competent than those with unattractive faces. A study of undergraduate students by Jussim and colleagues found that physical attractiveness, particularly facial beauty, best predicted the students' ratings of unfamiliar peers on measures of likeability and desirability as a dating partner. (See Jackson's chapter in this volume.)

IMPACT OF MALOCCLUSION ON SELF AND OTHERS' EVALUATIONS

Dental appearance, although only one component of the face, can independently influence others' perceptions of the individual's attractiveness. Children with normal dental appearance are evaluated as more attractive, more desirable as friends, and more intelligent by other children and even by adults. These findings are consistent with the literature on overall facial attractiveness, as described above. Dental malocclusion[*] is a common target of teasing in children. In particular, research by Shaw and colleagues in the United Kingdom, by Helm and colleagues in Denmark, and by Kilpelainen and colleagues in the United States has demonstrated that malocclusions in the anterior region, especially overjet (where the upper teeth project outward at an angle, rather than vertically, over the lower teeth by 7 mm or more), an extreme deep bite, as well as crowding of anterior teeth are most predictive of teasing by peers and also predict children's self-assessments of their facial appearance.

Many adults who have experienced overjet as children recall such teasing and its influence on their body image. Negative self-perceptions of one's face can have lifelong consequences. Feingold found that adults who have adopted a poor facial body image viewed themselves as less outgoing, less popular, and less socially skilled than those with a positive facial image. His research demonstrates that these perceptions are independent of objective judgments of the individual's facial attractiveness. In contrast, other researchers have found that severe overjet during childhood may have a negative impact on self-ratings of physical attractiveness but not on overall self-esteem.

Some researchers have reported that laypeople distinguish among types of malocclusion in rating others' appearance. Normal or Class I occlusion is evaluated most favorably, followed by open bite, overbite (i.e., upper teeth too far forward over lower teeth in resting position), Class III (i.e.,

---

[*]Malocclusions are generally less severe malformations of the teeth and jaws than conditions such as cleft lip and palate, and severe facial injuries. Malocclusions are also more common, estimated to affect 70–75% of the U.S. population, but varying in severity.

lower teeth too far forward of upper teeth in resting position), overjet, deep bite, and crowding. These differences are also associated with individuals' decision to seek orthodontic correction.

Nevertheless, it is noteworthy that objective clinical assessments of treatment need, based on the severity of each type of malocclusion described above, is not correlated with the individual's own perceptions of treatment need. Research with children in Florida by Wheeler and colleagues, and with teens by Soh and Lew in Singapore revealed a greater desire for treatment in females, in those of higher socioeconomic status, and in those living in urban settings. These differences have been observed in children's perceived need for treatment even when the same type and severity of malocclusion were involved. The study by Wheeler and colleagues and research by Kiyak and colleagues with ethnic minorities in the Pacific Northwest have demonstrated significant differences between Caucasian, African American, and Asian American children in dentofacial body image and perceived need for orthodontic treatment.

DEVELOPMENT OF FACIAL BODY IMAGE AND SELF-CONCEPT

What factors account for these subjective differences in self-ratings and desire for orthodontic correction when no objective differences in appearance exist? Self-concept, specifically one's body image, appears to be a critical variable in such perceptions and the consequent desire for dental intervention. It is widely agreed by developmental psychologists that the "reflected appraisal" of others plays a significant role in the development of a child's body image. Social comparisons with peers and implicit messages of acceptance or rejection by peers, parents, and teachers all influence the emergence of a child's body image and subsequent self-concept. Body image is perhaps the most directly influenced component of self-concept because it develops earlier and because the child's physical appearance is clearly evident and readily elicits the reactions of others. As noted earlier, facial attractiveness particularly evokes evaluations of intelligence and social competence, even in the absence of interpersonal contact.

In a recent publication on ethnic differences in orthodontic acceptance, Kiyak presented a theoretical model of the determinants of orthodontic treatment need. This model posits that the reflected appraisal of parents, teachers, and peers creates a subjective appraisal of one's appearance. Body image emerges from this emotional and evaluative judgment of one's appearance, combined with ethnic and cultural values about beauty and about the relative importance of beauty versus other characteristics (e.g., personality, intelligence). However, self-concept is multifactorial and includes body image as well as the individual's accomplishments in areas such as academics, athletics, and social skills. Children who succeed in school, athletics, music, and friendship formation, and those whose family and cultural values downplay the importance of physical attractiveness, can overcome negative messages about their dentofacial appearance from others, resulting in high self-esteem and self-acceptance. Their body image may or may not be high, but other strengths compensate for this area of dissatisfaction. Such children are less likely to desire orthodontic treatment. Conversely, children who feel less competent in the areas of academics, athletics, and interpersonal skills, and for whom physical appearance is a greater concern, are more likely to seek correction of the same severity of malocclusion.

MEASURING CHANGE IN DENTOFACIAL BODY IMAGE

As Cash describes in his chapter on evaluating body image states, assessing body image first requires an understanding of what facets of the body are critical for the research or clinical issue of interest. One can measure evaluative cognitions or emotions; one can obtain global evaluations or more specific judgments of particular physical attributes.

Three key measurement issues emerge in the area of dentofacial body image. First, it is important to examine specific components of the face, such as teeth, lips, mouth, and facial profile. Second, these components must be placed within the context of other body parts to assess the *relative* evaluation of dentofacial features compared to other facial and body components. Third, because most research on psychological aspects of dentofacial body image focuses on functional and esthetic *changes* resulting from trauma, pain, or elective treatment, it is important to select body image measures that are sensitive to such changes.

In our research with conventional and surgical orthodontic (or orthognathic surgery) patients over the past 20 years, as well as older adults undergoing dental implants, we have utilized a modified form of Secord and Jourard's Body-Cathexis Scale. The modification consists of adding five more items related to the lower face, mouth, and facial profile. With minor changes in some items, this scale has been adapted for use with children as young as 8 and adults as old as 78, and it can be administered to ethnically and culturally diverse groups. The Body-Cathexis Measure uses a 5-point response scale ranging from "Don't like, wish I could change it" to "I feel fortunate about this." In one study we decided to weight each response with the relative importance attributed to each body part by the respondent. Patients were asked to complete the Body-Cathexis Measure twice, once with the evaluative scale described above, and a second time with a 5-point scale of "Very important" to "Not at all important." At each assessment pre- and postsurgery, patients completed both measures. Two striking results emerged. First, responses on the two measures were highly correlated pretreatment, such that respondents who rated a particular body part as important were generally *less* satisfied with that feature. Second, there was little change in the relative importance of a body component postoperatively, even though patients' level of satisfaction with the part improved posttreatment. For example, if patients perceived their facial profile to have improved postsurgically, they rated their satisfaction higher than presurgery, but this item maintained its relative importance on the scale.

In another study, we compared adults who underwent surgical orthodontics with those who also needed a surgical correction of the upper or lower jaw in addition to the teeth but chose to undergo conventional orthodontics only, or no treatment. These three groups were assessed longitudinally, at points that corresponded to specific phases of orthodontic treatment. Several measures of psychological and functional characteristics were obtained at each assessment, including the Body-Cathexis Scale and the Tennessee Self-Concept Scale. Although self-concept did not differ across groups or over time, body image did. In particular, facial body image (average scores on eight items describing the lower face and chin) and facial profile (a single item) were lowest for surgery patients preoperatively, followed by orthodontics only, and no-treatment patients. By the 4- to 6-week assessment, and up to 24 months following surgery, these patients had significantly higher scores on both dimensions than their nonsurgical counterparts. It is noteworthy that the no-treatment group actually showed a *decline* in facial and profile body image, which may reflect a process of "second thoughts" or regret for not undergoing a recommended dental/surgical procedure. Indeed, the very act of completing a questionnaire on body image may have forced these no-treatment respondents to think through these issues more closely.

These findings of dramatic improvements in facial and profile body image following orthognathic surgery, with some improvement in generalized body image, have been supported by other studies. Some researchers have found that overall body image remains high along with the specific components affected by surgery, whereas others report a decline in overall body image to presurgical levels, but the dentofacial body image continues to be high. Still other researchers have focused on conventional orthodontic patients only, in whom skeletal discrepancies are minor or nonexistent. These studies also report significant improvements in dentofacial body image shortly after, and one year after, active treatment. Although overall body image also appears to improve in the short term, this change is transient, as seen with the orthognathic patients. Thus it appears that, in this patient population, the generalized "halo effect" of improved occlusion on one's physical identity following treatment gradually disappears, while satisfaction with one's dentofacial appearance continues.

MEASURING BODY IMAGE IN ADULTS WHO HAVE LOST TEETH

The Body-Cathexis Scale has also been administered to adults undergoing osseointegrated implants to permanently replace natural teeth that have been lost on the upper, lower, or both jaws. This procedure results in a more stable and natural appearing dentition than removable dentures because the teeth are placed on a titanium implant that becomes integrated with the supporting bone tissue. In our longitudinal study of 39 patients who underwent this procedure, several psychological measures were obtained before and after their phase I and phase II surgeries to place the implant, and again after their new prostheses were inserted into the implant. A total of six assessments were completed over 18–24 months. Significant improvements emerged on all body image scores over this time. However, the average change in overall body image was lower than for facial body image and especially for the individual items "mouth" and "teeth." In particular, mean scores on this latter item improved from 1.19 ($SD = 0.68$) on the 5-point response scale to 3.62 ($SD = 1.07$).

Other researchers have examined body image as part of a "health-related quality-of-life" measure among dental implant patients. Although less dramatic than changes in perceived function, perceived esthetics also improved significantly among patients following dental implant therapy. In a study by Rogers and colleagues in the United Kingdom, body image was measured with a body satisfaction scale among toothless patients ages 45–80. When patients who had undergone implant therapy were compared with those who received conventional removable dentures or no prosthetic replacement, the implant patients showed the most improvement in body satisfaction related to the face and head. Conventional denture patients, were in the second position, with the least satisfied the no treatment patients.

It is noteworthy that self-concept in adults undergoing implant therapy did not show any significant change; it remained high from pretreatment to postinsertion of the implant-supported prosthesis. These results are consistent with the findings reported earlier for orthodontic and orthognathic surgery patients. It appears that patients with malocclusion, dentofacial skeletal disharmony, and tooth loss perceive their facial, and especially their dentofacial, features negatively. Their facial body image is generally low but shows dramatic improvement with treatment. However, dissatisfaction with their dentofacial features does not generalize to their overall self-concept. As a result, while dental and surgical interventions improve dentofacial body image, they do not appear to have any impact on self-concept—which, for both patient populations, fell within the normal range for their age groups.

CONCLUSIONS

The research described in this chapter illustrates the significant influence of others on the development of body image. The earliest messages from others often pertain to one's physical appearance. Malocclusion is particularly apparent to others; some forms of malocclusion result in more teasing and ostracism than others. Body image may or may not influence the individual's overall self-concept, which is based on many other factors such as social competence, academic, athletic, musical, and occupational accomplishments. As described in the theoretical model to explain orthodontic treatment need, negative body image (overall or focused on a specific body part) need not prevent the development of a healthy self-concept. It appears that people who feel a sense of accomplishment in these other areas, and whose family or cultural values downplay the significance of physical appearance, are comfortable with the same severity of facial disharmony or malocclusion that can cause others to seek elective treatment.

This chapter also focused on the importance of measuring specific components of body image because treatment to change one body part may or may not influence one's perception of other body parts on the whole. As shown in several studies with orthodontic, orthognathic surgical, and dental implant patients, overall body image may improve slightly or transiently, but it is the specific body parts associated with the treatment and nearby features that show the greatest and most enduring change as a function of that procedure. These studies also demonstrate the importance of selecting a body image measure that is sensitive to change and can be applied to populations of diverse ages and cultural and ethnic backgrounds.

INFORMATIVE READINGS

Feingoid, A. (1988). Good-looking people are not what we think. *Psychological Bulletin*, *111*, 304–341.—Provides research and anecdotal evidence that objective and subjective assessments of facial attractiveness are not always correlated, and that subjective judgments of one's own appearance has a significant impact on self-concept, career, and personal choices.

Fitts, W. H. (1965). *Manual for the Tennessee Department of Mental Health Self-Concept Scale*. Nashville: Tennessee Department of Mental Health.—Provides a detailed description of a widely used measure of self-concept, including norms for a broad range of age, sex, racial, and educational groups on total and subscale scores.

Helm, S., Kreiborg, S., & Solow, B. (1985). Psychosocial implications of malocclusion: A 15–year follow-up study on 30–year-old Danes. *American Journal of Orthodontics, 87*, 110–118.—An excellent study of the long-term psychological impact of orthodontic treatment versus no treatment for severe malocclusions.

Jussim, L., Fleming, C. J., Coleman, L., & Kohlberger, C. (1996). The nature of stereotypes: A multiple process model of evaluations. *Journal of Applied Social Psychology, 26*, 283–

312.—Demonstrated that people make judgments of the acceptability of job applicants on the basis of their appearance and speech style than on their ethnicity, and that white judges evaluate African American job applicants more favorably than white applicants.

Kilpelainen, P. V., Phillips, C., & Tulloch, J. F. (1993). Anterior tooth position and motivation for early treatment. *Angle Orthodontist, 63*, 171–174.—Parents of children under age 16 sought treatment for their child primarily because of the appearance of the child's teeth, followed by the child's facial appearance. In particular, children with greater overjet of their front teeth were more likely to be a focus of parental concern than children with little or no overjet.

Kiyak, H. A. (2000). Cultural and psychologic influences on treatment demand. *Seminars in Orthodontics, 6*, 242–248.—Presents a useful model describing influences on body image and desire for orthodontic treatment; other articles in this issue of the journal report on other psychological outcomes associated with orthodontics and orthognathic surgery.

Kiyak, H. A., Beach, B. H., Worthington, P., Taylor, T., Bolender, C., & Evans, J. (1990). The psychological impact of osseointegrated dental implants. *International Journal of Oral and Maxillofacial Implants, 5*, 61–69.—The first longitudinal study of the psychological impact of dental implants, using standardized instruments; also assesses body image and its components in this population.

Kiyak, H. A., Hohl, T., West, R. A., & McNeill, R. W. (1984). Psychological changes in orthognathic surgery patients: A 24–month follow-up. *Journal of Oral and Maxillofacial Surgery, 42*, 506–512.—Describes the long-term effects of orthognathic surgery versus conventional orthodontics or no treatment on body image and self-concept.

Kiyak, H. A., McNeill, R. W., Hohl, T., West, R. A., & Heaton, P. J. (1986). Personality characteristics as predictors and sequelae of surgical and conventional orthodontics. *American Journal of Orthodontics, 89*, 383–392.—Compares changes in body image of patients undergoing surgical versus conventional orthodontics, using two different response scales for body image: satisfaction, and perceived importance of each body part.

Rivera, S. M., Hatch, J. P., & Rugh, J. D. (2000). Psychosocial factors associated with orthodontic and orthognathic surgical treatment. *Seminars in Orthodontics, 6*, 259–269.—An excellent review of the psychological variables measured in earlier studies of orthodontic and orthognathic surgery outcomes.

Rogers, S. N., McNally, D., Mahmoud, M., Chen, M. F., & Humphris, G. M. (1999). Psychologic response of the edentulous patient after primary surgery for oral cancer: A cross-sectional study. *Journal of Prosthetic Dentistry, 82*, 317–321.—Oral rehabilitation following oral cancer surgery appears to have significant psychological benefits for patients who elect to undergo these procedures, resulting in greater body satisfaction and self-esteem than for postcancer patients who decide not to have an implant-supported denture placed.

Secord, P. F., & Jourard, S. M. (1953). The appraisal of body cathexis: Body cathexis and the self. *Journal of Consulting Psychology. 17*, 343–347.—Provides the first systematic testing of a body image scale that has later been shown to have high reliability and validity for orthodontic and surgical patients.

Shaw, W. C., Meek, S. C., &, Jones, D. S. (1980). Nicknames, teasing, harassment, and the salience of dental features among school children. *British Journal of Orthodontics, 7*, 75–80.—One of many articles by the senior author on the impact of malocclusion on social acceptance.

Soh, G., & Lew, K. K. (1992). Assessment of orthodontic treatment needs by teenagers in an Asian community in Singapore. *Community Dental Health, 9,* 57–62.—Study of teenagers' perceptions of need for orthodontic treatment, demonstrating that perceived need is greater if facial appearance is rated less attractive and associated with gender and perceived need, but not with racial and income status.

Tung, A. W., & Kiyak, H. A. (1998). Psychological influences on the timing of orthodontic treatment. *American Journal of Orthodontics and Dentofacial Orthopedics, 113,* 29–39.—Supports the early development of body image and the distinction between body image and overall self-concept in children.

Wheeler, T. T., McGorray, S. P., Yukiewicz, L., Keeling, S. D., & King, G. J. (1994). Orthodontic treatment demand and need in third- and fourth-grade school children. *American Journal of Orthodontics and Dentofacial Orthopedics, 106,* 22–33.—Demonstrates the early development of self-judgments of treatment need, and the role of ethnicity and gender in determining need.

Body Image Issues in Obstetrics and Gynecology

LESLIE J. HEINBERG
ANGELA S. GUARDA

Obstetrics and gynecology (OB/GYN) are medical specialties that address women's reproductive and sexual functioning. Because yearly pelvic and breast examinations are recommended for all women of reproductive age, gynecologists are the most regular providers of women's health care. For sexually active women, contraception, sexually transmitted diseases, and obstetric care also result in frequent OB/GYN visits. These necessary visits are often experienced as anxiety-provoking events, associated with feelings of embarrassment, humiliation, vulnerability, discomfort, or shame. Body image discomfort is especially relevant during the gynecological exam, given its focus on breasts and genitalia, body areas that women are socialized from childhood to consider private and intimate. Associated thoughts, feelings, and behaviors may activate negative body image schemas, and apprehension about gynecological examinations may result from the vulnerability and loss of dignity inherent in the lithotomy (feet in stirrups) position. Gynecological and obstetrical exams also involve assessing weight, which makes the majority of women anxious. Indeed, Ogden and Evans found that mislabeling normal-weight women as overweight resulted in a drop in mood and self-esteem.

Women may avoid important preventive care and treatment because of these body image concerns as well as fears of cancer, sexually transmitted diseases, infertility, and moral judgments. Conversely, because of the intimacy and regular frequency of exams, women may have a closer rapport with their OB/GYN than with other health-care providers and be more likely to disclose body image concerns and related problems such as depression or eating-disordered symptomatology. Given these issues, it is surprising that so little empirical work has focused on body image issues in obstetrics and gynecology. This chapter reviews the extant literature related to body image and sexual and reproductive health, with a focus on new research directions.

GYNECOLOGICAL CARE

In 2000, Nusbaum and her colleagues surveyed 1,480 women and found that body image was their fifth most common concern when seeking gynecological care from their family practitioner. Clearly, women with elevated body dissatisfaction may experience above-average levels of discomfort with gynecological care. However, minimal research has addressed this issue, and information on body image is largely absent from the main OB/GYN or family practice resident training texts.

The menstrual cycle is often associated with body image concerns and premenstrual complaints involving water retention, such as bloating, breast tenderness, and weight gain. Research on the premenstrual syndrome (PMS), however, has been plagued by methodological flaws, including definitional problems and lack of prospective research. Also evident is a very high placebo response rate—often on the order of 50–80%—making double-blind controlled trials imperative. A longstanding association between PMS symptoms and water retention led to the rationale for using diuretics in treatment. However, strong support for premenstrual water retention or weight gain in the majority of women is lacking. Although women frequently describe these symptoms in the luteal phase of the menstrual cycle, consistent changes in weight or in body dimensions across different phases of the menstrual cycle have not been documented empirically.

Studies such as Altabe and Thompson's in 1990 have linked negative mood states, including those occurring during the premenstrual period, to increases in body dissatisfaction. Given that PMS sufferers have reported elevated psychopathology scores on measures such as the Eysenck Personality Questionnaire neuroticism scale and higher rates of affective illness, they may be at increased risk for body image dissatisfaction. Hormonally induced mood changes may also explain the increased frequency of body dissatisfaction and complaints of weight gain and bloating typical of the premenstruum. Finally, the smooth muscle relaxant effect of luteal progesterone may result in colonic distention and a perception of bloating or increased body size without change in weight or body dimensions.

Regular sexual activity, often the impetus for seeking initial gynecological care, is accompanied by concerns regarding contraception and sexually transmitted diseases. In 1984 McKinney and colleagues found that consistency in contraceptive use was correlated with a more positive body image. Type of contraceptive used has also been associated with body image concerns. In particular, compliance with the oral contraceptive pill and with depoprovera, two of the most effective methods of contraception, is easily affected by fears of weight gain. In 1987 Emans and colleagues found that 46% of adolescents believed that the pill increases risk of weight gain, and 56% of users had quit taking the pill by the 13-month follow-up. Adolescents who believed weight gain was a risk factor associated with use of the pill were statistically more likely to be noncompliant.

Several other studies have associated high adolescent noncompliance rates with typical exaggerated adolescent concerns regarding fears of acne or weight gain. In a recent comprehensive literature review, however, Gupta concluded that for most women, the combined oral contraceptive pill is not associated with an increased risk of weight gain. Although a small proportion of women experience small increases in body weight on the pill, controlled studies comparing oral contraceptive users to levonorgestrol implant or barrier contraceptive users have shown similar weight gain rates across groups. The weight gain seen in a small proportion of oral contraceptive users most likely reflects natural age-related weight increases rather than the consequences of hormonal treatment. In some uncontrolled studies, medroxyprogesterone acetate and the older oral contraceptive formulations were reportedly associated with increased risk of acne. Recent controlled studies, however, such as that by Gilliam and colleagues in 2001, have found that the new low-dose combination oral contraceptive pills, which reduce circulating androgen levels, are effective as a treatment for acne in adolescents. As primary sources of contraceptive information, gynecologists, primary-care providers and the media can contribute to dispelling the mistaken assumption that the combined contraceptive pill leads to weight gain or acne.

Sexually transmitted diseases (STDs), including herpes simplex, human papilloma virus (HPV), HIV, or hepatitis, affect self-esteem, sexuality, and body image. Contagion can be associated with a decreased sense of attractiveness, social isolation, and feelings of contamination, resulting in strong barriers to developing healthy intimate relationships. Worries about future rejection by prospective partners and about transmitting the disease are common.

Infertility, which affects 15% of couples of childbearing age, similarly has a strong impact on body image, sexuality, and self-esteem. Infertile individuals often feel damaged or defective and may develop fears of social unattractiveness, undesirability, and inadequacy as well as sexual performance problems. Surprisingly, however, little research has addressed these reactions in the infertile population. In a 1999 case control study of 281 patients, Oddens and colleagues found that both sexuality and self-perceived attractiveness were rated lower by infertility patients than by controls. Patients also had higher scores on depression and anxiety scales, with 25% scoring in the clinically depressed range. Independent of infertility or venereal disease, sexual performance problems have been repeatedly associated with poorer body image. (See the chapter by Wiederman in this volume.)

Breast and gynecological cancers can be especially devastating to body image. Even an abnormal PAP smear may be sufficient for the development of sexual dysfunction and body image disturbance. At the extreme, disfiguring radical pelvic surgery for recurrent cervical cancer has been associated with very high levels of body image disturbance. More attention has been paid to body image issues associated with mastectomy than with gynecological cancer. Hysterectomy and pelvic radiation result in less obvious disfigurement than mastectomy. However, Andersen and Jochimsen found that 82% of gynecological cancer patients had poor body image versus only 31% of a sample of breast cancer patients, making body image problems less prevalent than commonly believed in breast cancer patients but more prevalent in gynecological cancer patients. A positive relationship between perceived sexual functioning and body image in cancer patients was also evident in this study. (See chapter by White in this volume.) Hormonal changes associated with gynecological surgery may also be associated with body image problems. For example, in a 1993 study by Bellerose and Binik, untreated ovariectomized women were found to have poorer body image than ovariectomized women on estrogen replacement therapy.

OBSTETRICS

Pregnancy

A woman's body undergoes rapid physical changes during pregnancy. During a 9-month period, a woman will gain 25–35 pounds or more, experience significant increases in breast size, loss of waist definition, widening of the pelvis and hips, and both temporary and permanent skin changes. Even a woman's hair, nails, and shoe size are frequently altered. At no other time is a woman's weight and diet such a focus to herself, family, physicians, and even complete strangers. Thus it is not surprising that pregnancy is often marked by significant changes in body image satisfaction—both for the better and for the worse. Unfortunately, little empirical research has examined the impact of pregnancy on body image in normal women.

A number of studies suggest that pregnancy may provide a brief reprieve from the constant focus on weight, shape, and dieting that preoccupies many women. In general, women are less likely to diet during pregnancy, and extreme dieting behaviors are reportedly rare. However, Fairburn and Welch found that 25% of pregnant women reported overeating and an associated feeling of loss of control, and Abraham and colleagues found that number to be as high as 44%. Overeating is more common among women who were dieting prior to pregnancy, which is likely due to the increased hunger experienced during pregnancy, the established propensity to eat in response to negative mood, and overeating due to the abandonment of previous dietary restraint.

Early studies that focused on the perceptual aspects of body image found greater body size overestimation by pregnant women than by non-pregnant controls. Pregnant women's perceptual body image may also be sensitive to media exposure. In 1993 Sumner and colleagues demonstrated, in a small pilot study, that pregnant women's perceptions of their abdomen depth were influenced by their exposure to media images of fashion models throughout pregnancy.

In spite of significant changes to a woman's body that move her farther from the ideal shape than ever, body image researchers such as Clark and Ogden have found positive impacts associated with pregnancy. Women tend to abandon dietary restraint and strict body image ideals in favor of a more nurturing role. Davies and Wardle demonstrated that pregnant women have less dietary restraint, rate themselves as less overweight, have lower drive for thinness, and when BMI (body mass index) is controlled for, much lower body dissatisfaction scores than nonpregnant women. However, pregnant women's ideal body size generally remains the same as nonpregnant women's ideals. This suggests that women may be able to make specific cognitive and/or behavioral adjustments to their body image while pregnant, despite the presence of underlying negative body image and eating schemas.

The adjustment to a more positive body image may take time. Several researchers have suggested that women's perceptual and subjective body image is more positive later in pregnancy than earlier, when they are first gaining weight and changing shape. It may be that women are more uncomfortable with their shape when they do not clearly appear pregnant or when the experience of gaining weight is novel. Later in pregnancy, women may also receive positive attention for their changing appearance, leading them to embrace a maternal role rather than perceiving themselves as overweight.

Unfortunately, certain individuals may be at risk for increased body image disturbance and pathological eating behaviors during pregnancy. Baker and colleagues found that women who reported trying to lose weight prior to pregnancy may be at greater risk for dieting and preoccupation with body image during pregnancy. Pomerleu and colleagues found that women smokers with body image concerns have also been shown to gain much more weight during pregnancy and adopt smoking as a weight control strategy. Weight gains of 25–35 pounds are optimal for fetal health and decreasing mortality. However, fears of weight gain are especially intense among dieters and individuals with eating disturbances. Such body image issues clearly should be of concern for all health practitioners caring for pregnant women.

Postpartum

Pregnancy and the postpartum year are often viewed as periods of tumultuous change for mothers. Although almost all aspects of a woman's life are altered by the birth of a baby, concerns about weight gain and getting back to prepregnancy shape are among the most frequently expressed by postpartum women.

Strang and Sullivan have shown that body image dissatisfaction peaks in the postpartum period. Most women continue to look pregnant in the first few weeks following birth, and in the first few months the majority of new mothers continue to weigh more than their prepregnancy weight. During pregnancy this weight gain may have been perceived as a positive sign of the baby's health and development. However, it is generally not experienced as acceptable after giving birth, and quick weight loss is the expected goal. A number of researchers has demonstrated that postpartum body image concerns are greater than at preconception and that they may continue to increase for 6 months postpartum. In 1987 Hiser found that 75% of recent mothers studied were concerned about their weight, and Baker and colleagues demonstrated that 70% were still trying to lose weight 4 months postpartum.

It is important to remember that higher levels of body image dissatisfaction can lead to eating disturbances. Although the majority of women with eating disorders improve significantly during pregnancy, Lemberg and Philips found that about half of women relapsed in the first year postpartum. This relapse is often attributed to feeling fat and wishing to lose weight. Stein and Fairburn demonstrated an increase in eating-disordered symptomatology, including weight and shape concerns, during late pregnancy and at 3 months postpartum. This finding is especially critical, given recent evidence suggesting that disturbed maternal eating behavior during pregnancy, as well as lower weight gain and lower prepregnancy weight, predict infant growth retardation and interference with maternal–child feeding interactions.

Some degree of postpartum body image dissatisfaction may be due to unrealistic weight loss expectations. The majority of new mothers expect to return to their prepregnancy weight and shape by 6 weeks postpartum. In reality, most weight loss occurs during the first postpartum year, with decelerating loss occurring as the year progresses. Further complicating matters is the frequency with which permanent weight gain occurs: Harris and colleagues' 1999 research evidence suggests that, on average, approximately 2.2 pounds are retained after each pregnancy, with 10–30% of new mothers experiencing a permanent weight gain of 10 pounds or more. Although researchers have generally focused on weight- and shape-related body image, Jenkin and Tiggemann noted in 1997 that dissatisfaction with stretch marks, breast shape, pigmentation changes, and looseness of abdominal skin are common and have yet to be empirically investigated.

A few studies have explored the role of body image in the initiation and maintenance of breastfeeding. Qualitative studies have suggested that women who choose not to breastfeed consider it "distasteful" and fear an adverse effect on their body, particularly their breasts. Foster and colleagues found no relationship between BMI and intention to breastfeed. However, a woman's attitude toward her body, even after controlling for social class, predicted intention to breast- versus bottle-feed. Bottle-feeders had greater body shape-related concerns and less body image satisfaction. Similar findings were demonstrated by Barnes's 1997 epidemiological study of 12,000 women. Independent of depression scores, women who had no concerns over their body image were 1.25 times more likely to intend to breastfeed in the first week than women with marked body image concerns. Weight concerns also predicted breastfeeding at 4 months, with greater concern over weight resulting in a greater likelihood to bottle-feed. Ironically, breastfeeding is associated with more rapid weight loss and return to prepregnancy body shape.

FUTURE DIRECTIONS

The rich variety of body image experiences encountered in OB/GYN populations and the relative paucity of understanding makes this population ripe for future research. OB/GYNs and other providers of women's health are in a unique position to diagnose and treat body image concerns. Unfortunately, these health-care providers have not received adequate training in body image and eating issues and may be discouraged by a dearth of empirical studies. Very little work has focused on body image in relation to gynecological issues, particularly using a definition of body image that goes beyond weight issues. For example, outside of menarche, studies have not examined women's emotional reactions to, and experiences with, menstruation. The relation between overall comfort with one's body and compliance with OB/GYN care needs to be explored. For example, does body image impact compliance with regular gynecological visits, breast self-examinations, infertility treatment, or STD screening? Are women with poorer body image less likely to use contraceptive devices such as the diaphragm? Do concerns about weight and appearance lead to poor compliance with hormonally based contraceptives? It is hypothesized that as women feel greater body image distress, they are less likely to engage in health maintenance behaviors that increase focus on their bodies or put them at risk for change in body status (e.g., weight gain from contraception, breast biopsies, etc.). Further, studies examining these issues across the life cycle would be illuminating (e.g., the effect of hormone replacement therapy on body image during menopause).

Research suggests that pregnancy and the postpartum may be periods involving tremendous fluctuations in body image for women. Although women may relax the omnipresent pressure to achieve or maintain the ideal level of thinness, temporarily abandoning dietary restraint and unhealthy dieting behaviors during pregnancy, the postpartum period is one in which women are at high risk for body image and eating disturbances as they attempt to return quickly to their prepregnant weight. Studies have been hampered by a lack of body image measurement instruments specific to pregnancy and postpartum, and a dearth of empirical knowledge regarding other body changes that occur when having a child. In 2001 Kendall and colleagues developed a pregnancy-specific body image measure that should help illuminate these areas. Studies have not examined body image experiences during labor and delivery. Such a stressful experience, accompanied by a complete lack of modesty and privacy, may be particularly anxiety provoking for women who are already uncomfortable with their bodies. Body image distortions during labor and delivery have also not been examined. Research on body image in relation to pregnancy and postpartum focuses almost exclusively on weight and shape concerns; other bodily changes leading to dissatisfaction also need to be investigated. Future studies should further examine body image issues relating to infant caretaking behaviors, such as decisions regarding breastfeeding and infant weight gain. Finally, body image interventions for gynecological and obstetrical populations have yet to be developed or evaluated but may play an important role in increasing compliance and decreasing psychological and physical morbidity.

INFORMATIVE READINGS

Abraham, S., King, W., & Llewellyn-Jones, D. (1994). Attitudes to body weight, weight gain and eating behavior in pregnancy. *Journal of Psychosomatic Obstetrics and Gynecology, 15,* 189–195.—Prospective study of 100 women 3 days after birth of their first child that assessed weight control and body image attitudes during pregnancy.

Altabe, M., & Thompson, J. K. (1990). Menstrual cycle, body image, and eating disturbance. *International Journal of Eating Disorders, 9*(4), 395–401.—Prospective questionnaire study of undergraduates at three distinct phases of the menstrual cycle, revealing greater body image and eating disturbance during the perimenstrual than intermenstrual phase.

Andersen, B. L., & Jochimsen, P. R. (1985). Sexual functioning among breast cancer, gynecologic cancer, and healthy women. *Journal of Consulting and Clinical Psychology, 53*(1), 25–32.—Cross-sectional study of sexual behavior, sexual response, and body image in postoperative breast cancer and gynecological cancer patients and in routine clinic cancer-free controls.

Baker, C. W., Carter, A. S., Cohen, L. R., & Brownell, K. D. (1999). Eating attitudes and behaviors in pregnancy and postpartum: Global stability versus specific transitions. *Annals of Behavioral Medicine, 21*(2), 143–148.—Prospective study of 90 women in pregnancy and postpartum showing that global concerns remain stable but that specific attitudes and behaviors fluctuate.

Barnes, J., Stein, A., Smith, T., Pollock, J. I., & ALSPAC Study Team. (1997). Extreme attitudes to body shape, social and psychological factors and a reluctance to breast feed. *Journal of the Royal Society of Medicine, 90,* 551–559.—Large epidemiological study of 12,000 pregnant women showing that body image predicts intention to breastfeed.

Bellerose, S. B., & Binik, Y. M. (1993). Body image and sexuality in oophorectomized women. *Archives of Sexual Behavior, 22*(5), 435–459.—Cross-sectional interview/questionnaire and vaginal plethysmographic study. Compared to controls, women who underwent oophorectomy reported more sexual problems. Furthermore, untreated oophorectomized women reported greater body discomfort than did oophorectomized women on hormone replacement or control women.

Clark, M., & Ogden, J. (1999). The impact of pregnancy on eating behaviour and aspects of weight concern. *International Journal of Obesity and Related Metabolic Disorders, 23*(1), 18–24.—Cross-sectional study of 100 pregnant and nonpregnant women examining dietary restraint and weight concerns.

Davies, K., & Wardle, J. (1994). Body image and dieting in pregnancy. *Journal of Psychosomatic Research, 38*(8), 787–799.—Cross-sectional study demonstrating improved body image in pregnant women concurrent with no relaxation of their body image ideals.

Emans, S. J., Esthermann, G., Woods, E. R., Smith, D. E., Klein, K., & Merola, J. (1987). Adolescents' compliance with the use of oral contraceptives. *Journal of the American Medical Association, 257*(24), 3377–3381.—Prospective study of 209 adolescents, examining compliance with oral contraceptive over a 13-month period.

Fairburn, C. G., & Welch, S. L. (1990). The impact of pregnancy on eating habits and attitudes to shape and weight. *International Journal of Eating Disorders, 9*(2), 153–160.—One of the first studies of body image in pregnant women; qualitative interview methods were used to assess eating behaviors and attitudes toward weight and shape during pregnancy.

Foster, S. F., Slade, P., & Witson, K. J. (1996). Body image, maternal fetal attachment, and breast feeding. *Psychosomatic Research, 41,* 181–184.—Examined maternal fetal attachment, body satisfaction, and intention to breastfeed in 38 women. Women intending to breastfeed were more satisfied with their shape.

Gilliam, M., Elam, G., Maloney, J. M., Flack, M. R., Sevilla, C. L., McLauughlin-Miley, C. J., & Derman, R. (2001). Acne treatment with a low-dose oral contraceptive. *Obstetrics and Gynecology, 97*(4, Suppl.), 1:S9.—Multicenter placebo-controlled trial of Estrostep oral contraceptive in which Estrostep treated subjects had highly significant decrease in acne relative to controls.

Gupta, S. (2000). Weight gain on the combined pill—is it real? *Human Reproduction 6*(5), 427–431.—Comprehensive literature review addressing research on weight gain related to use of oral contraceptive pills.

Harris, H. E., Ellison, G. T., & Clement, S. (1999). Do the psychosocial and behavioral changes that accompany motherhood influence the impact of pregnancy on long-term weight gain? *Journal of Psychosomatic Obstetrics and Gynecology, 20,* 65–79.—Longitudinal study of 74 mothers examining weight gain during pregnancy and postpartum period.

Hiser, P. L. (1987). Concerns of multiparas during the second postpartum week. *Journal of Obstetric and Gynecological Neonatal Nursing, 16,* 196–203.—Qualitative study of 20 women interviewed 10 to 14 days postpartum. Significant proportion of the women were concerned about losing pregnancy weight.

Jenkin, W., & Tiggemann, M. (1997). Psychological effects of weight retained after pregnancy. *Women's Health, 25,* 89–98.—Prospective investigation of effect of retained weight following pregnancy in 115 women. Postnatal weight was the most important predictor of postnatal psychological well-being.

Kendall, A., Olson, C. M., & Frongillo, E. A. (2001). Evaluation of psychosocial measures for understanding weight-related behaviors in pregnant women. *Annals of Behavioral Medicine, 23,* 50–58.—First validated instrument designed to examine body image specifically in pregnant women.

Lemberg, R., & Phillips, J. (1989). The impact of pregnancy on anorexia nervosa and bulimia. *International Journal of Eating Disorders, 8,* 285–295.—Examination of 43 women with eating disorders experiencing first pregnancy. Although there was significant improvement in pregnancy, lasting benefit after birth was limited.

McKinney K., Sprecher S., & DeLamateur. J. (1984). Self-images and contraceptive behavior. *Basic and Applied Social Psychology, 5*(1), 37–57.—Telephone interview study of 967 men and women demonstrating that in women, body image and self-description are positively correlated with contraceptive use.

Nusbaum, M. R. H., Gamble, G., Skinner, B., & Heiman, J. (2000). The high prevalence of sexual concerns among women seeking routine gynecological care. *Journal of Family Practice, 49*(3), 229–232.—Cross-sectional mail survey reporting high levels of sexual and body image concerns in women seeking routine gynecological care.

Oddens, B. J., den Tonkelaar, I., & Nieuwenhuyse, H. (1999). Psychosocial experiences in women facing fertility problems—a comparative study. *Human Reproduction, 14*(1), 255–26l.—Multicenter questionnaire survey of women awaiting assisted reproduction treatment reporting decreased self-perceived attractiveness and sexual drive in this population.

Ogden, J., & Evans, C. (1996). The problem with weighing: Effects on mood, self-esteem and body image. *International Journal of Obesity, 20,* 272–277.—Experimental study of 74 normal-weight individuals examining the effect of overweight labeling on self-esteem, mood, and body image.

Pomerleu, C. S., Brouwer, R. J., & Jones, L. T. (2000). Weight concerns in women smokers during pregnancy and postpartum. *Addictive Behaviors, 25,* 759–767.—A retrospective study of women who were smokers when they became pregnant. Women smokers with high weight and body image concerns gained significantly more weight during pregnancy, in amounts that far exceeded maximum recommended weight gain, than did women with low concerns.

Stein, A., & Fairburn, C. G. (1996). Eating habits and attitudes in the postpartum period. *Psychosomatic Medicine, 58,* 321–325.—Prospective population study of 97 women studied during pregnancy and followed for 6 months postpartum. It was found that eating disorder symptoms increased markedly in the 3 months postpartum and then plateaued over the next 6 months.

Strang, V. R., & Sullivan, P. L. (1985). Body image attitudes during pregnancy and the postpartum period. *Journal of Obstetric, Gynecologic, and Neonatal Nursing, 14,* 332–337.—A seminal early study demonstrating improvement in body image during pregnancy and the deleterious effect of the postpartum.

Sumner, A., Waller, G., Killick, S., & Elstein, M. (1993). Body image distortion in pregnancy: A pilot study of the effects of media images. *Journal of Reproductive and Infant Psychology, 11,* 203–208.—Pilot study comparing body image distortion in 10 pregnant women to 10 nonpregnant controls after viewing photographs of models.

41

Body Image and Urological Disorders

STEVEN M. TOVIAN

Urology is the branch of medicine concerned with the urinary tract in both genders and with the male genital/reproductive system. The term "urogenital" refers to the urinary and genital organs. The urinary system includes those organs primarily responsible for cleaning and filtering excess fluid and waste material from the blood, including the kidneys, ureter, bladder, and urethra. The male urogenital tract includes the testes, penis, prostate gland, and efferent and ejaculatory ducts. Urinary system problems include kidney failure, urinary tract infections, kidney stones, prostate enlargement, and bladder control problems such as urinary incontinence (leakage of urine) resulting from decreased muscle strength of the sphincters around the bladder and pelvic area and from disease or injury. Some urological diseases include cancers of the bladder, penis, prostate, kidney, and testicle; male erectile dysfunctions (e.g., priapism, epididymitis); prostate enlargement (e.g., hyperplasia, prostatitis); kidney stones; and sexually transmitted diseases.

According to National Kidney Foundation estimates, kidney and urinary tract diseases are a major cause of illness and death in the United States and affect nearly 20 million Americans. More than 13 million people in the United States experience urinary incontinence (UI), with women twice as likely to develop it as men. UI may be chronic or temporary and result from underlying pathological, anatomical, or physiological conditions within the urinary system or elsewhere in the body. Symptoms can range from the discomfort of slight urine loss to severe, frequent wetting. Incontinence is not an inevitable result of aging, and though common in older people, does occur in the young. It is often caused by specific changes in bladder structure and function that may result from disease, medications, and/or trauma or illness. Often it is the first and only symptom of a urinary tract infection. Tovian, Rozensky, Sloan, and Slotnick (1994) reviewed the literature on UI and its effects of self-esteem.

COMMON BODY IMAGE PROBLEMS
AND DEVELOPMENTAL ISSUES

Body image and body experience are central to one's sense of self and how one relates to the world and to others; they are constantly evolving over the course of development and significantly influence our cognitive, emotional, and interpersonal experiences. Urological disorders can alter and distort one's body image and self-concept because the individual must adapt to many potential problems, including physical disfigurement and functional limitations such as use of an indwelling catheter, as well as pain. Many body image changes resulting from urological disorders may be partially due to limited mobility and social restriction as well as the subsequent cognitive distortion associated with these changes. Successful adaptation to a urological disorder entails integrating physical changes into one's restructured body image and self-perception. Unsuccessful adaptation is marked by symptoms that may include psychogenic pain, depression, anxiety, anger, and social withdrawal.

Body image can be described as the individual's mental image or cognitive representation of his or her own body, including outward appearance, internal organs, and physiological processes. Psychoanalytical theory sees body image as a crucial element in ego formation and, therefore, in all personality formation. According to this theory, the individual achieves differentiation from the world by distinguishing the bodily self from the non-self. (See the two chapters by Krueger in this volume.) The mental representation of the body changes and matures as the child passes through each psychosexual stage. If the child passes through each stage successfully, a mature body image and mature ego development result. Conflicts at any stage that result in fixation can alter body image and ego functioning. A physical illness, handicap, or deformity, whether acquired or congenital, can alter the course of developing a mature body image. The immature body image that results can interfere with personality functioning. With the body image playing a key role in ego development, body image distortions can impair such central ego-mediated processes as judgment and learning.

The body image of an adolescent with a urological disorder is thought to be particularly vulnerable. When the body image of an adolescent is different from that of his or her peers, this difference can interfere with identity formation and result in emotional dysfunction. (See Chapter 9 by Levine and Smolak in this volume.) Reiner (1999) studied 19-year-old males ($n = 14$), diagnosed with variations of congenital hypospadias (a condition in which testicles remain inside the body or pelvic area), who had received reconstructive surgery in the first year of life. This malformation affects both males and females and often involves a fusion of the abdominal wall over the bladder. Additionally, the urethra and the penis (or clitoris, in females) are split as if bisected. These subjects had penile deformities resulting in smaller erectile length and dorsal deviation. Using a semistructured psychiatric interview that included a sexual history, as well as measures of sexual knowledge and behavior problems, Reiner found evidence of psychosexual developmental delays, avoidance of normative experiences of nudity and masturbation in childhood and adolescence, as well as inhibited peer and dating relationships. Twelve out of these 14 boys had remained incontinent until age 6 out of fear of handling their penis. These findings illustrate the many medical, social, and emotional ramifications of urological conditions on development.

PSYCHOLOGICAL SEQUELAE

Emotional Response

Each patient with a urological condition responds uniquely. Tovian's (1997) review found agitated and retarded symptoms of depression to be the most commonly reported emotional response among individuals with urinary incontinence. The Federal Agency for Health Care Policy, in its Urinary Incontinence Guideline Panel (AHCPR Publication No. 92-0038), estimates that 25% of patients with UI view life as not worth living because of their incontinence. Actual embarrassment and/or fear of possible public embarrassment from "accidents" or others noticing urine wetness on clothes or urine odor are very pertinent emotional sequelae in managing incontinence. Directly associated with managing incontinence are feelings of loss of control, helplessness, insecurity, and despair that often cast gloom over other life domains. It is a common clinical observation that the loss of control in personal hygiene secondary to UI leads to feelings of self-doubt, shame, humiliation, and a damaged self- and body image (see review by Tovian and colleagues; Tovian, Rozensky, Sloan, & Slotnick, 1994). For example, patients with an indwelling catheter tend to be constantly aware of its presence and are often fearful of noticing the odor of urine.

Perhaps one of the most psychologically damaging emotional sequelae associated with urinary disorders are anticipated or real experiences with isolation, loneliness, and abandonment. Many patients with such symptoms tend to deny their emotional distress and focus their dissatisfaction on their physical symptoms. For example, Yarnell and colleagues (1982), reporting in the *Journal of Epidemiology and Community Health*, found that women who reported incontinence tended to appear more concerned with somatization issues on the Minnesota Multiphasic Personality Inventory (MMPI) relative to other medical populations. Government consensus panels assert that roughly one-third of the estimated 13 million incontinent patients would benefit from psychological intervention.

Social Response

Some people with urological disorders find it difficult to obtain and keep employment. For example, Tovian and colleagues reported patients losing their jobs or changing employment due to restriction of activities because of UI. Concerns regarding leakage and/or odor, for example, can impair work performance.

Many individuals rearrange their physical and social environments to accommodate the effects of urological disorders. Incontinent individuals often report that feelings of isolation are reinforced due to self-induced social withdrawal in response to fears of being "found out." Ouslander and colleagues (1987), reporting in the *Journal of Gerontology*, found that nursing home residents with UI felt they had fewer close friends or that they talked with friends less often but, in actuality, engaged in activities as frequently as others. (See Cash and Fleming's chapter on body image and social relations in this volume.) Patients who do not stay isolated or cannot mask their symptoms may be subject to gossip, hostile actions, and other forms of social ostracism and discrimination. Such social responses occurring in adolescence, when peer group acceptance and developing body awareness are particularly salient issues, can be especially damaging.

One often unavoidable consequence of urological disorders such as incontinence is a dependency resulting from difficulties with daily activities such as shopping, housekeeping, and hygiene. This is especially true for the elderly, who need more help from spouses and other family members. Many individuals with urinary disorders fear entering into marriage due to fear of rejection by a potential spouse once he or she learns of the urinary disorder or because of possible awkwardness in sexual relations.

Living with a person who suffers from a urological disorder can also have negative effects on family relations. The tasks involved in caring for the individual with incontinence, for example, are tiring, difficult, and often upsetting. Those who experience urinary disorders are often reluctant to talk openly about their condition. For this reason, caregivers are often unsure as to whether or not they are caring properly for their relative.

Sexual Functioning

Sexual functioning and body image are intimately related. (See Wiederman's chapter in this volume.) Myths and taboos have long existed about the genitals and sexual practices. Children are often admonished not to touch their genitals, and questions about sexual topics are often responded to with embarrassment. Such messages about sexuality and the genitals may (1) produce a lack of open discussion about sexual concerns, (2) distort perceptions of genitalia and sexuality, and (3) inhibit sexual pleasure.

This context of silence and conflict occurs in relation to urogenital disfigurement or dysfunction, either congenital or acquired, which engenders the emergence of destructive myths, such as the following: Penis size affects sexual pleasure; disabled persons are not sexual; the genitals and female breasts are the sole organs of sexual expression; one's masculinity or femininity is contingent on the number of people sexually attracted to one and the frequency of intercourse. Such myths, as well as negative views held by the affected individual regarding his or her sexual desirability and sexual competence, in combination with the real physical limitations, can impact sexual functioning.

The sexual and body image effects of these conditions may be influenced by the visibility or extent of the physical problem. However, changes in a person's body image are not always directly proportional to physical changes in appearance or function. Diagnosis of a urological disorder can leave a patient feeling stigmatized, even though little physical evidence of disease can be seen. The degree of impairment in a person's body image depends on a myriad of beliefs and feelings. Reviewing the cognitive-behavioral model of body image functioning described by Cash (in this volume) provides one very productive way of understanding the wide range of variables influencing how patients with urological conditions adapt to body image changes, in general, and to sexual changes, in particular.

Urological disorders often interfere with lovemaking skills. Some patients must adjust to making awkward preparations for sexual activity, including performing bladder care. For example, a male with an internal catheter inserted through the penis must fold the catheter back on the penis in order to apply a condom. A woman may elect to tape the catheter to the lower abdomen, using care not to tug or put tension on the catheter when taping it, lest irritation occur to the urinary opening.

Finally, despite the preservation of the capacity for erotic sensation, the psychological impact of penectomy (partial or total surgical amputation of the penis) or the presence of a penile prosthesis (such as a penile implant) can be devastating. The disfigurement that occurs almost inevitably leads to a vastly altered body image, lowered self-esteem, embarrassment, and dysphoria. The primary therapeutic goal following such radical surgery is to provide emotional support, accurate information, and to help the man reestablish the affection that may have existed prior to surgery. Rushing to establish sexual satisfaction prior to resolving the profound psychological distress can be counterproductive.

EVALUATION AND TREATMENT

Assessment

The clinical interview is the most important and common method of gathering diagnostic information from urology patients. Patients should be asked open-ended questions about their attitudes toward their urological disorder. These questions should elicit the behavioral, affective, and cognitive implications of the disorder; the degree of change and/or impairment involving social, sexual, occupational, leisure, and familial spheres; and degree of body image changes. Assessment questions should focus on whether the patient is maintaining a reasonable emotional balance, a satisfactory self-image, and a sense of competency and mastery. In addition, the patient should be asked whether he or she is preserving relationships with family and peers, and how he or she is preparing for a possibly uncertain future with the disorder. The patient's significant other as well as other family members should be asked how the urological disorder has affected his or her coping and body image functioning. Assessment of body image issues should parallel changes in urological symptoms and the implementation of any new treatments.

Shumaker and colleague (1994) developed an assessment instrument specific to urinary incontinence, the Incontinence Impact Questionnaire (IIQ), and a symptom identification and severity inventory, the Urogenital Distress Inventory (UDI), designed to assess quality of life issues associated with lower urinary tract and genital dysfunction. The Psychological Adjustment to Illness Scale (PAIS) developed by Derogatis in 1986 can be used to assess affective reactions and social and vocational concerns with respect to urological conditions when used with renal patient norms. Assessment of specific body image effects are, however, quite limited when using these measures. For example, in both the IIQ and UDI only one item assesses changes in the appearance of the vagina and/or penis secondary to UI; one item on the PAIS-R Emotional Distress subscale evaluates the degree of body image distortion secondary to renal disease. However, a number of body image measures described in the present volume can be used to evaluate the body image effects of urological conditions. In particular, Cash and Fleming's Body Image Quality of Life Inventory may be particularly applicable.

Interventions

Individual or group psychotherapy utilizing a coping skills approach could facilitate body image improvement by training patients in specific cognitive, behavioral, and affective competencies for managing the disruptive effects of urinary disorders. Tovian suggests the use of self-instruction techniques to help individuals with urinary incontinence learn constructive self-talk and avoid negativistic thinking. Tovian also proposes that patients engage in stress inoculation training, problem-solving strategies, assertiveness training, and progressive relaxation approaches, any or all of which can be applied in the midst of distressing social situations. Learning both cognitive and behavioral coping strategies may enhance adjustment and body image by expanding coping repertoires and increasing self-perception of control. To date, there have been no published studies on the effectiveness of using these approaches with specific body image dysfunctions. However, Cash and Strachan (in this volume) describe the efficacy of similar interventions for body image treatment in other contexts.

FUTURE RESEARCH

Further investigation of body image as it relates to urological disorders is clearly merited. However, even the relationship between urological disorders and body image requires clarification and specification. For example, health professionals fail to distinguish between the subjective body image experiences and the objective and definitive effects of the urological disorder itself. Similarly, there have been few attempts to discern the relative effects of self-concept and social response on body image and overall psychological adaptation. Making such distinctions is necessary to expand our understanding of how the quality of life of patients with urological conditions is mediated by psychological and body image functioning.

Studies are needed to identify specific body image problems associated with specific types of urological disorders. This specificity requires the development of body image assessment instruments that address and are normed with urological populations. (See Pruzinsky and Cash's chapter on quality-of-life assessment in medical settings in this volume.) More longitudinal studies are also needed to evaluate body image dysfunction over time.

Many additional questions remain, including: Are there gender and age-related differences in body image dysfunction specific to different types urological disorders? What are considered "normal" versus "abnormal" body image adaptations to urological disorders? Which type of psychological treatment is most effective with which type of body image dysfunction? The guidance provided by other chapters in the book—for example, Cash and Strachan's chapter on the efficacy of cognitive-behavioral interventions for body image disorders—is particularly helpful in addressing such questions.

INFORMATIVE READINGS

Abel, G. C., & Blendinger, D. E. (1986). Behavioral urology. In J. L. Houpt & H. K. Brodie (Eds.), *Consultation–liaison psychiatry and behavioral medicine* (pp. 163–174). New York:

Basic Books.—A review of behavior therapy techniques in the treatment of urological disorders.

Agency for Health Care Policy and Research, Public Health Service, U.S. Department of Health and Human Services. (1996, March). Urinary Incontinence Guideline Panel. *Urinary incontinence in adults: Clinical practice guidelines* (AHCPR Pub. No. 92-0038). Rockville, MD: Author.—A decision-tree model for assessment and treatment options with urinary incontinence.

Backman, M. E. (1989). *The psychology of the physically ill patient: A clinician's guide*. New York: Plenum.—A description of the psychological aspects of coping with medical illness.

Cash, T. F., & Fleming, E. C. (2002). The impact of body image experiences: Development of the Body Image Quality of Life Inventory. *International Journal of Eating Disorders, 31*, 455–460.—Presents information on the psychosocial impact of body image experiences including affects on social relations.

Cash, T. F., & Pruzinsky, T. (Eds.). (1990). *Body images: Development, deviance, and change*. New York: Guilford Press.—This volume covers the many diverse aspects of body image.

Derogatis, L. (1986). The Psychological Adjustment to Illness Scale (PAIS). *Journal of Psychosomatic Research, 30*, 77–91.—A 46-item semistructured interview designed to evaluate and quantify the level of adjustment along seven dimensions of a chronically ill medical patient to his or her disease.

Gartley, C. B. (1985). *Managing incontinence*. Ottawa, IL: Jameson Books.—This book covers the many diverse aspects of urinary incontinence.

Livneh, H., & Antonak, R. F. (1997). *Psychosocial adaptation to chronic illness and disability*. Gaithersberg, MD: Aspen.—A description of the psychological aspects of rehabilitation in the context of medical illness and physical disabilities.

Ouslander, J. G., Morishita, L., Blaustein, J., Orzeck, S., Dunn, S., & Sayre, J. (1987). Clinical, functional, and psychosocial characteristics of an incontinent nursing home population. *Journal of Gerontology, 42*, 631–637.—A profile of demographics, functional capacities, and psychological factors of urinary incontinent individuals living in a nurshing home.

Reiner, W. G. (1999). Psychosexual dysfunction in late adolescent males with genital anomalies. *Journal of American Academy of Child and Adolescent Psychiatry, 15*, 1040–1054.—A study identifying psychosexual problems among late adolescent males with genital abnormalities several years postsurgery.

Schover, L. R., & Jenson, S. B. (1988). *Sexuality and chronic illness: A comprehensive approach*. New York: Guilford Press.—A description of sexual problems and interventions with patients having chronic medical illnesses.

Shumaker, S. A., Wyman, J. F., Ubersax, J. S., McClish, D. K., & Fantl, J. A. (1994). Health-related quality of life measures for women with urinary incontinence: The Incontinence Impact Questionnaire and The Urogenital Distress Inventory. *Quality of Life Research, 3*, 291–306.—A 30-item and a 19-item questionnaire, respectively, which assess quality-of-life factors among women with urinary incontinence and genital dysfunction.

Tovian, S. M. (1996). Health psychology and the field of urology. In R. J. Resnick & R. H. Rozensky (Eds.), *Health psychology through the life span: Practice and research opportunities* (pp. 289–312). Washington, DC: American Psychological Association.—A review of the interface between health psychology and urological disorders from a developmental perspective.

Tovian, S. M. (1997). Urological disorders. In P. M. Camic & S. J. Knight (Eds.), *Clinical handbook of health psychology: A practical guide to effective interventions* (pp. 439–480). Seattle, WA: Hogrefe & Huber.—A review of psychological interventions with urological disorders such as incontinence, erectile dysfunction, and urethral syndrome.

Tovian, S. M., Rozensky, R. H., Sloan, T. B., & Slotnick, G. M. (1994). Adult urinary incontinence: Assessment, intervention, and the role of clinical health psychology in program development. *Journal of Clinical Psychology in Medical Settings, 1,* 339–362.—A review of psychological assessment and interventions with urinary incontinence.

Wincze, J. P., & Carey, M. P. (2001). *Sexual dysfunction: A guide for assessment and treatment* (2nd ed.). New York: Guilford Press.—A clinician's guide to sex therapy, with chapters on patients with chronic medical illness.

Yarnell, J. W., Voyle, G. J., Sweetnam, P. M., Milbank, J., Richards, C. J., & Stephenson, T. P. (1982). Factors associated with urinary incontinence in women. *Journal of Epidemiology and Community Health, 36,* 58–63.—A correlational study comparing social demographics and psychological factors among women with urinary incontinence.

42

Body Image Issues in Endocrinology

JANE GILMOUR

This chapter explores the nature of body image and other psychosocial concerns that may develop for some individuals with a select number of endocrine disorders, including short stature, growth hormone deficiency, precocious puberty, as well as Turner's and Cushing's syndromes. Because these disorders negatively affect physical appearance, it is reasonable to hypothesize that they will also negatively affect overall self-esteem and body image functioning. Unfortunately, however, much of the endocrine disorder literature does not specifically evaluate body image functioning, though there are numerous studies describing general psychosocial dysfunction in the form of depression, social isolation, and anxiety. While these psychosocial problems might be secondary to body image concerns, many other possible explanations for such symptoms must be considered, especially the role of biological variables that are particularly relevant to consider in the context of endocrine function.

Body image experiences are also clearly influenced by social factors, as documented in the chapters in this volume by Tiggemann, Kearney-Cooke, Tantleff-Dunn and Gokee, as well as Cash and Fleming. There is increasing evidence that the psychological responses to endocrinological conditions such as "normal short stature" and Turner's syndrome may also reflect the negative views of family members, peers or partners. Such negative social responses can easily result in negative self-concept, body image concerns, and social isolation, each of which can have profoundly negative effects on many areas of psychological and social functioning and overall quality of life.

On the other hand, in some (admittedly rather rare) cases, there may be positive social biases associated with the physical anomalies resulting from endocrinological conditions. For example, some prepubertal children of short stature appear to enjoy the "cute personality" assigned to them on the basis of their height. Such personality assignation is clearly the result of social stereotyping, but the experience, nonetheless, seems to be positive for some individuals and illustrates how physical anomalies are not invariably associated with negative psychological experiences.

AGE- AND GENDER-SPECIFIC BODY IMAGE CONCERNS

To clearly understand the nature of body image concerns for individuals with endocrine disorders, it is necessary to know how their psychological development is similar to and different from individuals not affected by such disorders. For example, we know that body image concerns are often exacerbated for adolescents (see Chapter 9 by Levine and Smolak in this volume), and that physical appearance becomes increasingly less important through adulthood (see the chapter by Whitbourne and Skultety in this volume). We also know that, in general, men report higher self-esteem and a more positive body image than women, particularly in adolescence.

Unfortunately, however, a significant proportion of the research on endocrine disorders does not include adequate comparison groups to allow for conclusions to be drawn regarding the relative impact of gender or age on the development of psychological problems, in general, or body image concerns more specifically. For example, although social stereotypes lead us to believe that it is a greater social handicap for males to be of short stature than females, this observation has not been adequately documented. Similarly, while hirsutism would appear to be socially less acceptable for females than for males, there is, once again, little empirical documentation of this stereotype.

SHORT STATURE—MIXED ETIOLOGY

There is some scientific documentation of the psychological profile of individuals with various conditions that cause short stature (including growth hormone insufficiency and Turner's syndrome). Unfortunately, however, in this research literature all individuals with short stature are considered as one group, irrespective of etiology. Therefore, these data have only limited value, as it is often difficult to determine if some diagnoses are disproportionately represented in the mixed etiology groups. Further, there may be specific factors associated with conditions included in these samples that have an effect on body image, such as depression.

Individuals who are significantly shorter than "normal" (usually defined as being at or below the third population centile for height) but who have no identified endocrine condition, such as growth hormone insufficiency, are described as having normal short stature (NSS). NSS may more accurately be considered a variation on the normal continuum, as opposed to a medical condition requiring treatment. Nevertheless, because of the importance of height in social and personal evaluations, NSS is interesting and important to study in terms of its influence on body image functioning. Additionally, individuals with NSS have neither hormonal imbalance nor dysmorphic features. Therefore, any body image difficulties that may develop for these individuals are likely to be the result of short stature alone.

General adjustment problems, such as low confidence and self-esteem, have been reported for both children and adults with short stature. However, these studies included individuals with short stature of mixed etiology, not just those with NSS. More recent accounts in epidemiological studies using homogeneous groups—for example, the study conducted by Downie and colleagues—indicate that prepubertal children with NSS have good general adjustment and largely positive self-concept. This finding also holds for children attending growth clinics, who are likely to have greater awareness of, and possibly concern about, their stature, and is therefore a robust test of the hypothesis that these children have no demonstrable adjustment problems. Nevertheless, some prepubertal children with NSS are described by parents and teachers as having behavioral difficulties, as reported by Voss and colleagues in 1991, for example. The study by Gilmour and Skuse indicates that much of the maladjustment variance is explained by general cognitive ability. In other words, children with a proportionately lower IQs (though still within normal limits) are more likely to be described as having adjustment problems

It is characteristic of the general population, irrespective of age or gender, to overestimate one's own height. The findings of Skuse and Gilmour's 1997 study documented that the majority of children with NSS correctly recognize that they are shorter than their peers, though interestingly they tend to underestimate the relative degree of difference as compared to their peers of average height. They do, however, express a wish to be taller. Indeed they aspire to be taller than the population average. This finding has implications for patient satisfaction with treatment in that patient expectations may be too high. In sum, it is true that prepubertal children with NSS are dissatisfied with their body image, because they clearly wish to be taller, but this preference does not constitute an adjustment problem, per se, for the majority. Once again, however, it is important to note that these investigators have not specifically used measures of body image functioning, and therefore we cannot draw definitive empirical conclusions regarding the body image concerns of these individuals.

The influence of parental views on children's body image is becoming increasingly well documented. (See chapter by Kearney-Cooke in this volume.) Gilmour and Skuse asked children with NSS and comparison subjects to describe the body shape and size they believed their parents would like them (the children) to be. Both groups reported that they believed their parents' ideal was for their children to be of average height. It is fair to conclude, then, that children with NSS have a sense of their parents' dissatisfaction with their body size. This dissatisfaction might feasibly constitute a risk factor for future adjustment problems. It may be that during childhood, children of short stature expect that because they are still growing, they will eventually catch up with their peers. There may also be a cumulative effect of negative social evaluations of short stature over time, in which short children absorb and internalize peers' and significant others' views of their appearance. Data reviewed by Siegel, Clopper, and Stabler in 1991 indicated that individuals with short stature have positive perceptions of their social relationships early on, but develop more negative interpersonal perceptions later. Adult males with NSS report feeling less satisfied with their height than men of average or tall stature. In contrast to the prepubertal children with NSS who may be perceived as "cute," there is clear evidence from studies, such as those by Martel and Biller in 1987 and Schumacher in 1982, that people have frankly negative perceptions of short men in personal, social, and professional contexts. The little longitudinal data that do exist support this observation of the social disadvantages men of short stature encounter. Holmes and colleagues described individuals with NSS who were well adjusted in middle childhood but who showed decline in social competence in adolescence. Large-scale longitudinal studies currently being conducted (such as the Wessex Growth Study in the United Kingdom and the National Co-operative Growth Study in the United States) will add valuable data to the developmental profile of individuals with NSS.

GROWTH HORMONE DEFICIENCY

Investigations of body image and growth hormone insufficiency (GHI) should distinguish between isolated growth hormone deficiency (IGD) and multiple pituitary hormone deficiencies (MPHD), though many studies fail to do so. Individuals with MPHD characteristically have lower levels of general cognitive ability than those with IGD. Low general cognitive ability is associated with poor self-concept in individuals of average stature. Therefore, there is every indication that this relationship may apply to some individuals with GHI. Given the high correlation between overall self-concept and body image, it seems warranted to investigate the relationship between these variables and cognitive ability in patients with all forms of GHI.

In contrast to the general population, both male and female adults with growth hormone deficiency tend to underestimate their body size, in some instances, by a significant margin, and also have low self-esteem. Earlier studies described many general psychosocial problems associated with GH deficiency, including a negative body image. More recent data (e.g., Carroll and colleagues' 1997 study) indicate that these individuals have primary psychological problems caused by lack of GH, in contrast with those who have adjustment problems secondary to negative perceptions and societal expectations. How these primary psychological disturbances affect body image remains unclear. However, it is likely that adaptation problems and body image dissatisfaction will have numerous biological and psychosocial causes.

GH therapy increases ultimate adult height when it is administered to children with GHI. In some cases, adults with GHI are offered GH therapy, even if they underwent it in childhood. When given in adulthood, GH therapy influences body composition and metabolism, though it no longer affects stature or the recipients' underestimation of body size. There is consistent evidence, based on studies employing double-blind methodologies (including the 1997 study described by Carroll and colleagues), that GH therapy in adulthood has a positive effect on general psychosocial adjustment. However, one needs to cautiously interpret even the most rigorously designed study, because the physical effects associated with GH therapy, such as the reduction of body fat and increase in lean tissue, make it very unlikely that individuals cannot be entirely unaware of their treatment condition. The mechanism causing the apparent improvement in well-being is not known. However, a number of different hypotheses exist, including one positing that GH therapy increases beta-endorphin levels or alters levels of homovanillic acid, which are known to affect mood.

PRECOCIOUS PUBERTY

Traditionally, precocious puberty is identified in girls less than 9 years old and boys less than 10 who show signs of pubertal onset. Idiopathic precocious puberty is much less common in males, which may explain the lack of data describing their adjustment, though in their 1994 review, Ehrhardt and colleagues hypothesized that the issues are similar across both genders. In young adulthood, there is evidence of minor general adjustment difficulties. However, young women who have had precocious puberty do not have particularly negative perceptions of their body. Although they tend to be of relatively short stature in adulthood, they describe no marked dissatisfaction with their height, and they accurately describe themselves as having developed faster and looking older.

TURNER'S SYNDROME

Turner's syndrome (TS), the complete or partial absence of one X chromosome, is a sex chromosomal disorder affecting only females. TS has several cardinal endocrinological features, including short stature, though the precise mechanism of growth disorder is debated in the literature. Affected females also lack sex hormones. There is good evidence that GH therapy, with the addition of estrogen substitution to induce puberty, increases adult height. There are fairly consistent reports, including one by McCauley, Ito, and Kay in 1986, indicating that women with TS are dissatisfied with their physical appearance relative to comparison groups. Like children with NSS, prepubertal girls with TS believe that they are taller than they really are and have unrealistic expectations about the final height they can achieve following GH treatment.

Girls and women with TS have a greater chance than the non-TS female population of developing anorexia nervosa (AN), a disorder in which body image is characteristically distorted. The oral–motor problems associated with TS, which include poor lip muscle tone and chewing skills, may precipitate poor appetite to some degree, though some affected females have a tendency to be overweight. It is unclear if AN is more likely to occur in girls with a history of poor appetite or those who tend to be overweight. However, in the general population, a slightly elevated body mass index is linked to the onset of AN. (See chapter by Garner in this volume.)

Nicholls and Stanhope suggest that there is an interaction between girls' social cognition and pubertal hormonal treatment that precipitates AN. Females with TS have marked visuospatial difficulties—specifically, relating and locating aspects of visual information—which might feasibly affect body perception. Though it is speculative, one might consider how such visuospatial and social-cognitive difficulties could influence body image perception. That is, the body image distortions that develop in this population may not be completely the result of the actual physical anomalies that exist, but may be partially the result of these visuospatial and social-cognitive deficits as well as hormonal influences. There is also evidence that women and girls with TS have marked difficulties interpreting social cues such as facial expression. These social-cognition problems seem to be partly secondary to their visuospatial deficits. Studies have shown that social perception (and peer perception, in particular) predicts satisfaction with self-perception. Therefore, it may be that, to some degree, those with TS have developed a negative body image because they tend to misinterpret social signals, though no empirical data exist to support such a relationship.

CUSHING'S SYNDROME

Individuals with Cushing's syndrome (CS) have elevated levels of cortisol. The features of the condition, which include obesity, a "moon face," hirsutism (excess body hair) in females, and a "buffalo hump" (a mound of fat between the shoulders), suggest that affected individuals may be particularly vulnerable to body image problems. Unfortunately, there is a lack of empirical data describing body image in people with CS. However, we do know that a significant proportion of individuals with CS have psychiatric disorders, the most common being depression. Estimates indicate that between one half to two-thirds of those with CS have a depressive illness. There is also good evidence, provided by Kelly in 1996, for example, that these psychiatric conditions are a primary effect of the hormonal imbalance characteristic of CS. However, older studies, such as the 1970 paper by Gifford and Gunderson, suggested that they are secondary to the same stressful life events that precipitate the condition itself. It is clear that depression affects the ability to objectively evaluate oneself, the world, and the future. Whatever the nature of the cause of the depression in these individuals, it may very well be that they have a negative and potentially distorted self and body image, as a general consequence of having a depressive illness. These issues illustrate two distinct variations of body image problems that need to be considered during patient assessment: that is, the distinction between body dissatisfaction and perceptual distortion, in which the perception may be different from objective evidence. In other words, individuals with CS may feel dissatisfied with their body because they are objectively obese. These same people may have, in addition, a distorted negative body image secondary to a depressive illness and therefore perceive themselves to be more obese than objective data indicate. Understanding this distinction is crucial if we are to develop effective interventions aimed at the specific mechanisms that contribute to body image problems.

INTERVENTION

Current treatment for many forms of endocrinological disorders has focused on the use of hormonal therapy. For example, GH therapy in childhood increases adult height for some conditions, such as TS and GHI. GH therapy also accelerates the growth trajectory of children with NSS, though it does not affect final adult height. One may question if such a potentially disruptive, painful, and expensive treatment is warranted for children with NSS, given the lack of evidence of psychosocial disturbance throughout childhood. Boulton and colleagues described children with NSS who received GH treatment over 2 years. After 6 months both the treatment and placebo groups had similar views about their growth and stature. Following the 6-month period, the placebo group was also offered treatment for the remainder of the study. All participating children described a more positive attitude toward their stature after 2 years. It is unclear if the improved attitude is linked to increased stature or a developmental effect during prepuberty; however, that body image attitude was measured at all is a remarkable feature of this study. Patient perception and report is surely a key outcome variable in treatment evaluation, whether intervention is psychological or endocrinological.

The efficacy of future treatment packages may be increased by including a psychological treatment component. Adding such a component is particularly important in view of the evidence that both children and parents have unrealistic exceptions about the effects of GH therapy. Treatment efficacy of endocrine disorders should be multifactorial, including psychological and body measurement appraisal.

Psychological interventions, particularly cognitive-behavioral approaches, are effective in positively modifying body image functioning in domains such as eating disorders. (See Cash and Strachan's chapter in this volume.) Currently, there are no systematic trials, as far as I am aware, assessing the efficacy of such interventions for individuals with endocrine conditions. However, given the range of potential body image concerns in this population, it seems reasonable to evaluate if such psychosocial interventions could help improve the quality of life of these individuals. Also especially needed are measures specific to the appearance and body image concerns of this population. Currently available body image measures, with their focus on weight and body shape, do not evaluate those variables of particular concern to this patient population (see chapter in this volume by Pruzinsky and Cash on the assessment of body image and quality of life in medical settings). The development of disease-specific measures will enhance assessment of patients' quality of life as well as the efficacy of biological and psychological interventions.

INFORMATIVE READINGS

Boulton, T. J. C., Dunn, S. M., Quigley, C. A., Taylor, J. J., & Thompson, L. (1991). Perceptions of self and short stature: Effects of two years of growth hormone treatment. *Acta Pediatrica Scandinavica, 377*, 20–27.—One of the few studies to include *child's attitude* as a treatment outcome variable.

Carroll, P. V., Littlewood, R., Weissberger, A. J., Bogalho, P., McGauley, G., Sonksen, P. H., & Russell-Jones, D. L. (1997). The effects of two doses of replacement growth hormone on the biochemical, body composition and psychological profiles of growth hormone-deficit adults. *European Journal of Endocrinology, 137*, 146–153.—An informative double-blind study.

Dowdney, L., Woodward, L., Pickles, A., & Skuse, D. (1995). The Body Image Perception and Attitude Scale for Children: Reliability in growth retarded and community comparison subjects. *International Journal of Methods in Psychiatric Research, 5*, 29–40.—A good visual analogue measure of body size suitable for children.

Downie, B., Mulligan, J., Stratford, R. J., Betts, P. R., & Voss, L. D. (1997). Are short normal children at a disadvantage?: The Wessex growth study. *British Medical Journal, 314*, 97–100.—Valuable data from a large-scale epidemiological longitudinal study.

Ehrhardt, A., Meyer-Bahlburg, H., Bell, J., Cohen, S., Healey, J., Stiel, R., Feldman, J., Morishima, A., & New, M. (1984). Idiopathic precocious puberty in girls: Psychiatric follow-up in adolescence. *Journal of the American Academy of Child Psychiatry, 23*, 23–33.—A wide-ranging psychosocial assessment of girls experiencing precocious puberty .

Gifford, S., & Gunderson, J. G. (1970). Cushing's disease as a psychosomatic disorder. *Medicine, 49*, 397–409.—A series of 10 case studies concluding that Cushing's disease and its associated psychiatric features were secondary to the adverse life events, as opposed to primary hormonal imbalance.

Gilmour, J., & Skuse, D. (1996). Short stature: The role of intelligence in psychosocial adjustment. *Archives of Disease in Childhood, 75*, 25–31.—A study describing a homogeneous group of clinic-referred children with NSS.

Holmes, C. S., Karlsson, J. A., & Thompson, R. G. (1986). Longitudinal evaluation of behaviour patterns in children with short stature. In B. Stabler & L. E. Underwood (Eds.), *Slow grows the child: Psychological aspects of growth delay* (pp. 1–12). Hillsdale, NJ: Erlbaum.—One of the few longitudinal studies of individuals with short stature.

Kelly, W. F. (1996). Psychiatric aspects of Cushing's syndrome. *Quarterly Journal of Medicine, 69*, 545–551.—A case comparison retrospective study describing the temporal relationship between psychiatric illness and Cushing's syndrome.

Martel, L. F., & Biller, H. B. (1987). *Stature and stigma: The biopsychosocial development of short males.* Lexington, MA: DC Heath.—Men of average-range height and short stature using questionnaire data, report their levels of confidence in different social situations.

McCauley, E., Ito, J., & Kay, T. (1986). Psychosocial functioning in girls with Turner's syndrome and short stature: Social skills, behaviour problems and self-concept. *Journal of the American Academy of Child Psychiatry, 25*, 105–112.—A comprehensive description of functioning in girls with TS.

Nicholls, D., & Stanhope, R. (1998). Turner's syndrome, anorexia nervosa and anabolic steroids. *Archives of Disease in Childhood, 79*, 1–2.—A paper hypothesizing why AN occurs disproportionately in girls and women with TS; includes clinical case studies.

Schumacher, A. (1982). On the significance of stature in human society. *Journal of Human Evolution, 11*, 697–701.—An interesting study showing that once confounding factors are controlled, taller people have higher-status jobs.

Siegel, P. T., Clopper, R., & Stabler, B. (1991). Psychological impact of significantly short stature. *Acta Paediatrica Scandinavica, 377*(Suppl.), 14–18.—A review of the literature describing cognitive and psychosocial adjustment in children with short stature of mixed etiology.

Skuse, D., & Gilmour, J. (1997). The quality of life of children with Normal Short Stature. *Clinical Pediatric Endocrinology, 6*, 29–37.—A case comparison study including children's reports of their own body perceptions and their understanding of their parents' aspirations of body shape.

Voss, L. D., Bailey, B. J. R., Mulligan, J., Wilkin, T. J., & Betts, P. R. (1991). Short stature and school performance—the Wessex Growth Study. *Acta Pediatrica Scandinavica, 377*(Suppl.), 29–31.—An excellent epidemiological study of short stature in the population.

43

Body Images in Oncology

CRAIG A. WHITE

Cancer and cancer treatments can significantly change appearance and bodily integrity, particularly in some cancers. Much of the literature on body image and cancer is observational, atheoretical, and anecdotal. Though more empirical research has recently emerged, it is often of poor quality, resulting in inconsistent findings.

Interpreting results has been difficult due to use of poorly validated measures. Definitions of body image have often been tautologous (e.g., "positive," "negative," "secure," "insecure"), and distinctions among multiple body image dimensions have not been made. Additionally, the term "body image" has been used to refer to related constructs, such as sexuality, self-esteem, stigma, and self-consciousness, and has been defined too broadly to permit meaningful investigation.

These problems have compromised assessment and treatment of body image problems in oncology patients. It is clear, nevertheless, that many people with cancer experience appearance and body integrity concerns. Fortunately, researchers are beginning to specify in greater detail the psychological constructs necessary for understanding how body image is affected by oncological conditions.

COMMON CANCER-RELATED BODY IMAGE CONCERNS

Appearance-Related Changes

For some people the distress associated with cancer centers on appearance-related changes that may act as persistent reminders of the disease. Such distress can trigger preexisting vulnerabilities to psychological disorders and

379

adjustment problems. Appearance changes are particularly traumatic when accompanied by functional changes (e.g., loss of speech).

Some cancers have clearly observable appearance effects (e.g., disfigurement from head and neck cancer). Less observable appearance changes—for example, the effects of lymphedema (i.e., swelling caused by drainage failure in the lymphatic system)—can also have a significant negative impact on appearance and can influence clothing choice for some patients.

The speed with which appearance changes occur can also influence psychological adjustment. A patient who experiences gradual loss of hair over the course of a week has some time to adjust, whereas the surgical loss of a body part happens suddenly. The degree to which the change in appearance is permanent can also affect patients' responses. Some patients cope well only because they are told that the changes are temporary (e.g., in the case of temporary ileostomy). Many appearance changes are reversible or can be minimized. Some patients now undergo immediate surgical reconstruction, thus avoiding the need to adjust to dramatically altered appearance. For example, approximately one-third of women who undergo mastectomy opt for immediate breast reconstruction.

Sensory-Related Concerns

In addition to appearance changes, cancer and its treatment may result in sensory changes, including auditory (e.g., changes in speech production for patients with laryngeal cancer, or the noises produced by an artificial limb used to replace an amputated limb due to osteosarcoma), olfactory (e.g., colorectal tumors result in placement of a stoma), or tactile changes(e.g., alterations in breast sensation in breast reconstruction patients). These sensory changes can also influence how others respond to the patient and may be viewed as important as appearance-related changes to both patient and close others.

Body Image Concerns Specific to Cancer Treatment

In addition to tumor removal, surgery may also result in removal of a body part (e.g., removal of an eye due to an intraocular tumor). Though it appears that most surgical treatments have short-term effects on self-image, some can significantly reduce body satisfaction (e.g., cystectomy for bladder cancer). Additionally, the physical effects often last much longer, such as the body image discomfort reported by women with breast cancer up to 2 years postdiagnosis.

Surgery to an internal body part, although not visible, can cause significant body image distress because of its particular psychological importance—for example, the removal of a testicle. Scarring resulting from surgery, as occurs when a bowel resection is done, can also be distressing. Interestingly, a small portion of patient consider themselves to be "incomplete" as a result of cancer surgery, a factor associated with increased risk of psychopathology.

Body image concerns may also be focused on external devices, such as when a stoma or an external feeding device is needed. Some women who undergo mastectomy without reconsturuction report having difficulty adjusting to breast prostheses. Indeed, many women report more problems adjusting to the prostheses than to the surgical change in appearance (e.g., mastectomy scars).

Chemotherapy can also affect appearance, for example, by causing hair loss or by requiring the presence of catheters. Additionally, corticosteriods may cause changes in facial appearance, and cancer may result in pallor or postural changes associated with fatigue. Women with breast cancer may experience weight gain because of treatment-induced menopause, hormone treatments, changes in endocrine function, overall activity level, and possibly overeating. Radiation treatment can be associated with visible dermatological changes, and the body marking used for treatment planning concerns some patients.

These appearance-related changes resulting from treatment are often ranked as more severe than side effects such as nausea, insomnia, breathlessness, and fatigue. Patients' responses to such changes, though not always apparent, can significantly affect their self-confidence and overall well-being and therefore warrant careful consideration. In some instances, diminished self-confidence does not return to pretreatment levels, even when prior appearance is restored.

Body Image Concerns of Children and Adolescents

Varni and colleagues found that children with cancer who perceive their physical appearance more positively tend to be less depressed, less socially anxious, and have higher self-esteem. The positive view of appearance seems to be mediated by self-esteem, which influences perceived adequacy and competency.

Children and adolescents may find it more difficult to deal with cancer-related appearance changes than the pain associated with the disease or its treatment. Adolescent cancer survivors tend to have more negative perceptions of their bodies than controls who have not had cancer, even when objective assessment of attractiveness reveals no between-group differences. Despite these problems, adolescents with cancer appear less inclined to report such difficulties—an important trend to consider when evaluating body image concerns in this population. Younger patients tend to have greater concern about their appearance than older patients, though this is not invariably the case.

ASSESSING CANCER-RELATED BODY IMAGE VARIABLES

Body image assessment within oncology is still primitive. Assessment methods have included open-ended questions, semistructured interviews, and self-report measures. Some assessments consist of single-item evaluations, and most questionnaires lack adequate standardization, have poor psychometric properties, and/or are insufficiently validated. Some measurement strategies may have variable sensitivity to assessing body image change (e.g., when comparing results from a semistructured interview with those from questionnaires). (See chapter by Pruzinsky and Cash regarding body image assessment in medical contexts.)

The content of many currently available and well-validated body image measures is not suitable for use in oncology because the focus is on weight-related appearance. However, some measures, such as the Appearance Schemas Inventory and the Situational Inventory of Body-Image Dysphoria, are readily applicable with little or no modification. Additionally, a few oncology-specific measures have emerged, such as the Body Image Scale (BIS), which, though not tumor site-specific, evaluates behavioral and satisfaction variables as well self-consciousness, physical attractiveness, and physical integrity. The BIS was developed by Hopwood and colleagues and is compatible with the quality-of-life assessments developed by the European Organization for Research and Treatment of Cancer Quality of Life Group. Additionally, Kopel and colleagues developed the Body Image Instrument for use with adolescents; it evaluates patient perception of appearance, reactions of others to appearance, and the value placed on appearance. Carver and colleagues devised the Measure of Body Apperception to assess attitudes reflective of investment in appearance and body integrity.

CONCEPTUALIZATION OF BODY IMAGE IN ONCOLOGY

Prevailing models of body image in cancer have been oversimplistic (i.e., focusing on negative/positive or secure/insecure dimensions) and limiting. However, a heuristic, multidimensional model of body image in oncology was developed by White (see Figure 43.1).

From the perspective of this model, clinicians and researchers need to understand the value attached to the body part affected by cancer. Patients should be asked about appearance concerns, and if these exist, be given the opportunity to describe their thoughts, feelings, behaviors, life experiences, and beliefs related to appearance.

People who have greater levels of investment in body parts affected by cancer are more likely to experience psychological problems related to appearance change. However, Carver and colleagues demonstrated that patients with greater investment in appearance were more resilient when it

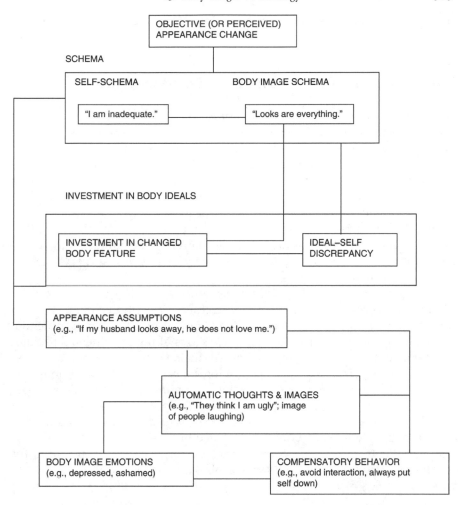

FIGURE 43.1. A heuristic model of important body image dimensions. From White (2000). Copyright 2000 by John Wiley & Sons Limited. Reprinted by permission.

came to self-perceptions of general attractiveness, femininity, and sexual desirability. They also found that investment in body integrity had an adverse effect on social and recreational functioning and produced greater self-alienation. Although these findings are limited by the use of an unvalidated measure, they reinforce the critical observation that we should not assume that high levels of appearance investment invariably have a globally deleterious effect on other psychological variables. Additionally, the intensity of investment in appearance is likely to change as a function of time, status of cancer, emotional functioning, and social network and relationship quality.

To fully understand body image functioning in oncology, each of these variables must be assessed.

BODY IMAGE AND CANCER TREATMENT DECISIONS

People with decisions to make about appearance-changing cancer treatment need support when evaluating how their thoughts, beliefs, and feelings about appearance may influence their decisions. For example, women who choose lumpectomy over mastectomy usually have more anticipatory anxiety concerns about appearance, and breast-conserving surgery does seem to have fewer negative body image effects. Although women are likely to place more importance on survival when it comes to deciding about cancer treatments, there may be a minority for whom appearance is so important that they opt for a medically less desirable alternative. Some patients may refuse any treatment rather than undergo extremely disfiguring surgery, such as radical vulvectomy.

Surgery may also be offered to women who have a high genetic risk of developing cancer (e.g., risk-reducing mastectomy or oophorectomy). Women considering this form of surgery are often quite concerned about the potential impact on appearance and subsequent reactions of their partners. Although the majority of women who undergo risk-reducing mastectomy and breast reconstruction experience positive psychological benefits, a proportion report negative effects on appearance and feelings of femininity. Some patients experience skin necrosis, nipple loss, infection and pain, as well as the perception that the breast feels unnatural when touched, which increases likelihood of dissatisfaction. In general, body image outcomes are hard to predict. For example, patients who undergo reconstructive surgery and/or are fitted for prostheses often experience the same levels of satisfaction as those who have had not.

DELIVERING SENSITIVE CARE

Delivery of psychological care for people with cancer would be greatly enhanced if all clinical staff were knowledgeable and competent in assessing body image variables such as body satisfaction, level of investment in appearance, and recognition of problems requiring assessment by specialists in psychosocial oncology. These specialists can evaluate a range of related psychosocial variables, including appearance schemas and compensatory behavior, and provide appropriate intervention.

Ideally, cancer centers should ensure equitable access to specialists in psychological assessment and intervention for body image problems. This addition is particularly essential for those professionals who treat cancers that have a major negative impact on appearance and function. In the future, protocols should be developed that clearly outline how body image variables will be considered in treatment decision making (e.g., when planning risk-reducing mastectomy).

FUTURE RESEARCH QUESTIONS

There is an urgent need for consensus on what constitutes clinically significant body image disturbance in cancer survivors. Additionally, psychological interventions that have demonstrated effectiveness for body image problems in other patient groups should be evaluated in cancer settings. Given their intensive patient contact, oncology nurses may be in a particularly advantageous position to apply an improved understanding of body image variables in cancer assessment and treatment. Similarly, more work is needed to apply mainstream body image research to cancer. For example, Cash and Szymanski's research on self–ideal discrepancies may be particularly informative. In general, taking a multidimensional approach to research and treatment that is informed by current body image theory is also essential. Fortunately, some of these developments are occurring. Recent publication of cancer-specific body image assessment tools will likely assist in establishing validated models that can be used to guide assessment, psychological and medical treatment, and outcome evaluation within cancer care settings.

INFORMATIVE READINGS

Carver, C. S., Pozo-Kaderman, C., Price, A. A., Noriega, V., Harris, S., Derhagopian, R. P., Robinson, D. S., & Moffat, F. L (1998). Concern about aspects of body image and adjustment to early stage breast cancer. *Psychosomatic Medicine*, 60(2), 168–174.—A prospective evaluation of the role of appearance investment and body integrity in a group of women with early stage breast cancer.

Cash, T. F., & Szymanski, M. L. (1995). The development and validation of the body-image ideals questionnaire. *Journal of Personality Assessment*, 64(3), 466–477.—A description of the validation of a questionnaire to assess the extent to which an individual's ideals vary from his or her actual appearance. A key figure of the questionnaire is that responses are weighted according to perceived importance of appearance attributes.

Hopwood, P., Fletcher, I., Lee, A. & Al. Ghazal, S. (2001). A body image scale for use with cancer patients. *European Journal of Cancer*, 37, 189–197. —A description of the development and psychometric properties of a brief assessment scale for body image variables in cancer.

Kopel, S. J., Eiser, C., Cool, P., Grimer, R. J., & Carter, S. R. (1998). Brief report: Assessment of body image in survivors of childhood cancer. *Journal of Pediatric Psychology, 23*(2), 141–147.—An outline of the development of the Body Image Instrument, a 28-item measure of general appearance, body competence, others' reaction to appearance, value of appearance, and self-consciousness.

Piff, C. (1998). Body image: A patient's perspective. *British Journal of Theatre Nursing, 8*(1), 13–14.—A personal account of the psychosocial impact of disfiguring cancer.

Price, B. (1998). Cancer: Altered body image. *Nursing Standard, 12*(21), 49–55.—A series of self-guided learning exercises to increase understanding of contributors to altered body image and the delivery of assessment and care.

Varni, J. W., Katz, E. R., Colegrove, R., & Dolgin, M. (1995). Perceived physical appearance and adjustment of children with newly diagnosed cancer: A path analytic model. *Journal of Behavioral Medicine, 18*(3), 261–277.—A well-executed study that tests a conceptual model of the contribution of perceived physical appearance to depressive symptoms, self-esteem, and social anxiety.

White, C. A. (2000). Body image dimensions and cancer: A heuristic cognitive behavioural model. *Psycho-Oncology, 9*, 183–192.—A review that argues for integration of mainstream body image research with body image research in cancer care.

44

Rehabilitation Medicine and Body Image

BRUCE D. RYBARCZYK

JAY M. BEHEL

Rehabilitation medicine is a broad field that provides a range of inpatient and outpatient services to enhance the overall health and functioning of individuals with various chronic diseases and disabilities. The same breadth is found in *rehabilitation psychology*, which encompasses the study and application of psychosocial principles on behalf of persons who have physical, sensory, cognitive, developmental, or emotional disabilities. For this chapter we narrow the scope of discussion to the disability groups that rehabilitation psychologists have the most experience serving: those who are admitted to an inpatient rehabilitation unit with an *acquired disability*. Common acquired disabilities in this setting include traumatic brain injury, spinal cord injury, stroke, amputation, and various neurological conditions that result in physical impairment and/or chronic pain.

Rehabilitation psychologists frequently cite body image changes as a central issue in the adjustment process faced by individuals with an acquired disability. Body image is generally viewed by clinicians as a critical element of an individual's overall self-concept. Sometimes body image plays a central role in the adjustment process, and other times it is secondary to more global adjustments in self-concept (e.g., from nondisabled to disabled, "independent" to "dependent," employed to unemployed, etc.). These more fundamental changes in self-concept may take precedence over changes in body image, and body image changes may not be fully integrated until these other issues are addressed. In other cases, a focus on body image changes may serve as a diversion from less tangible and more anxiety-provoking concerns about one's changed role or purpose in life.

The impact of a given medical condition and consequent disability on self-concept and body image runs the gamut from catastrophic to positive, depending on a wide range of factors. In the sections that follow, drawing from both research findings and our own clinical experience in rehabilitation medicine, we review the impact of disability-related, psychological, developmental, and sociocultural factors on body image.

DISABILITY-RELATED FACTORS

For most people who experience an acquired disability, the factors that most immediately impact self-concept, and thus most strongly affect body image, are those related to the disability itself. The most basic factor to consider is the actual impact of the disability on the individual's physical appearance. Such changes range in scope from small surgical scars to profound changes such as the loss of a limb. Although the degree of alteration in appearance is one marker for associated changes in body image, it must be considered in its proper context. Developmental, psychological, and sociocultural factors all play crucial roles in shaping an individual's response, diminishing the impact of a disability for some and magnifying it for others. Furthermore, clinical examples of incongruous responses are not difficult to find. One person may psychically magnify a small scar to disfiguring proportions, whereas another may experience the loss of a limb as an unimportant cosmetic change relative to the life-threatening medical conditions that necessitated the amputation.

Individuals' internal representations of their appearance tend to attach different cognitive-affective values to different parts of the body. Consequently, the area of the body affected by a disability can have important implications for the process of integrating the disability into one's self-image. Body image changes associated with facial changes typically manifest as frank concern about appearance, whereas changes associated with other parts of the body are apt to be more subtle and diffuse. The loss of a hand or arm, because of its highly symbolic and multifunctional nature, is known to be more traumatic than the loss of a leg. Grunert and colleagues have found that individuals who have sustained hand and arm injuries report high rates of posttraumatic stress disorder (PTSD) symptoms as well as body image and social acceptance concerns. This finding underscores how disabilities that threaten body image and cannot be easily concealed with a prosthesis may present a more challenging psychological adjustment than conditions that are equally disabling and disfiguring but have fewer public acceptance implications.

Although the body's appearance while static is a core component of body image, one's sense of one's body in motion, performing activities both routine and extraordinary, also is an essential aspect of body image. This kinetic aspect of body image, while frequently overlooked, is central to the rehabilitation process. Although restoring the individual to his or her previous level of functioning is the primary goal of rchabilitation, and complete recovery is viewed as ideal, the pragmatics of the rehabilitation process often require that patients be instructed in the use of adaptive equipment (e.g., a cane or walker), alternative postures, and a slower pace. Although excellent as a means of returning functional mobility, these function-over-form approaches typically result in gross changes in kinetic presentation. Therefore, the reconciliation of "old" kinetic representations of the self with the new ways of functioning may be a critical aspect of the psychologist's role in the rehabilitation process.

Adaptive equipment, for example, can trigger powerful negative associations in the minds of some rehabilitation patients. Many of these negative associations revolve around the fears of the social stigma attached to disability in our culture. Other associations involve fears of growing old and feeble. Wheelchairs, walkers, canes, braces, and even orthopedic shoes can be laden with symbolism for many individuals. Not surprisingly, many patients choose to discard such items after discharge from a rehabilitation treatment program. A frank discussion with patients, in which their feelings about these devices are elicited, can avert some of these problems by articulating the underlying beliefs and attitudes.

The cause of a disability can have a substantial impact on the individual's response to, and ultimate ability to cope with, the disability and the attendant changes in body image. Identical disabilities (e.g., the loss of a leg) can be experienced, interpreted, and managed in drastically different ways, depending on the proximal cause of the disability. Disabilities that are incurred during accidents, through medical mismanagement, or due to personal neglect are likely to be viewed as random, unnecessary, and unfair. In such circumstances, people may blame themselves or someone else. Body image changes associated with this type of disability may be characterized by an idealization of the former appearance and may be closely associated with unresolved feelings of anger, resentment, and self-blame. This response pattern may become entrenched, making it difficult to progress beyond the initial feelings of loss.

On the other hand, disabilities incurred during the course of medically necessary, life-saving interventions frequently are associated with altogether different response patterns. This type of disability may be viewed as the price of being saved from a life-threatening condition or an opportunity to resume a life interrupted by a protracted, painful illness. Such adaptive responses are not uncommon and are typically associated with positive rehabilitation outcomes. However, it is important to be sensitive to the fact that individuals may express feelings of gratitude, relief, or renewal because they perceive such feelings to the socially sanctioned response. Consequently, it is important to evaluate patients for masked signs of distress.

Sensory changes, particularly pain, associated with a disability can significantly impact body image by serving as potent and, in some cases, constant reminders of the disability and the attendant changes in physical presentation. Moreover, as a sensory experience, pain typically is associated with illness and disability and may act as an ongoing agent for negative changes in body image, long after medical and functional changes have been adaptively integrated into one's self-concept.

Detailed discussions of the complex interrelation between cognition and body image and the role of rehabilitation in addressing changes in cognitive functioning are well beyond the scope of this chapter. Nevertheless, given the prevalence of brain injuries in the rehabilitation setting, two salient points should be noted. First, neurological changes can impact the system responsible for representations of the self and the world, including body image. Second, such fundamental alterations in information processing can limit one's ability to adapt to other aspects of disability, including changes in function and appearance.

PSYCHOLOGICAL FACTORS

The process of physical rehabilitation is paralleled by a psychological process during which the individual transitions from the "sick" role to recovery. Sense of self, particularly sense of one's physical self, is at the heart of this process. In fact, psychological rehabilitation may be conceptualized as a feedback loop in which the predisability self-image/body image is continuously presented with challenging new information about the self to which it must adapt. This new information may include both increasing awareness and understanding of the disability itself as well as ever-changing feedback regarding the recovery process.

Ideally, this is a fluid, evolutionary process in which the predisability body image is constantly undergoing revision, during which a sense of integrity is preserved through an appropriate balance of assimilation and accommodation, even as body image is transformed to accurately reflect ongoing changes. However, this equilibrium rarely is achieved without some degree of distress, and different response styles are associated with different recovery trajectories. Some individuals respond to disability by attempting to accommodate all cognitive and affective information about their disability instantaneously. In other words, these individuals attempt to effect an instant transformation in their self-concept by trying to adopt the role of an adjusted disabled person prematurely. This response style runs the paradoxical risks of either overwhelming the patient with an unmanageable amount of distressing information or allowing him or her to process information about the disability only superficially, thereby postponing genuine adjustment to the new physical and psychic reality.

Others attempt to preserve their predisability sense of self by assimilating, or forcing, all information about their disability into their old schemas. For example, someone who loses the use an arm following a stroke may overassimilate by focusing on predisability limitations ("I wasn't very good with my hands anyway") and minimizing the extent to which they have changed. These individuals often have a distorted sense of reality and are poorly prepared to meet the challenges of their disability.

Finally, some individuals react by distancing themselves from their disability by either explicitly viewing it as separate from themselves or suppressing it outright. Cognitively, the response pattern is characterized by either a failure to process and classify disability-relevant information or an attempt to process information about the disability as self-irrelevant. Emotionally, the response pattern may manifest as frank denial of the disability and its impact, extreme avoidance of disability-related information, and/or emotional collapse when the reality of the disability becomes unavoidable. This response pattern closely parallels the posttraumatic response cycle delineated by Horowitz, and not surprisingly, it often is accompanied by delayed traumatic responses and psychiatric complications.

Over the course of time, some people with acquired disabilities develop relatively stable negative self-perceptions resulting from their altered body. For example, in one study (Rybarczyk and colleagues, 1995) individuals who had undergone amputation of a limb many years previously continued to express embarrassment, shame, or even revulsion about their own bodies as a consequence of the amputation. We view this pattern as a form of self-stigmatization, in the sense that an individual is internalizing the social stigma that often is applied to individuals who are viewed as abnormal in some significant way. In a milder form, other people reported that they did not like to look at their prosthesis or leg and did not like it when others ask about their amputation. These negative self-perceptions were significantly predictive of depression and lower overall quality of life. Typically, these individuals often choose to avoid social situations where they are exposed to the public, thereby reducing potential sources of physical activity and social support. In a 1995 study, for example, Williamson found that greater self-consciousness in public situations was significantly correlated with activity restriction among older adults with amputations.

In spite of the potential adjustment problems outlined above, the majority of individuals who acquire a disability ultimately integrate these changes and develop a healthy self-concept and body image. Beatrice Wright has provided enlightening research on how individuals make such a positive adjustment by focusing on the changes that take place in their value system. These value shifts include moving away from basing one's worth on either physical qualities or comparative value (e.g., "I am a worthy person because

I'm physically fit"). Positive adjustments occur when the individual shifts to basing his or her self-worth on nonphysical qualities and a sense of intrinsic value (e.g., "I'm as important as any other person because of my uniqueness"). This intrinsic value perspective is present when, for instance, the individual comes to see his or her wheelchair in a positive light because of what it enables him or her to do rather than in a negative light because of its inferiority to walking or the way it is viewed by the public.

DEVELOPMENTAL FACTORS

The developmental timing of an acquired disability is a central factor in the effect is has on body image. For example, several studies of children suggest that younger children cope relatively well with the loss of a limb and that adapting to limb loss becomes more difficult as children become older. Body image is a prime concern among adolescents, and physical changes during these sensitive developmental years can have a profound impact on social functioning. For example, increased high school dropout rates have been reported due to concern over cosmetic appearances among teenagers with upper-limb amputations. These problems notwithstanding, some evidence suggests that prospects for normal long-term adjustment and integration of body image changes during these formative years may be even more promising than when similar changes occur during early and middle adult years.

At the other end of the lifespan, older adults (age 65+), compared to younger adults, are generally less prone to adjustment problems and body image concerns following an acquired disability. We have hypothesized that older adults do not have as strong a reaction as younger adults because they view the acquired disability and attendant changes in mobility and body image as an undesirable but relatively "on-time" event (i.e., common for their age). Events that are perceived as normative are far less likely to elicit a negative reaction. In addition, various developmental theorists, such as Erikson, have posited that older adults reach a level of psychological maturity that allows them to view such changes in appearance with greater perspective and less ego involvement. Indeed, Rybarczyk and colleagues (1995) found a significant relationship between older age and fewer body image concerns following an amputation. (See also chapter by Whitebourne and Skultety in this volume.)

SOCIOCULTURAL FACTORS

The process of rehabilitation often occurs in the protected environment of a rehabilitation hospital or outpatient center. In this setting, newly disabled individuals are surrounded by similarly impaired people and professionals whose job it is to assist their return to independence. This protected subculture allows individuals to form important, mutually supportive relationships and often introduces them to the increasingly vast network of support groups, advocacy organizations, and publications available to disabled individuals. When accessed, this system of supports often forms a *de facto* community for the disabled person, and within this community one is exposed to revised norms for attractiveness and independence. This exposure provides newly disabled people with vital information with which they can begin to reconstruct their sense of self.

On the other hand, the protected environment of the rehabilitation setting shields patients from unpleasant realities that they must ultimately confront and overcome. Specifically, our culture retains an implicit bias against disabled people, with particularly odious stigma attached to certain disabilities. Consequently, one may successfully establish a renewed, positive sense of self during rehabilitation only to have it assailed by prejudices and negative expectations upon returning to the outside world. Rehabilitation psychologists must begin to directly address the biases that newly rehabilitated people are likely to encounter and to assist in the development of a self-image/body image that is not dependent upon the approbation of a prejudiced world.

SUMMARY

There are several research steps that need to be taken to further our understanding of the role of body image in rehabilitation medicine. First, the body image construct needs greater precision through the development of a rehabilitation-specific measure and studies testing its relationship to more established constructs (e.g., acceptance of disability, locus of control, optimism). In contrast to more general measures of body image, a rehabilitation-specific measure should tap into changes in body image (e.g., "as a result of my disability, I see myself as less attractive"). Research by Rybarczyk and colleagues (1992, 1995) suggests that such measures are likely to account for more variance than general measures (see Pruzinsky and Cash's chapter on assessing body image and quality of life in medical settings in this volume). Second, longitudinal and path analysis studies are needed to establish whether body image concerns are a direct causal factor in adjustment or serve a mediating or moderating role. Third, future studies should also explore the relationship between body image and perceived social stigma. Based on earlier findings, Rybarczyk and colleagues (1995) hypothesized that individuals who report high levels of perceived social stigma (e.g., "most people are 'turned off' by my amputation") may be projecting their own difficulties with integrating body image changes. Finally, studies need to establish whether cognitive-behavioral treatments designed to directly address body image concerns in individuals with acquired disabilities can be effective in promoting psychological, social, and sexual functioning.

It is important to emphasize that rehabilitation psychologists are continually struck by the remarkable resilience of most individuals who experience life-altering acquired disabilities. In this new era of *positive psychology*, there is much to be learned from individuals who face adversity and grow stronger and more mature as a result. Our training sometimes leads us to place too much emphasis on searching for psychopathology when the focus should be on empowering individuals to cope with a social world that frequently denies access and dignity to those who are physically different.

INFORMATIVE READINGS

Horowitz, M. J. (1986). *Stress response syndrome*. New York: Jason Aronson.—A comprehensive review of stress response syndrome.

Grunert, B. K., Devine, C. A., Matloub, H. S., Sanger, J. R., Yousif, N. J., Anderson, R. C., Roell, S. M. (1992). Psychological adjustment following work-related hand injury: 18–month follow-up. *Annals of Plastic Surgery, 29*, 537–542.—A study of the significant psychological adjustment problems experienced by individuals with hand injuries.

Grunert, B. K., Hargarten, S. W., Matloub, H. S., Sanger, J. R., Hanel, D. P., & Yousif, N. J. (1992). Predictive value of psychological screening in acute hand injuries. *Journal of Hand Surgery, 17A*, 196–199.—A report on the clinical value of screening for adjustment difficulties following a hand injury.

Rybarczyk, B., Nyenhuis, D. L., Nicholas, J. J., Cash, S., & Kaiser, J. (1995). Body image, perceived social stigma, and the prediction of psychosocial adjustment to leg amputation. *Rehabilitation Psychology, 40*, 95–110.—A follow-up study showing that a negative body image and perceived social stigma were predictive of poor adjustment to an amputation.

Rybarczyk, B., Nyenhuis, D. L., Nicholas, J. J., Schulz, R., Alioto, R. J., & Blair, C. (1992). Social discomfort and depression in a sample of adults with leg amputations. *Archives of Physical Medicine and Rehabilitation, 73*, 1169–1173.—A study demonstrating that social discomfort pertaining to body image was related to poorer adjustment.

Rybarczyk, B., Szymanski, L., & Nicholas, J. J. (2000). Limb amputation. In R. G. Frank & T. Elliott (Eds.), *Handbook of rehabilitation psychology* (pp. 29–47). Washington, DC: American Psychological Association.—An overview of the topic of adjustment to an amputation.

Williamson, G. M. (1995). Restriction of normal activities among older adult amputees: The role of public self-consciousness. *Journal of Clinical Geropsychology, 1*, 229–242.—A study that delineates the relationship between activity restriction and public self-consciousness/body image concerns.

Wright, B. A. (1983). *Physical disability: A psychological approach*. New York: Harper & Row.—A classic text on adjustment to a disability.

Yuker, H. E. (Ed). (1988). *Attitudes toward persons with disabilities*. New York: Springer.—A review of the literature on social biases and stigma.

45

Body Image Issues among Individuals with HIV and AIDS

ELIZABETH CHAPMAN

Individuals with HIV and AIDS encounter many body image problems. The most common are the visible manifestations of HIV on the skin, loss of weight, and treatment side effects. However, there are also less visible problems related to media representations of HIV and the way it is transmitted. These representations are likely to affect the way one feels about one's body and may lead to perceptions of the body as "at-risk," "contaminated," or "dangerous." Body image issues usually begin with the HIV test, which people take because they fear that they have put their body at risk in some way. They probably look and feel healthy and may have no physical symptoms of HIV or AIDS. However, they are aware that their body's boundaries have been potentially breached, perhaps through unsafe sex or needle usage. A second context in which people go for HIV tests is when physical symptoms arise and a doctor is concerned that immune system depletion is responsible. In this case it is likely that the body has been infected with HIV for a while. The first context is more likely to occur in the Western world; the second context is more likely in countries such as Africa.

This chapter focuses on the issues applicable for people living in the Western world. These issues are discussed chronologically, dealing first with changed social and personal attitudes toward the body stemming from the impact of the HIV test, followed by discussion of the physical signs and symptoms that increasingly emerge with the progression from HIV to AIDS.

ATTITUDINAL ASPECTS OF BODY IMAGE IN HIV

An HIV test has the potential to redefine someone as sick when he or she may not be experiencing any symptoms. An early HIV test for members of at-risk groups is encouraged to enhance prevention. The person now redefined as "HIV-positive" faces the daunting task of coming to terms with the fact that his or her body contains a potential life-threatening condition waiting to break out. The phenomenological state of the body as "taken-for-granted" is disrupted. This diagnosis moves the person from a state of health to a state of being "at-risk," even in the absence of symptoms and signs of illness. It also creates a category of illness that would otherwise remain unknown for years. From the moment the person knows he or she is infected with HIV, it becomes necessary to think about and adopt anti-contagion measures in everyday activities to ensure that HIV is not transmitted. Just as it is impossible to become uninfected, the awareness of the diagnosis never goes away.

Social representations of HIV have a considerable influence on an infected person's feelings about his or her body. Sontag's work suggests that how we feel about our bodies is not only a matter of physical symptoms but of how we internalize prevailing social metaphors. Given that the metaphors of HIV largely focus on *plague, punishment, contamination, bodies out of control, fear,* and *death,* as illustrated in Gilman's work, there is a likely negative body image impact. An amplifying factor comes from the association of HIV/AIDS with discredited groups and the stigma of its transmission through morally reprehensible activities. Not only are people seen as being fatally ill but as members of social groups who have been pilloried and harassed for their different beliefs and sometimes illegal practices.

The metaphor of contamination can be clearly linked to the reality of the disease in that every blood cell contains the potential to transmit the virus. Due to concern about HIV being passed on to other bodies, and because being HIV-positive defines someone as potentially dangerous, the boundaries of the body are symbolically significant. HIV is represented as entering into the body and breaching the boundaries through some sex practices or drug use. These boundaries then have to be closely guarded to stop others from becoming infected. When these symbolic issues are combined with the physical contagion and prevention aspects of HIV (safer sex practices and vigilance regarding accidentally infecting others through blood spills), there is a further impact on body experience. If there are both real and symbolic reasons to consider bodily fluids as contaminated, then the potential to feel negatively about one's body is greatly increased. As Chapman notes, a cognitive representation of the body as contaminated or polluted can further impact the way HIV-positive people interact with others. Chapman's study examined body image and touch contacts in a group of HIV-positive participants and their close supporters and found that members of the HIV-positive group felt very differently about their bodies after receiving their diagnosis. These individuals felt that their bodies were contaminated; they also felt that they were not receiving as much tactile contact from others as they would have liked. This experience of "body as contaminated" can be further reinforced by overly cautious social reactions and discriminatory practices of health-care workers toward the body of someone with HIV, such as those seen in the early years of the epidemic. McCann suggested that these discriminatory practices still occur, whereas Lupton, in 1999, suggested that they may be moderating over time. However, moral judgments about people with this illness are now based not so much on how they acquired the virus but on how they deport themselves once ill. These moral judgments can continue to have an impact on the way affected individuals feel about themselves and how others perceive them.

For some people, having a positive HIV test could result in discrimination, insurance, or employment problems. It also means that inferences may be made about their sexuality. Many people with a positive HIV test therefore keep it secret for as long as they can. For the person with HIV, it is especially important that his or her body does not betray this knowledge to others, and self-monitoring of the body for early signs and symptoms of HIV is common. Adam and Sears illustrate many of these issues particularly clearly.

The person's continued awareness of HIV following the test may be amplified by the need for regular T-cell monitoring as a marker of immune system functioning. Medical understanding of how HIV works is constantly increasing. Previously it was assumed that the virus remained dormant in the body for many years until AIDS symptoms manifested. It is now understood that there is no latency period in the HIV continuum and that HIV and the body's immune system have been fighting each other for years before the immune system starts to lose the battle and HIV has an impact on health. Soon after HIV is acquired, it replicates in both the lymph nodes and blood, making an average of 10 billion new viruses daily and frequently producing new mutations. The optimum treatment strategy to minimize replication is to introduce antiretroviral medication soon after a positive test. Regular monitoring of viral load is necessary to assess whether a different combination of medication is required. These checks, although essential, also act as a constant reminder of the virus's action within the body. Therefore, even when physically fit and apparently well, it is hard to forget that the HIV virus is inside the body relentlessly attempting to overcome the body's natural defense system.

At this stage the body may be perceived as unpredictable. Although viral load can be held at "undetectable" levels for long periods of time with virtually no external manifestations by antiretroviral medication, the virus is still within the body, hidden deep in areas of the brain, lymph nodes, or testicles and has the potential to resurrect itself. For the combination therapies to work, medication has to be taken according to a strict and complex regimen. If the challenge of medication compliance is not met, drug-resistant variants of HIV arise and can be transmitted.

PHYSICAL ASPECTS

It has become increasingly apparent that certain protease inhibitor drugs, currently being used successfully to lower viral load, may be implicated in changes in body fat distribution (lipodystrophy). Lipodystrophy is associated with the growth of atypical fat-like tissues in the stomach, upper back, and neck area, breast enlargement, and wasting of facial and limb tissue (lipoatrophy). Taking these powerful antiviral drugs may prolong the lives of people with HIV but at some cost to quality of life and appearance. Patients may have to decide whether the positive impact of the drugs on viral load (which is not visibly apparent in the asymptomatic stage) is worth the appearance-changing side effects. Current research on this topic is very limited and it is hard to advise patients, though there is growing understanding of the metabolic changes associated with this phenomenon. U.S. and U.K. guidelines differ on the best time to start this therapy, which needs to be continued indefinitely. However, there is growing evidence that the longer a person takes these medications, the more likely he or she is to experience these changes in appearance. However, not all individuals are susceptible to changes in body fat, and there are different patterns of body fat redistribution depending on the medications taken.

Body image issues vary depending on the stage of the HIV cycle. In early stages patients focus on trying to forget about or conceal HIV status and are vigilant for the first signs and symptoms of immune suppression—a cough or cold perhaps being wrongly interpreted as an early sign of an AIDS-related pneumonia. Once the inevitable effects of immune depletion start to occur, however, many problems can develop that have more tangible effects on body image, as they often affect the external body boundary, the skin. Immune depletion may lead to conditions that cause the skin to break down and erupt with visible manifestations of the HIV virus, and affect the genitals. For example, opportunistic infections that arise in the absence of a functioning immune system may lead to Kaposi's sarcoma tumors (often occurring in the genital region), molluscum (a mildly contagious skin infection that occurs on the face and neck), or bacterial angiomatosis (reddish purplish skin lesions) on the skin. Other visible signs of the illness include coughing resulting from pneumonias or chest infections. When HIV causes a visible sign on the body, expected or actual fearful reactions from others may lead the infected person to withdraw from social and/or tactile contact or to feel uncomfortable in public places. It is common for patients to try and conceal these skin conditions, often with the use of cosmetics, with varying degrees of success.

Weight loss from wasting syndrome also has an impact on quality of life and self-perception in people living with HIV, as reviewed by Miller and Gorbach. The Centers for Disease Control and Prevention define AIDS wasting as involuntary weight loss of more than 10% of body weight, plus more than 30 days of either diarrhea, or weakness and fever. However, weight loss as a clinical problem in HIV is seen in more cases than those categorized by this definition alone.

Weight loss can be secondary to opportunistic infections such as pneumonia, where the loss is often rapid and acute. Studies show that weight can sometimes be partially regained following such episodes. Weight loss may also be related to difficulty in eating because of a painful mouth and throat caused by oral thrush or skin lesions. Oral thrush causes significant mouth and throat irritation and is due to an overgrowth of a naturally occurring fungus that may occur when the immune system is damaged. Several antifungal drugs are effective against oral thrush. Where wasting is the result of chronic gastrointestinal disease, the loss of weight may be progressive. Patients' weight is regularly monitored and, when necessary, patients are given nutritional supplements or enteral feeding. Steroid treatment or human growth hormone therapy may also be offered.

The visible manifestations and weakness associated with such weight loss are a significant problem for people with HIV, as shown by Tate and George in 2001. Their study examined the implications of weight loss in a group of HIV-positive gay men. Results showed that these visible signs of their illness had implications for degree of stigmatization experienced and for the quality of social interactions with family members, who may not have been aware of the man's HIV status. The HIV-positive individual may sometimes avoid people due to concerns about social reactions to his or her weight loss. The participants in this small qualitative study also described how emaciation brought with it bodily discomfort and acute personal and social recognition of increasing illness. Furthermore, although recent studies show that initiation of highly active antiretroviral therapy (HAART) is often associated with rapid weight gain, this weight may be composed of fat rather than lean tissue.

DIFFERENT RISK GROUPS—DIFFERENT IMPLICATIONS FOR THE BODY

Sexual Transmission

Many people infected with HIV have contracted it through sexual means and, as such, the disease may be linked in their minds with sexuality. For some, the link between disease and sex is strong enough to make them give up sex and physical contact altogether. For those who continue to engage in sexual relations, there are many problems. Not only do they have to fight the dominant social belief that it is unsuitable for people with HIV to desire or engage in sex, they also must be careful about when and how to disclose their status to a potential partner for the first time.

The impact that HIV status has on sexual practices can affect crucial dimensions of self-identity. This effect has been observed most frequently in populations of gay men, whose cultural identity revolved around the free expression of sexuality and where sexual restrictions resulted in feelings of loss and depression; such experiences are discussed by Schönnesson and Ross. These problems may vary as a function of age since younger gay men may not have considered sex with multiple partners as constituent of their identity in the same way as older men.

Gender-Related Differences in HIV-Related Concerns

In 1992 Richardson and Bollé noted the gender differences in how men and women talk about HIV in their bodies, specifically their use of metaphors when talking about how the body fights HIV. For women, there are specific issues relating to transmitting HIV to infants through childbirth and breast-feeding, and the monthly concern surrounding menstrual blood. For men, the knowledge that HIV is present, in heavy concentrations, in semen can influence how they think about sex and sexual practices.

There are also particular illnesses in the later stages of HIV that affect men and women differently. For women, there are increased gynecological problems associated with advancing HIV disease, especially an increased incidence of cervical cancer. These concerns, which are addressed by Johnson and Johnstone, are particularly threatening to body image because of their intimate connection to sexual functioning.

Kaposi's sarcoma (KS) is more likely to affect gay men. This previously rarely occurring cancer behaves differently in people with HIV, in whom internal and/or external tumors form, often several at a time and, though treatable, are often unsightly. KS tumors are characteristically black or purple spots, commonly appear on the skin, genitals, and face, and can be a distinguishing feature of HIV infection. They can sometimes be concealed with makeup or removed surgically. Again, Tate and George briefly review the particular body image issues relevant to gay men.

UNRESOLVED ISSUES

As combination therapy has become the optimum means of keeping viral replication low, significant body shape changes have been observed in patients. It is still not clear whether these changes are due to adverse side effects of treatment or are a function of increasing survival times in people with HIV. Findings of body fat redistribution are relatively recent and the natural history has yet to be confirmed, but early data suggest that the syndrome is progressive unless there are changes in treatment. However, when treatment is initiated early on, these effects can occur in the absence of pronounced AIDS symptoms. Treatment side effects that lead to the patient having the appearance of someone with AIDS may well be unacceptable, despite the therapeutic effects.

A key issue that remains unaddressed is the impact of these problems on HIV-infected individuals and to what extent treatments such as steroids, human growth hormone, exercise, or cosmetic surgery can help. No strategy has yet proven wholly effective for the treatment of lipodystrophy, lipoatrophy, and the related metabolic changes that occur in people on HAART. Stopping treatment may not be a realistic option, yet the visible side effects that are widely reported are also stigmatizing.

It is clear that HIV has many different effects on the body, yet there is no validated scale for assessing problems in the clinic, and the literature, in general, on body image issues for people with HIV is small. In a clinical setting, patients should be given ample opportunity to express their body image concerns in general terms and specifically as related to HAART treatment. Given the increasing quality-of-life and health issues facing patients with HIV, some clinicians have questioned the need to treat lipodystrophy if patients' viral load remains low. Yet a more compassionate view suggests that these anxieties must be noted and research into treatment for the side effects continued.

INFORMATIVE READINGS

Adam, B. D., & Sears, A. (1996). *Experiencing HIV: Personal, family and work relationships.* New York: Columbia University Press.—Provides a sociological perspective and includes chapters discussing intimacy and sex, discourse and identity, and managing symptoms.

Bartlett, J. G., & Finkbeiner, A. K. (1998). *The guide to living with HIV infection* (4th ed.). Baltimore: Johns Hopkins University Press.—A clearly written book with chapters on how HIV affects the body and how to handle different stages of the illness.

Chapman, E. (2000). conceptualization of the body for people living with HIV: Issues of touch and contamination. *Sociology of Health and Illness, 22*(6), 840–857.—Reports that people with HIV consider their bodies to be contaminated and that this perspective affects tactile contact with supporters.

Gilman, S. L. (1995). *Health and illness: Images of difference.* London: Reaktion Books.—One chapter focuses on the negative depiction of people with HIV in the early stages of the epidemic.

Johnson, M. A., & Johnstone, F. D. (Eds.). (1993). *HIV infection in women.* London: Churchill.—Specifically addresses issues related to HIV infection in women.

Lawless, S., Kippax, S., & Crawford, J. (1996). Dirty, diseased and undeserving: The positioning of HIV positive women. *Social Science and Medicine, 43*(9), 1371–1377.— Discusses the way that HIV-positive women are seen and treated in society, particularly focusing on the stigma and discrimination they experience in the hands of health professionals.

Lupton, D. (1999). Archetypes of infection: People with HIV/AIDS in the Australian press in the mid 1990s. *Sociology of Health and Illness, 21*(1), 37–53.—An interpretative analysis of representations of people with HIV/AIDS in the Australian press between 1994 and 1996. Three major achetypes were uncovered: the AIDS victim, AIDS survivor, and AIDS carrier. These are discussed in the context of contemporary approaches to HIV/AIDS, general notions of morality and self-control, and previous representations of HIV.

McCann, T. V. (1999). Reluctance amongst nurses and doctors to care for and treat patients with HIV/AIDS. *AIDS Care, 11*(3), 355–359.—Discusses the responses of health-care workers and comments on the blaming and discriminatory practices that coexist with stigma.

Miller, T. L., & Gorbach, S. L. (Eds.). (1999). *Nutritional aspects of HIV infection*. London: Arnold.—Comprehensive, medically oriented book covering weight loss and related issues in HIV, including several chapters on wasting and fat redistribution syndrome.

Richardson, A., & Bollé, D. (1992). *Wise before their time: People with AIDS talk about their lives*. London: Fount.—Based on interviews with people with HIV/AIDS. Uncovers gender differences in how men and women with HIV talk about how their bodies fight the virus and their use of metaphor.

Schönnesson, L. N., & Ross, M. W. (1999). *Coping with HIV infection: Psychological and existential responses in gay men*. New York: Klewer Academic.—Based on longitudinal clinical experiences of gay men in psychotherapy in Sweden, including chapters on the impact of chronic and terminal illness, HIV testing, HIV-related threats, and the "shattered"self.

Sontag, S. (1989). *AIDS and its metaphors*. London: Penguin Press.—Discusses two powerful metaphors about illness seen in AIDS; as enemy invader destroying from inside, and the metaphor of plague and punishment because of the sexually transmitted nature of HIV.

Tate, H., & George, R. (2001). The effect of weight loss on body image in HIV-positive gay men. *AIDS Care, 13*(2), 163–169.—Describes a small qualitative study looking at HIV-related weight loss and body image for gay men. Problems of self-consciousness and bodily comfort were identified.

VII

Changing the Body: Medical, Surgical, and Other Interventions

46

Weight Loss and Changes in Body Image

GARY D. FOSTER
PATTY E. MATZ

Rosen (1995) has described body image as "a person's mental image and evaluation . . . of appearance and the influence of these perceptions and attitudes on behavior" (p. 369). Discontent with one's body (image) has been labeled in various ways, including negative body image, body image disturbance, and body image dissatisfaction. For the purposes of this chapter, we call this phenomenon negative body image, and we limit our discussion to the affective and evaluative aspects of body image rather than its perceptual dimensions.

Negative body image is most often related to body weight and weight-sensitive body parts (e.g., abdomen, waist line) and is often higher in overweight than nonoverweight people, particularly women (see Schwartz and Brownell's chapter in this volume). Surprisingly, variability in body image among overweight persons is not related to the degree of overweight. Negative body image (or concern about appearance) is an important factor in deciding to lose weight and in selecting how much weight to lose. Given that changes in body image are an expected benefit of weight loss treatment, it is disturbing that the effects of weight loss on body image have not been well studied. Such information is necessary to help patients and practitioners make informed choices about the most effective methods to improve body image in those who are overweight or obese.

This chapter discusses three issues related to weight loss and body image in overweight persons: (1) the effects of weight loss and weight regain on body image; (2) the effects of body image treatments, either as adjunctive to, or separate from, weight loss treatment; and (3) the implications for future research.

THE EFFECT OF WEIGHT LOSS AND WEIGHT REGAIN ON BODY IMAGE

Weight Loss and Body Image

Weight loss, by a variety of methods, is associated with significant improvements in body image. In a representative study by Foster and colleagues, a 19.4 kg weight loss was associated with significant body image improvements after 24 weeks. Changes in body image did *not* correlate with the amount of weight loss. Weight losses ranging from 9 kg to 25 kg resulted in similar body image improvements. This finding suggests the possibility of a threshold effect in which smaller weight losses confer improvement in body image, with further reductions in weight offering no additional benefit. Cash found similar body image improvements after a 21.8 kg weight loss. In both of these samples, the body image ratings following weight loss were similar to nonoverweight controls. By contrast, Adami and colleagues' (1998, 1999) studies of severely obese patients following bariatric surgery suggest that, though improved, negative body image was still greater than that of nonobese controls.

Adami et al.'s (1998, 1999) findings support the notion of a "phantom fat" phenomenon, which was originally reported in a sample of undergraduate females by Cash and colleagues in 1990. They found that formerly overweight people experience greater negative body image than weight-matched, never-overweight controls. Recently, Milkewicz and Cash studied a community sample of overweight, formerly overweight, and never-overweight women and found that negative body image was greater in the first two groups than in the latter. Other findings (Foster et al. and Cash) do not confirm this phenomenon. Discrepant results may be due to differences among the samples in initial weight, weight loss, age, and setting (i.e., treatment seekers vs. community samples). In addition, most studies that have supported the phantom fat phenomenon have been cross-sectional, whereas those not supporting it have been prospective.

Despite significant improvement in body image after weight loss, it is important to note individual variability. Our clinical experience suggests that some patients, even after a significant weight loss, retain negative feelings about their bodies. Rather than just asking, "Does weight loss improve body image?" the field needs to investigate, "For whom and under what conditions is body image affected by weight loss?" For example, one cross-sectional study by Adami et al. (1998) suggested that those with childhood-onset obesity had greater negative body image after surgical weight loss than did those with adult-onset obesity. It is also possible that any lack of improvement in body image might be explained by disappointment with less than expected weight losses. It is clear that the weight losses patients desire (30% reductions in initial weight) are typically not achievable with nonsurgical methods. These unmet expectations may exacerbate negative body image in some patients even after significant (10%) weight loss. Alternatively, some aspects of body image may represent a subjective, psychological experience that is independent of weight status and, thus, not affected by weight loss.

Body Image and Treatment Outcome

In addition to the effects of weight loss on body image, initial levels of negative body image may affect obesity treatment outcomes, such as weight loss and attrition. Several studies have found that more positive ratings of body image before treatment were associated with greater weight losses, although at least one study has not. In terms of attrition, Ramirez and Rosen observed that initially higher levels of negative body image were associated with greater attrition. Cash reported that smaller improvements in body image early in treatment were associated with greater attrition, independent of weight change, and that lower pre- to posttreatment improvements in fitness orientation related to attrition during the maintenance phase. These findings suggest that both baseline levels of negative body image and changes early in treatment may influence important outcomes in the treatment of obesity.

Effects of Regaining Weight

As might be expected, weight regain partially reverses the improvements in body image that accompany weight loss; indeed, even small weight gains (2–3 kg) have been reported to diminish improvements in body image. Foster and colleagues found that regaining 3.5 kg of a 19.4 kg weight loss from 24 to 48 weeks was associated with small but significant increases in negative body image. Cash also noted that, with weight regain, improvements in appearance evaluation diminished. In a 3-year follow-up study, Wadden and colleagues found that body image was among the factors cited as most negatively affected by weight regain. The effects of full weight regain, including weight cycling, on body image have not been well studied and represent an important gap in our current knowledge about how regaining weight affects body image.

Summary

Weight loss is associated with significant improvements in body image that approximate levels of nonobese controls in most studies. Surprisingly, the improvement in body image does not appear to be related to the amount of weight loss. The improvement, however, is fragile, diminishing with minimal weight regain. No study has examined the effects of full weight regain. Because complete weight regain is the expected long-term outcome for many, body image improvements induced by weight loss may be particularly temporary. Thus, weight loss may not be the most effective long-term method to treat negative body image in obese people.

BODY IMAGE TREATMENT FOR OVERWEIGHT PEOPLE

Treatment for overweight people has generally focused on weight loss, with little or no attention given to ameliorating the body image concerns that motivate weight loss treatment. To address these concerns, treatment for negative body image could either be conducted independently as an obesity treatment alternative or integrated into weight loss programs. In advocating body image treatment, we are neither minimizing the health risks associated with obesity nor suggesting that body image treatment and weight control efforts are antithetical.

Body Image Treatment as Obesity Treatment Alternative

Given the fleeting nature of weight loss, efforts to enhance body image that are not contingent upon weight loss may be more helpful in the long term. Most but not all nondieting approaches produce favorable improvements in body image without weight loss. These approaches focus on issues of overall health, self-esteem, and body image that are independent of weight (change). The magnitude of changes in body image produced by these nondieting approaches is similar to that achieved by weight loss programs.

Rosen and colleagues employed a comprehensive manual-based cognitive-behavioral treatment for negative body image (with no effort to change eating habits, exercise, or weight) in overweight women seeking treatment for negative body image (not weight loss). Although not nondietary in nature, treatment included modifying distressing body image thoughts, challenging stereotypes about obesity and beliefs about the importance of physical appearance, exposure to avoided body image situations, and eliminating body checking behaviors that promote appearance preoccupation. Participants were neither encouraged to, nor discouraged from, losing weight. In fact, weight loss was not discussed in the treatment sessions, because it was viewed as a method to improve body image. In this study, body image was significantly improved after an 8-session treatment program and improvements were maintained at a 4-month follow-up. Approximately equal numbers of participants lost, gained, or maintained their weight during treatment; the improvement in body image was not related to the change in weight. The lack of weight change, on average, suggests that a salient concern of patients and clinicians—that body image treatment will promote weight gain through abandonment of weight control efforts—was not borne out. This study demonstrated that body image in overweight women can be enhanced without weight loss. This finding needs to be replicated and extended to determine if such changes are more sustainable than those achieved with weight loss.

Body Image Treatment as an Obesity Treatment Component

Cash and Strachan's chapter in this volume provides a review and discussion of cognitive-behavioral body image therapy. Reasons for integrating body image treatment into obesity treatment include the need for addressing the body image concerns of obese patients and promoting the acceptance of a realistic body size that parallels the current emphasis on reasonable expectations for weight loss.

Recently, Ramirez and Rosen conducted the first study comparing weight loss treatment alone with combined body image/weight loss treatment. They hypothesized that combined treatment would yield greater body image improvement in the short term and protect participants from the negative body image increase typically associated with weight regain. Neither prediction, however, was supported. After the 16-week program, negative body image had improved in both conditions from the above-normal to normal range, with no differences between conditions. Both groups lost similar amounts of weight (9–10%). At a 1-year follow-up, both groups had experienced similar amounts of weight regain and deterioration of their body image improvement. In sum, adding body image treatment to a standard weight loss program did not result in significantly greater improvements in body image, nor did it buffer participants from the increase in negative body image at 1-year follow-up. It is important to note that the follow-up in this study was measured 1 year later, at which point participants in both conditions had regained some weight but still had a net weight loss. Body image treatment might attenuate negative body image increases if measured at a longer-term follow-up point (e.g., 5 years), when weight losses typically have been completely regained. Greater long-term follow-up is needed to measure any sustained effects of combined body image and weight loss treatment.

Summary

Numerous studies of nondieting approaches make it clear that weight loss is not required for body image improvements in overweight and obese persons. It is less clear whether these treatments have a better long-term effect than those based on weight loss, because they have not been studied over long periods of time. The only study to evaluate the effects of combining body image and weight loss treatments found no added benefit for either body image or weight loss. Perhaps addressing body image before weight loss may have produced different results. It is possible that the highly observable and externally reinforcing benefits of weight loss may have made participants less likely to develop the cognitive and behavioral skills necessary for changes in body image that are independent of weight.

DIRECTIONS FOR FUTURE RESEARCH

Many questions regarding the effects of weight loss and other treatments on negative body image in overweight and obese persons remain unanswered. There are several areas of investigation that may be helpful in answering these questions.

Body Image as a Primary Outcome

Because negative body image is a principal motivator of weight management efforts, body image should be a primary outcome in all weight loss studies. This includes affective, cognitive, and behavioral components of body image throughout treatment and follow-up. It is particularly important to document whether cognitive and affective improvements translate into behavioral changes (e.g., going to the beach, wearing more revealing clothing, engaging in previously avoided activities). Such data would enable clinicians to provide clients with realistic expectations regarding weight loss and associated body image changes.

Addressing Heterogeneity

Greater attention needs to be focused on the heterogeneity of body image changes in overweight and obese persons. For example, as Schwartz and Brownell point out in this volume, most research on overweight people and body image has been conducted with adult female treatment-seekers, limiting generalization. It is necessary to give greater attention to the effects of gender, sampling (i.e., community vs. clinic samples), weight category (i.e., overweight, obese, superobese), ethnicity, socioeconomic status, and age. Additionally, factors such as age of obesity onset, internalization of cultural appearance ideals, and history of weight-related teasing may mediate the relationship between body image and weight loss.

The body image construct is multidimensional in conceptualization, definition, and assessment. This heterogeneity makes it difficult to compare results across studies. Conceptual agreement among researchers and standardization of assessment measures would advance our understanding of body image and its association with weight control. Even with standardized assessment, however, the multidimensional nature of body image may lead to differential improvements after weight loss. For example, one may have more favorable feelings about the body, in general, but continue to have concern about shape and weight.

Given the large variation in individual response to obesity treatment, better characterization of responders and nonresponders might help target those receptive to body image interventions and the development of new treatments. Body image might predict response to obesity treatment, both in terms of attrition and treatment outcomes, and thus deserves further study. It is possible, for example, that pretreatment improvements in body image would increase weight loss and decrease attrition. Body image treatment might be particularly helpful to certain subgroups of overweight persons. Specifically, as Schwartz and Brownell discuss in this volume, those subjected to negative verbal commentary, those who have binge eating disorder, and those who had juvenile-onset obesity may be at greater risk for negative body image. It is important to ascertain the effects of negative body image treatment on body image and weight loss outcomes in such individuals.

Clinical Significance

It is unclear whether, or for whom, negative body image is a clinically significant phenomenon (i.e., associated with significant impairment in daily functioning). Also undetermined is the nature and extent of body image improvements needed to make a difference in day-to-day affective and behavioral status. Thus, in addition to assessing changes in body image before and after treatment, attention should be focused on measures of clinical significance related to body image (e.g., mood, self-esteem, quality of life). It is important to know whether the changes produced by treatment are improvements within a normal range or changes from clinical to nonclinical levels. In his chapter on the epidemiology of negative body image, Cash discusses this issue of the clinical relevance of typical body image assessments.

CONCLUSION

Despite the fact that negative body image motivates weight control efforts, body image is rarely assessed in obesity treatment studies. Body image should be a principal efficacy outcome for all obesity treatment studies. Significant improvements in body image can be attained through weight loss and do not require reductions to ideal weight. Some individuals, however, do not improve in body image after weight loss, and the examination of only mean values obscures these important cases. Moreover, weight regain increases negative body image, suggesting that weight loss does not promote permanent body image improvement. As such, negative body image treatment that is not contingent upon weight loss might be more effective than weight loss in promoting permanent body image change, although long-term studies would be needed to investigate this possibility. The only study to date that has combined body image and weight loss treatments did not find additional benefits on body image or weight loss; however, the sequencing of treatments has not been studied. We hope that greater attention to the issues described above will give health-care professionals and overweight or obese individuals more informed expectations about the relative benefits of weight loss, nondieting, and cognitive-behavioral treatments of body image.

INFORMATIVE READINGS

Adami, G. F., Gandolfo, P., Campostano, A., Meneghelli, A., Ravera, G., & Scopinaro, N. (1998). Body image and body weight in obese patients. *International Journal of Eating Disorders, 24,* 299–306.—Cross-sectional analysis comparing body image in obese patients, postobese patients, and nonobese controls that suggested early-onset obesity may be a factor when body image is not ameliorated by weight loss.

Adami, G. F., Meneghelli, A., Bressani, A., & Scopinaro, N. (1999). Body image in obese patients before and after stable weight reduction following bariatric surgery. *Journal of Psychosomatic Research, 46*(3), 275–281.—Describes the nature and extent of body image changes associated with weight loss surgery.

Cash, T. F. (1994). Body image and weight changes in a multi-site comprehensive very-low-calorie diet program. *Behavior Therapy, 25,* 239–254.—Prospective study documenting body image changes associated with weight loss following a very-low-calorie diet.

Cash, T. F., Counts, B., & Huffine, C. E. (1990). Current and vestigial effects of overweight among women: Fear of fat, attitudinal body image, and eating behaviors. *Journal of Psychopathology and Behavioral Assessment, 12*(2), 157–167.—Compared body image in never-overweight, formerly overweight, and currently overweight college females and found that formerly and currently overweight shared similar body image concerns on some measures.

Foster G. D., & McGuckin, B. G. (2002). Nondieting approaches: Principles, practices, and evidence. In T. A. Wadden & A. J. Stunkard (Eds.), *Handbook of obesity treatment* (pp. 494–512). New York: Guilford Press.—A comprehensive review of nondieting approaches, including their effects on body image.

Foster, G. D., Wadden, T. A., & Vogt, R. A. (1997). Body image in obese women before, during, and after weight loss treatment. *Health Psychology, 16*(3), 226–229.—Prospective analysis of body image changes associated with weight loss and regain.

Milkewicz, N., & Cash, T. F. (2000). *Dismantling the heterogeneity of obesity: Determinants of body images and psychosocial functioning.* Poster presented at the convention of the Association for Advancement of Behavior Therapy, New Orleans.—Compared body image in a community sample of overweight, formerly overweight, and never-overweight women, and found greater negative body image in the first two groups than in the last.

Ramirez, E. M., & Rosen, J. C. (2001). A comparison of weight control and weight control plus body image therapy for obese men and women. *Journal of Consulting and Clini-*

cal Psychology, 69, 440–446.—A randomized controlled trial that found body image treatment plus weight loss treatment was not superior to weight loss treatment alone in improving body image.

Rosen, J. C. (1995). Assessment and treatment of body image disturbance. In K. D. Brownell & C. G. Fairburn (Eds.), *Eating disorders and obesity: A comprehensive handbook* (pp. 369–373). New York: Guilford Press.—A concise, helpful review of the multiple causes affecting the link between body image and obesity.

Rosen, J. C. (1996). Improving body image in obesity. In J. K. Thompson (Ed.), *Body image, eating disorders, and obesity* (pp. 425–440). Washington, DC: American Psychological Association.—Reviews many aspects of body image in obese people and presents an overview of body image treatment that targets this population.

Rosen, J. C., Orosan, P., & Reiter, J. (1995). Cognitive behavior therapy for negative body image in obese women. *Behavior Therapy, 26,* 25–42.—Tested a body image treatment program for obese women and suggested that negative body image could be improved without weight loss.

Sarwer, D. B., & Thompson, J. K. (2002). Obesity and body image disturbance. In T. A. Wadden & A. J. Stunkard (Eds.), *Handbook of obesity treatment* (pp. 447–464). New York: Guilford Press.—A comprehensive overview of the relationship between body image and obesity, focusing on prevalence, specificity, clinical significance, and treatment of body image dissatisfaction.

Wadden, T. A., Stunkard, A. J., & Liebschutz, J. (1988). Three year follow-up of the treatment of obesity by very-low-calorie diet, behavior therapy, and their combination. *Journal of Consulting and Clinical Psychology, 56*(6), 925–928.—Follow-up study of weight loss treatments, with attention to the psychological consequences of weight regain.

47

Fitness Enhancement and Changes in Body Image

KATHLEEN A. MARTIN
CATHERINE M. LICHTENBERGER

Over the past two decades, a growing body of research has attempted to validate the notion that improvements in physical fitness are associated with improvements in body image. To date, much of this research has consisted of correlational and cross-sectional studies that have compared body image between exercisers and nonexercisers. Not only have these studies produced equivocal results, but the nature of their designs has been inappropriate for drawing conclusions about the effects of exercise-induced fitness change on body image change. In order to draw conclusions, the effects of systematic exercise interventions on *both* fitness *and* body image need to be examined. Only a handful of published studies have done so. The results of these studies are summarized in this chapter, which examines fitness change and other potential mediators of the exercise–body image relationship. The chapter also discusses potential moderators of the exercise–body image relationship, and the implications of the current state of knowledge for developing exercise interventions and advancing research.

THE EFFECTS OF EXERCISE TRAINING ON FITNESS AND BODY IMAGE CHANGE

There seems to be an inherent assumption within the exercise and body image literature that exercise produces changes in fitness, which, in turn, lead to changes in body image. "Fitness" encompasses level of cardiorespiratory endurance (or aerobic fitness), muscular strength and endurance, flexibility,

414

body composition, and ability to perform functional activities such as those associated with daily living. "Fitness-enhancing interventions" can be defined as any program of aerobic (e.g., walking, jogging, dance) or anaerobic activity (e.g., weight training, stretching) that is designed to improve one or more fitness components. Although most intervention studies have utilized exercise programs of sufficient intensity, duration, and frequency to improve *multiple* fitness components, the vast majority of studies have examined body image change in relation to change in just a *single* fitness component— body composition (e.g., skinfold thickness, body weight, body fat).

Changes in body composition appear to be a significant predictor of body image change following an exercise intervention. However, the effects of improved body composition are fairly modest and generally account for less than 10% of the variance in body image scores. Moreover, some studies have failed to show a significant relationship between changes in body composition and changes in body image. Thus greater decreases in body weight are not necessarily associated with greater improvements in body satisfaction, and relatively small alterations in body composition can lead to a substantial enhancement of body image. Improvements in strength and/or cardiovascular endurance also account for only modest variance in body image change. As with body composition, it is possible that the secondary appearance-related changes that are associated with improved fitness (e.g., improved muscle tone, clothing fits better) might trigger improvements in body image rather than changes in fitness, per se. In sum, it is unclear whether fitness enhancement, per se, plays a distinct role in the exercise–body image relationship, or whether secondary, appearance-related changes account for the modest association between fitness change and body image change. Moreover, because only a couple of studies have conducted followups, it is uncertain whether systematic fitness interventions produce lasting body image change.

Are certain types of fitness interventions more conducive to facilitating changes in body image than others? Within the body image literature, most exercise intervention studies have utilized aerobic exercise training (e.g., walking) or a combination of aerobic exercise plus strength training. There are relatively few studies of the effects of strength training alone on body image. Based on the limited research in this area, the emerging picture is that while both aerobic exercise and strength training can lead to body image change, strength training—weight training, in particular—produces the greatest improvements in body image. Weight training may be superior to walking or jogging because improvements in strength emerge more quickly and tend to be larger than improvements in aerobic capacity (especially for the novice exerciser). Strength can improve 10–30% within the first 6–8 weeks of a weight training program simply as a result of neuromuscular adaptation and learning the technique of weightlifting. In contrast, improvements in aerobic capacity are dependent upon physiological adaptations that occur at a slower rate (especially in a walking program) and may be less noticeable in terms of changes in body composition.

MEDIATORS OF THE EXERCISE–BODY IMAGE RELATIONSHIP

Changes in *objective* indices of physical fitness cannot fully explain the effects of exercise on body image. Therefore there must be other mechanisms by which exercise exerts its influence. One possibility is that the effects of exercise are mediated by changes in *subjective* perceptions of one's physical fitness and competence. According to Sonstroem and Morgan's expanded Exercise and Self-Esteem Model, exercise-induced changes in physical self-efficacy fuel exercise-related changes in body image. "Physical self-efficacy" refers to beliefs about one's capabilities for *specific* physical tasks (e.g., confidence in one's ability to run 5 miles or to lift 100 pounds) and beliefs about one's physical fitness and functioning *in general* (e.g., beliefs about one's level of strength, agility, and physical condition).

Although it seems intuitively likely that one must experience changes in physical fitness before change in physical self-efficacy can occur, this is not always the case. Sometimes exercise training can significantly increase physical self-efficacy for tasks such as lifting and running, in the absence of significant objective changes in strength and cardiovascular fitness. Thus, although exercise training may sometimes fail to generate *statistically meaningful* improvements in strength and fitness, exercisers may perceive real or imagined yet *personally meaningful* improvements in their physical functioning that significantly enhance self-efficacy. According to the Exercise and Self-Esteem Model, these increases in self-efficacy result in more positive feelings about one's body.

In addition to enhancing efficacy, exercise may improve body image by making people more aware of their physical capabilities, while reducing focus on their physical appearance. Research on exercise motives indicates that although many people start an exercise program with the goal of altering their appearance, motives for exercise tend to shift over time toward improving physical functioning and psychological well-being. Thus long-term participation in regular exercise can divert attention from appearance-related body image concerns.

This shift in values may be particularly relevant to women, who, unlike men, tend to place greater value on physical appearance than on physical functioning and who are motivated to start exercising to improve their appearance rather than to enhance their functioning. Ironically, it is virtually impossible for most women to achieve today's ultrathin, aesthetic body image ideal through exercise (or even through exercise plus dieting). Women who embark on an exercise program with a perfectionistic goal of attaining the aesthetic ideal are setting themselves up for failure and continued body dissatisfaction (see Davis's chapter in this volume). It is possible, however, for most women to improve their *physical conditioning* through exercise training. When women exercise to improve their fitness, they are more likely to experience success and satisfaction than when they exercise for appearance-related reasons. This finding may explain why women who exercise for fitness-related motives express greater body satisfaction than those who exercise for appearance-related motives. Because society does not have strictly defined ideals for fitness (i.e., in terms of how fast a woman should be able to run, or how much weight she should be able to lift), women who focus on improvement along these dimensions are not constantly comparing themselves and coming up short against an unattainable standard.

WHO BENEFITS FROM EXERCISE INTERVENTIONS?

The positive effects of exercise training on body image have been demonstrated in both men and women and in younger adults as well as those who are middle-aged and older. People with the poorest initial body image tend to show the greatest improvement. As such, women tend to show greater improvement than men, and older people may show greater improvement than younger people, particularly on measures of body image that assess satisfaction with physical function. Thus, although exercise interventions can have a positive effect regardless of one's age or gender, these variables can moderate the magnitude of the effects. Unfortunately, there has been virtually no examination of other individual differences that may moderate the body image outcomes of exercise interventions.

If those with the poorest body image have the most to gain from exercise interventions, then it follows that exercise training could be particularly beneficial to people whose body image may be threatened by disease or illness. Although few controlled studies have examined the effect of exercise interventions on body image in such individuals, extant data are promising. For example, exercise training has been associated with increased body satisfaction among women recovering from breast cancer, men and women with paraplegia and quadriplegia, adolescents with postural deformities, and women classified as obese. These findings speak to the robustness of exercise for improving body image within a variety of populations.

EXERCISE INTERVENTIONS IMPROVE OTHER ASPECTS OF PSYCHOSOCIAL WELL-BEING

Body image is not the only aspect of psychological well-being that can be improved through exercise training. Exercise has also been shown to relieve symptoms of depression and anxiety, improve mood and affect, and bolster aspects of self-concept and self-esteem. There is also some evidence to suggest that exercise training can buffer against stress and depression.

However, just as changes in aerobic fitness and strength may not be prerequisites for changes in body image, changes in these physical fitness components may not be necessary for changes in psychological well-being to occur. For example, most aerobic exercise interventions that have resulted in improved psychological well-being have consisted of moderate-intensity programs that were not necessarily performed at a level conducive to improving cardiovascular fitness. In addition, there has been inconsistent support for a dose–response relationship between the amount of exercise performed and the amount of change incurred along psychosocial dimensions. The absence of a dose–response relationship suggests that when the objective is to improve psychological well-being through exercise, *more* is not necessarily *better*. In fact, too much exercise can actually be indicative of psychological dysfunction (see Davis's chapter in this volume). Thus, to borrow the Nike motto, when it comes to using exercise to improve psychological well-being, the most important thing may be that people "just do it."

IMPLICATIONS FOR DEVELOPING
BODY IMAGE INTERVENTIONS

Whereas "just doing it" may improve other aspects of psychological well-being, our review of the literature suggests that when the goal is to improve body image, attention should be paid to at least three programmatic aspects of an exercise intervention. First, in terms of exercise prescription, studies suggest that in order to see significant gains in body image, exercise intensity and duration should be moderate to high—perhaps because this level of exercise is most likely to generate the greatest improvements in physical function, fitness, and appearance. Moreover, if enhanced perceptions of physical competence mediate changes in body image, then successful, difficult, high-intensity workouts will result in a greater sense of self-efficacy and body image change than successful, easier, low-intensity workouts. With regard to exercise type, weight training seems to be the type of exercise most conducive to facilitating changes in body image.

Second, some evidence suggests that people who enjoy their workouts more show bigger improvements in body image. Perhaps the cumulative effects of mood-enhancing exercise bouts lead to a more positive state of mind, in general, which leads to better feelings about oneself and one's body. It may also be that people who enjoy their workouts exercise harder and more effectively than those who don't enjoy exercising, thus reaping greater improvements in fitness, function, and appearance. Exercise programmers can enhance enjoyment by creating opportunities for exercisers to socialize with one another, by adding variety to workouts, and by ensuring that the program's fitness leaders are positive and encouraging.

Third, we suggest that exercise programs focus on improving physical function, strength, and endurance rather than on changing physical appearance. Programs that help people set realistic and attainable goals and that teach people how to monitor progress in terms of functional fitness improvements will have a more positive impact on body image than programs emphasizing "building buns of steel" and "fighting flabby abs."

FUTURE RESEARCH DIRECTIONS

To date, the exercise and body image literature is largely comprised of studies involving well-educated Caucasian women between the ages of 17 and 65. Although there have been some studies of exercise and body image in men, most of this research, surprisingly, has focused on older men (over 45 years old) and given little attention to the effects of exercise on body image among younger cohorts. As such, the generalizability of the literature remains questionable. Studies of other cultural groups and across a broader sociodemographic spectrum are needed. Other questions and topical areas that warrant research attention are summarized below:

- How should exercise be prescribed when the goal is to improve body image? What is the optimal exercise frequency, intensity, and duration? How long does it take for body image improvements to emerge? Can an acute bout of exercise influence body image?
- How long do the effects of exercise on body image last? Do the effects of weight training last longer than the effects of aerobic exercise? Does exercise provide a buffer against the effects of minor weight gain and other potential threats to body image?
- Given the increasing rate of body image disturbances in young boys and girls, exercise should be explored as both a preventive measure against the development of body dissatisfaction and as a treatment strategy for improving body image in children and teenagers. In a similar vein, healthy, moderate exercise may play a role in both the treatment and prevention of body image disturbances associated with eating disorders.
- What role do changes in perceived improvements in fitness and function play in relation to objective changes in fitness and function?
- An understanding of the mechanisms by which exercise improves body image has been hindered by a lack of theory-driven research. Bandura's self-efficacy theory and the Exercise and Self-Esteem Model are potential frameworks in which future research might be situated. Appropriate statistical methods (e.g., mediational analyses, structural equation modeling) should be used when testing these models and examining variables that mediate and moderate the effects of exercise on body image.

- Do individual differences along dimensions such as perfectionism, neuroticism, extroversion, depression, and exercise motives and beliefs influence the exercise–body image relationship?
- Does goal-setting and goal-attainment mediate the effects of exercise on body image?
- What is the relationship between body image change and changes in mood and affect? Does one precede the other? Is it possible that exercise-related biochemical changes vis-à-vis mood-enhancement (e.g., endorphin release) also play a role in body image enhancement?
- Most research has focused on exercise-related changes along cognitive and affective dimensions of body image (e.g., satisfaction with appearance, social physique anxiety). Additional studies are needed to determine the effects of exercise on perceptual aspects of body image (e.g., effects on self-estimates of body size) and on behavioral aspects (e.g., effects on the type of clothing one chooses to wear).

CONCLUSIONS

Based on the limited research to date, it appears that exercise is an effective intervention for improving body image in college-age and older men and women. Weight training seems to produce greater increases in body satisfaction than aerobic training, and those with the lowest baseline levels of body satisfaction seem to reap the largest gains from exercise training. Changes in objective indices of physical fitness play a minor role in changing body image. Rather, what seems to be important is that exercisers *perceive* improvements in their fitness, function, and appearance. Fitness-enhancing interventions may promote the greatest amount of body image change when careful attention is paid to the exercise prescription as well as to the goals and social environment of the exercise training. Given the relatively small number of controlled studies of exercise and body image, many questions about the nature of this relationship remain unanswered. The effect of exercise on body image is an area that is ripe for investigation.

INFORMATIVE READINGS

Bandura, A. (1997). *Self-efficacy: The exercise of control.* New York: W. H. Freeman.—An exhaustive analysis of the concept of self-efficacy and related research in fields such as health, physical activity, and aging.

Bane, S. M., & McAuley, E. (1998). Body image and exercise. In J. Duda (Ed.), *Advances in sport and exercise psychology measurement* (pp. 311–322). Morgantown, WV: Fitness Information Technology.—A comprehensive review of body image measures used in exercise and other types of research.

DiLorenzo, T. M., Bargman, E. P., Stucky-Ropp, R., Brassington, G. S., Frensch, P. A., & LaFountaine, T. (1999). Long-term effects of aerobic exercise on psychological outcomes. *Preventive Medicine, 28,* 75–85.—Examines the short- and long-term psychological effects of a 12–week fitness program on 82 men and women.

Fox, K. R. (1997). *The physical self: From motivation to well-being.* Champaign, IL: Human Kinetics.—A reflection on the importance of the physical self as a determinant or motivator of behaviors, including exercise, and as a contributor to mental health and well-being.

Martin, K. A., Leary, M. R., & Rejeski, W. J. (2000). Self-presentational concerns in older adults: Implications for health and well-being. *Basic and Applied Social Psychology, 22,* 169–179.—A comprehensive review of the implications of self-presentational concerns and impression management strategies for the physical and psychological well-being of older adults.

McAuley, E. (1994). Physical activity and psychosocial outcomes. In C. Bouchard, R. J. Shephard, & T. Stephens (Eds.), *Physical activity, fitness, and health: International proceedings and consensus statement* (pp. 551–568). Champaign, IL: Human Kinetics.—Overview of research examining the relationships between physical activity and psychosocial outcomes, including self-esteem, self-efficacy, and psychological well-being.

Sidney, K. H., & Shephard, R. J. (1976). Attitudes towards health and physical activity in the elderly. Effects of a training program. *Medicine and Science in Sports, 8,* 246–252.—Describes attitude change following a 3-month exercise intervention and the most effective combination of exercise intensity and frequency for improving body image.

Sonstroem, R. J. (1997). The physical self-system: A mediator of exercise and self-esteem. In K. R. Fox (Ed.), *The physical self: From motivation to well-being* (pp. 3–26). Champaign, IL: Human Kinetics.—Describes and provides evidence for the Exercise and Self-Esteem Model.

Sonstroem, R, J., & Morgan, W. P. (1989). Exercise and self-esteem: Rationale and model. *Medicine and Science in Sports and Exercise, 21,* 329–337.—A summary of self-esteem theory and presentation of a model that can be used to examine exercise and self-esteem interactions.

Tucker, L. A., & Maxwell, K. (1992). Effects of weight training on the emotional well-being and body image of females: Predictors of greatest benefit. *American Journal of Health Promotion, 6,* 338–371.—A controlled study of the effects of weight training in college-age women.

Tucker, L. A., & Mortell, R. (1993). Comparison of the effects of walking and weight training programs on body image in middle-aged women: An experimental study. *American Journal of Health Promotion, 8,* 34–42.—An experimental study demonstrating the superiority of weight training for improving body image in middle-aged women.

Williams, P. A., & Cash, T. F. (2001). The effects of a circuit weight training program on the body images of college students. *International Journal of Eating Disorders, 30,* 75–82.—A controlled study confirming the effectiveness of weight training, independent of aerobic activity, in the improvement of body image, social physique anxiety, and physical self-efficacy.

Cosmetic Surgery and Changes in Body Image

DAVID B. SARWER

The American Society of Plastic Surgeons reports that more than 1.3 million Americans underwent cosmetic surgery in 2000, an increase of more than 225% since 1992. While staggering, these statistics underestimate the number of cosmetic procedures performed annually, as physicians from a variety of medical specialties now offer cosmetic medical treatments. The five most popular procedures in 2000 were liposuction (removal of fat), breast augmentation, blepharoplasty (eyelid surgery), Botox injections (to reduce wrinkles), and facelifts. These procedures are no longer reserved for the wealthy and elite; women and men across age, racial, and socioeconomic groups now seek cosmetic surgery to improve their appearance and, ultimately, their body image.

This chapter provides an overview of the relationship between cosmetic surgery and body image. It begins by reviewing psychological studies of cosmetic surgery patients and discussing the theoretical relationship between body image and cosmetic surgery. Studies directly investigating the body image concerns of cosmetic surgery patients are also reviewed. The relationship between body image psychopathology and cosmetic surgery is discussed. The chapter concludes with an overview of patient assessment procedures for mental health professionals who encounter cosmetic surgery patients.

PSYCHOLOGICAL STUDIES OF COSMETIC SURGERY PATIENTS

Interest in the psychological aspects of cosmetic surgery dates back more than 50 years. With few exceptions, clinical reports and formal studies have investigated the psychological issues of adult women, who represent the vast majority of cosmetic surgery patients. Thus, little is know about the psychological characteristics of the increasing number of men and adolescents who now seek cosmetic surgery. (Readers interested in learning about cosmetic surgery for adolescents are referred to a chapter by Sarwer that is listed in the Informative Readings.)

Studies of women who seek cosmetic surgery attempt to answer two basic questions. First, do these women share a common psychological profile? Second, do they experience positive psychological changes postoperatively? As my colleagues and I have discussed in our previous reviews of this literature (Sarwer et al., 1998b; Sarwer et al., 2000), results of these studies are equivocal. Preoperative interview-based investigations of cosmetic surgery patients have typically described high rates of DSM Axis I and Axis II disorders among patients. In contrast, investigations utilizing psychometric measures have found far less psychopathology. Both types of studies have reported mixed results postoperatively, with some reporting modest improvements in psychological symptoms and others reporting no change. Unfortunately, numerous methodological problems with both sets of studies raise questions about the validity of the results and, in our opinion, leave the two most basic questions investigated by the research largely unanswered.

Nevertheless, my colleagues and I (Sarwer et al., 1998b) hypothesized that cosmetic surgery patients likely exhibit certain personality traits as compared to individuals who do not seek surgery. One such characteristic may be body image dissatisfaction. This dissatisfaction may serve as a defining characteristic of those who seek to alter their appearance through cosmetic surgery.

BODY IMAGE AND COSMETIC SURGERY

Body image has long been considered central to understanding the psychological characteristics of cosmetic surgery patients. Clinical reports have suggested that cosmetic surgery patients express increased dissatisfaction with their bodies preoperatively and experience body image improvements postoperatively. Only recently, however, has the relationship between body image and cosmetic surgery become the focus of theoretical discussion and empirical study.

A Theoretical Model of the Relationship between Body Image and Cosmetic Surgery

Borrowing heavily from existing theories of body image, my colleagues and I (Sarwer et al., 1998b) proposed a theoretical model of the relationship between body image and cosmetic surgery, in which both physical and psychological factors influence the decision to seek this elective surgery. The physical reality of one's appearance provides the foundation for an individual's subjective body image. Perceptual, developmental, and sociocultural experiences also play an important role. Perceptual influences account for an individual's ability to accurately assess the physical characteristics (e.g., size, shape, texture) of a given body part. Developmental experiences (such as the occurrence of appearance-related teasing) and sociocultural factors (particularly mass media depictions of physical beauty) also may influence an individual's decision to seek cosmetic surgery.

We believe that body image attitudes, as they pertain to cosmetic surgery, have at least two dimensions. The first consists of *valence*, defined as the degree to which body image is important to one's self-esteem. People with a high body image valence are thought to derive much of their self-esteem from their body image and thus may be more likely to identify and enact behaviors that might improve their body image. Furthermore, body image has a *value*, which can be thought of as the degree of dissatisfaction with appearance. Dissatisfaction with appearance is thought to serve as the motivational component for the pursuit of many appearance-enhancing behaviors, such as weight loss, exercise, cosmetic and clothing purchases, as well as cosmetic surgery. The interaction between body image valence and body image value ultimately influences the decision to pursue cosmetic surgery.

Body Image Dissatisfaction Prior to Cosmetic Surgery

Our initial empirical study (Sarwer et al., 1998a) investigated the nature of body image dissatisfaction in cosmetic surgery patients. Women who sought a variety of cosmetic procedures preoperatively completed two measures of body image. The Multidimensional Body Self-Relations Questionnaire (MBSRQ), developed by Brown, Cash, and Mikulka in 1990, was used to assess the overall body image, particularly the degree of investment (as assessed by the Appearance Orientation subscale) and the degree of dissatisfaction (the Appearance Evaluation subscale). Patients also were asked to complete Rosen and Reiter's 1996 Body Dysmorphic Disorder Examination—Self-Report (BDDE-SR), which quantifies the degree of dissatisfaction with the specific feature for which the patient is seeking surgery. This measure also allowed for an assessment of body dysmorphic disorder. Compared to the norms provided with these measures, prospective patients reported heightened dissatisfaction with the specific body feature for which they were pursuing surgery but did not report a greater investment or increased dissatisfaction with their overall body image. These findings supported the role of body image dissatisfaction in the decision to pursue surgery but did not support the role of body image valence.

Subsequent investigations have provided additional information on the body image concerns of women who seek cosmetic surgery. Breast reduction patients, as compared to breast augmentation patients, reported significantly greater dissatisfaction with both their breasts and overall body image.

The majority of women in both groups, however, reported having negative feelings about their breasts, avoiding being seen undressed by others, and camouflaging the appearance of their breasts with clothing or special bras. Greater than 20% of both groups also reported increased symptoms of anxiety and depression. Breast augmentation patients, as compared to small-breasted women not seeking surgery, reported significantly greater dissatisfaction with their breasts, more appearance-related teasing, and greater use of psychotherapy in the previous year. These studies not only confirm that cosmetic surgery patients experience increased body image dissatisfaction but suggest that this dissatisfaction may be related to more general dysphoria. This later finding, however, awaits confirmation by future studies.

Changes in Body Image Following Cosmetic Surgery

We have recently investigated changes in body image following cosmetic surgery (Sarwer et al., 2002). Compared to their preoperative assessment of body image, cosmetic surgery patients reported a significant reduction in dissatisfaction with the specific feature altered by surgery. More specifically, they reported significantly less embarrassment about the feature in public areas, social settings, or when others noticed the feature. They also reported a significant reduction in the use of camouflaging behaviors. These women, however, reported no significant improvements in the degree of investment or dissatisfaction with their overall appearance. These results indicate that individuals who undergo cosmetic surgery may experience an improvement in dissatisfaction with the feature altered by surgery, but these improvements may not generalize to the overall body image. Thus cosmetic surgery may be an appropriate body image treatment for individuals with specific concerns about their appearance.

BODY IMAGE PSYCHOPATHOLOGY IN COSMETIC SURGERY PATIENTS

Given the relationship between body image and cosmetic surgery, it is likely that many different types of body image disorders occur among cosmetic surgery patients. Eating disorders and body dysmorphic disorder (BDD) may be of greatest concern.

Eating Disorders

Although formal prevalence studies have not been completed, anorexia and bulimia may be disproportionately represented among those who seek liposuction to alter the shape of their bodies. Many people assume that liposuction results in weight loss, when, in fact, the amount of fat removed typically results in little body weight change. Thus it is not considered an acceptable weight reduction treatment. Eating disorders also may be a concern for women interested in breast augmentation surgery. These patients are frequently of low-average or below-average weight, suggesting that some of them may be at risk for eating disorders. Women with both anorexia and bulimia who have undergone breast augmentation or liposuction frequently report an exacerbation of their eating-disordered symptoms postoperatively. Interestingly, Losee and colleagues reported that four of five breast reduction patients (who are often overweight or obese) with bulimia experienced an improvement in their bulimic symptoms postoperatively.

Body Dysmorphic Disorder (BDD)

People with BDD frequently attempt to treat their appearance concerns with cosmetic medical treatments (for a detailed discussion of BDD, see the chapter by Phillips in this volume). In a sample of 188 individuals with BDD, Phillips and Diaz found that 131 sought and 109 received cosmetic surgical, dermatological, dental, or other medical treatments. Only recently has the prevalence of BDD among people who seek these treatments been established. Sarwer and colleagues (1998a) found that 7% of cosmetic surgery patients met diagnostic criteria for BDD. Phillips and colleagues found that 12% of dermatology patients screened positive for BDD.

BDD is often difficult to identify in patients who seek cosmetic surgery. Many cosmetic surgeons are likely unfamiliar with the disorder. The goal of cosmetic surgery—to improve "slight defects" in an otherwise "normal" appearance—also makes diagnosis difficult. Given the inherent ambiguity and subjectivity in defining the disorder in terms of appearance, we have suggested that the degree of emotional distress and behavioral impairment, rather than the size or nature of the physical defect, may be more accurate indicators of BDD in these patients.

The vast majority of persons with BDD do not benefit from cosmetic medical treatments. In two retrospective studies of BDD patients who received these treatments (Phillips and Diaz, as well as Veale), more than three-fourths reported dissatisfaction with the outcome as well as an exacerbation of, or no change in, their BDD symptoms. In response to these outcomes, some patients perform "do it yourself" surgeries or become violent toward themselves or the surgeon. These reports suggest that BDD may contraindicate cosmetic surgery.

PSYCHOLOGICAL ASSESSMENT OF COSMETIC SURGERY PATIENTS

Mental health professionals may encounter cosmetic surgery patients in a variety of contexts. Patients in a psychotherapy practice who have body image concerns may have considered or undergone cosmetic surgery. Cosmetic surgeons also may refer patients to a mental health professional to assess psychological functioning pre- or postoperatively.

Preoperative Consultations

The majority of cosmetic surgery patients probably do not require a psychological assessment prior to surgery. Patients with existing psychopathology, or those in whom a body image disorder (such as an eating disorder or BDD) is suspected, warrant psychological evaluation. In addition to the basic principles of psychological assessment, the evaluation should focus specifically on patients' body image concerns.

Psychological assessment of cosmetic surgery patients often begins with discussing motivations for surgery. To assess the source of patients' motivations, it may be useful to ask when they first started thinking about changing their appearance and why they are interested in doing so at this particular time. Patients should be able to articulate "internally" based motivations (e.g., "I am having the surgery because I am self-conscious about my love handles when I am undressed in front of my partner."). Those who articulate "externally" based motivations (e.g., "I need a facelift to help me get a new job.") may be less likely to meet their goals for surgery.

The assessment should include a discussion of patients' postoperative expectations. Pruzinsky categorized postoperative expectations as surgical, psychological, and social: Surgical expectations represent patients' specific concerns about their appearance; psychological expectations include the potential benefits to self-esteem, body image, and quality of life postoperatively; social expectations address the effects of cosmetic surgery on patients' social interactions. Cosmetic surgery patients frequently report improvements in their appearance postoperatively. These improvements, however, may not lead to career advancement or enhanced relationships. To assess patients' postoperative expectations, they should be asked how they anticipate their lives being different following surgery. Patients who can articulate realistic expectations may be more likely to be satisfied with the postoperative result.

A comprehensive assessment of body image concerns is perhaps the most central task of the assessment. Prospective patients should be able to articulate specific appearance concerns, which should be readily visible. For example, an appropriate patient may say "I dislike this bump on my nose," and the bump is easily seen by the professional. In contrast, a patient inappropriate for cosmetic surgery might say, "My nose makes me grotesquely ugly," and the professional sees nothing abnormal about the person's nose. The consultant also should assess the degree of body image dissatisfaction by asking patients about the amount of time they spend thinking about or addressing their appearance. Patients also should be asked if their appearance concerns lead them to avoid certain activities. Those patients who are markedly distressed about slight defects that are not readily visible, those who report spending more than 1 hour per day on their appearance, and those who report disruption in daily activity due to appearance-related concerns should be assessed further for BDD. This assessment can be augmented with measures of body image dissatisfaction, such as the MBSRQ or BDDE-SR, which may help quantify the degree of body image dissatisfaction.

In addition to assessing body image concerns, consulting professionals should conduct a thorough assessment of current and past psychological functioning. The presence of a particular psychiatric disorder may not be a contraindication for surgery, particularly if the disorder is unrelated to body image concerns. Patients with a positive psychiatric history should be assessed to determine if there is a need for psychiatric treatment prior to surgery. Those currently in mental health treatment should receive clearance from their provider prior to surgery. Most cosmetic surgeons will not operate on a patient who is actively psychotic, manic, or severely depressed.

Postoperative Consultations

Cosmetic surgeons also may refer their patients to mental health professionals postoperatively. Referral typically occurs when patients are unhappy with the postoperative result or experience an exacerbation of psychopathology that was not detected preoperatively. Patients in both of these categories should be assessed in a manner similar to that for preoperative patients. These patients frequently struggle with guilt and shame regarding the decision to have surgery, believing that their "vanity" brought about the unsatisfying result. Cognitive-behavioral models of body image psychotherapy (see chapter by Cash and Strachan in this volume) are often useful with these individuals, although more diagnosis-specific treatments also may be required.

CONCLUSION

More people than ever before are now changing their bodies though cosmetic surgery. For decades, both surgeons and mental health professionals have been interested in the psychological functioning of these individuals, but only recently has increased attention been directed toward investigating the relationship between cosmetic surgery and body image. Body image dissatisfaction, particularly dissatisfaction with the specific feature for which surgery is being considered, is thought to motivate the pursuit of surgery. Preliminary findings suggest that the majority of patients experience body image improvements postoperatively. Furthermore, extreme body image dissatisfaction, categorized by BDD, occurs in a significant minority of both cosmetic surgical and dermatological patients.

These studies, however, have just begun to shape our thinking about the relationship between body image and cosmetic surgery. At present, we know little about the effect of developmental and sociocultural influences on body image and the resulting decision to seek cosmetic surgery. Similarly, little is known about the relationship between preoperative body image dissatisfaction and postoperative long-term improvements in body image. It is unclear if individuals who request repeated cosmetic procedures, either on the same or different features, have greater body image dissatisfaction than those who only seek a single cosmetic procedure. Finally, we need to explore further the relationship between body image disorders, such as eating disorders and BDD, and cosmetic surgery. The increasing number of people who pursue cosmetic surgery are likely to teach us a great deal about body image in the near future.

INFORMATIVE READINGS

American Society of Plastic Surgeons. (1999). *2000 plastic surgery procedural statistics.* Arlington Heights, IL: Author. Available online: *plasticsurgery.org/mediactr/stats-06.pdf*—Provides up-to-date statistics on the number of plastic surgery procedures performed by members of the American Society of Plastic Surgeons.

Brown, T. A., Cash, T. F., & Mikulka, P. J. (1990). Attitudinal body image assessment: Factor analysis of the Body Self-Relations Questionnaire. *Journal of Personality Assessment, 5*, 135–144.—A principal-components analysis of the MBSRQ that supports the conceptual components of the measure.

Losee, J. E., Serletti, J. M., Kreipe, R. E., & Caldwell, E. H. (1997). Reduction mammaplasty in patients with bulimia nervosa. *Annals of Plastic Surgery, 39*, 443–446.—Report of five women with bulimia nervosa who underwent breast reduction.

Phillips, K. A., & Diaz, S. F. (1997). Gender differences in body dysmorphic disorder. *Journal of Nervous and Mental Diseases, 185*, 570–577.—A retrospective study of 188 persons with BDD that provides data on the use of nonpsychiatric medical treatments.

Phillips, K. A., Dufresne, R. G., Wilkel, C. S., & Vittorio, C. C. (2000). Rate of body dysmorphic disorder in dermatology patients. *Journal of the American Academy of Dermatology, 42*, 436–441.—First study to establish the rate of BDD among dermatology patients.

Pruzinsky, T. (1996). Cosmetic plastic surgery and body image: Critical factors in patient assessment. In J. K. Thompson (Ed.), *Body image, eating disorders, and obesity: An integrative guide for assessment and treatment* (pp. 109–127). Washington, DC: American Psychological Association.—Contains a detailed description of the psychological assessment of cosmetic surgery patients.

Rosen, J. C., & Reiter, J. (1996). Development of the body dysmorphic disorder examination. *Behaviour Research and Therapy, 34*, 755–766.—Discusses the development of the Body Dysmorphic Disorder Examination as a measure of the symptoms of body dysmorphic disorder.

Sarwer, D. B. (2001). Plastic surgery in children and adolescents. In J. K. Thompson & L. Smolak (Eds.), *Body image, eating disorders, and obesity in children and adolescents: The-*

ory, assessment, treatment and prevention (pp. 341–336). Washington, DC: American Psychological Association.—Discusses the body image issues of children and adolescents who undergo plastic surgery.

Sarwer, D. B., Bartlett, S. P., Bucky, L. P., LaRossa, D., Low, D. W., Pertschuk, M. J., Wadden, T. A., & Whitaker, L. A. (1998). Bigger is not always better: Body image dissatisfaction in breast reduction and breast augmentation patients. *Plastic and Reconstructive Surgery, 101,* 1956–1961.—Empirical study that compared the body image concerns of breast reduction and breast augmentation patients.

Sarwer, D. B., Nordmann, J. E., & Herbert, J. D. (2000). Cosmetic breast augmentation surgery: A critical overview. *Journal of Women's Health and Gender-Based Medicine, 9,* 843–856.—Reviews both the medical and psychological literature on cosmetic breast implants.

Sarwer, D. B., Wadden, T. A., Pertschuk, M. J., & Whitaker, L. A. (1998a). Body image dissatisfaction and body dysmorphic disorder in 100 cosmetic surgery patients. *Plastic and Reconstructive Surgery, 101,* 1644–1649.—First empirical study of body image dissatisfaction and BDD in cosmetic surgery patients.

Sarwer, D. B., Wadden, T. A., Pertschuk, M. J., & Whitaker, L. A. (1998b). The psychology of cosmetic surgery: A review and reconceptualization. *Clinical Psychology Review, 18,* 1–22.—Provides a historical review of the literature and proposes a model of the relationship between body image and cosmetic surgery.

Sarwer, D. B., Wadden, T. A., & Whitaker, L. A. (2002). An investigation of changes in body image following cosmetic surgery. *Plastic and Reconstructive Surgery, 109,* 363–369.—Found that women report improvements in the degree of dissatisfaction with the feature altered by cosmetic surgery but not in the overall body image.

Veale, D. (2000). Outcome of cosmetic surgery and "DIY" surgery in patients with body dysmorphic disorder. *Psychiatric Bulletin, 24,* 218–221.—Reported that 76% of patients with BDD reported dissatisfaction with the results of cosmetic surgery.

Optimizing Body Image in Disfiguring Congenital Conditions
Surgical and Psychosocial Interventions

NICHOLA RUMSEY

A visibly disfiguring condition poses considerable challenges to the process of building and maintaining a positive body image and self-esteem (see chapter by Rumsey in Part IV). The pressures that lead affected individuals to seek surgical, medical, and/or psychosocial interventions come from a variety of possible sources: social context, peers and/or family, as well as from personal beliefs. Certainly, this society has well-entrenched standards regarding physical appearance, and the media and advertising exert persistent pressures to correct any and all flaws (see chapter by Tiggemann in this volume). Thompson and colleagues note that, as normalizing technologies become more accessible and it becomes more acceptable and even expected for people to change their appearance, pressure mounts on people with visible disfigurement to "fix" their features.

Clearly, individual differences in the degree of vulnerability to sociocultural influences are ubiquitous. Harter maintains that levels of appearance-related stress in the general population are affected by the extent to which individuals' body image and self-esteem are dependent upon appearance and the perceived importance of cultural standards as a source of comparison. Recent research on disfigurement focuses on the attribute of "resilience"—comprised of positive self-beliefs, effective social skills, and social support—which buffers an individual against the stresses and strains of living with a visible difference. This chapter addresses these components of resilience in the context of considering how to optimize the body image of individuals with congenital disfigurement.

TYPES OF INTERVENTION

Surgical and Medical Interventions

Patients undergoing reconstructive surgery are obviously motivated to change their appearance. In addition, they have psychological and social outcome expectations (e.g., improved body image, self-esteem, social relations). It seems paradoxical, therefore that the prevailing forms of intervention focus solely on changing physical appearance. The assumption is that treatment (surgery, lasers, medications) will indirectly result in these psychosocial benefits. Normalizing appearance can clearly benefit psychosocial functioning. However, care providers are, in effect, colluding with the simplistic myth that quality of life necessarily improves when appearance is enhanced. Research suggests that, in reality, the picture is much more complex.

Patients with a congenital abnormality often undergo multiple surgeries; there is always the possibility of revising scars or submitting to new techniques. However, the majority of people with visible congenital defects express the desire to be "normal" and "unremarkable" rather than perfect. Therefore, we should avoid assuming that individuals with residual congenital deformity invariably want to undertake all possible forms of intervention.

Interventions for congenital conditions can be carefully planned and timed to take into account pertinent physical (e.g., growth) and social (e.g., the desirability of normalizing appearance before joining a different social group, such as a new school) factors. Some patients may require only one operation. For others, however, multiple surgical procedures are the norm. For the more commonly occurring conditions, the existence of rigid treatment protocols may make it difficult for the affected person to participate fully in treatment decisions. In cleft care, for example, surgery to the jaw is often planned for early adolescence. At this stage, the patient might be more concerned with another aspect of appearance (for example, the nose), but may not wish to offend the care team by expressing wishes that are at odds with the normal pattern of care.

Psychosocial Interventions

In contrast to the increasing accessibility of surgery, psychosocial support and interventions are not routinely available. Although some treatment teams have access to a psychologist or psychiatrist, interventions tend to be problem-focused (offered after difficulties have been identified) rather than preventive, and many are offered by professionals who have no specialized knowledge of disfigurement.

Because many of the difficulties reported by people with visible differences concern problems that involve social interaction (see chapter by

Rumsey in Part IV), Robinson and colleagues documented the effectiveness of using group social interaction skills training (SIST) with adults. Similarly, Kapp-Simon highlighted the relevance of social skills training for adolescents affected by a cleft.

Although SIST results in positive changes in a range of psychosocial variables, including body image, more recent interventions are based more explicitly on cognitive-behavioral therapy (CBT) principles. These interventions focus on relevant aspects of behavior (e.g., initiating social interaction), emotions (e.g., promoting positive feelings about the self), and thoughts (e.g., changing how social information is processed). Some interventions are specific to a particular abnormality—for example, the difficulties associated with a progressive condition. However, many components are applicable to a range of disfiguring conditions as well as to nondisfigured appearance-related concerns. CBT interventions that are specific to body image (see Cash and Strachan's chapter in Part VIII) effectively complement SIST techniques but have yet to be systematically applied in this population.

Information, support, and intervention can be preventive and/or problem-focused and can be delivered in many formats to individuals, families, and peers. CBT interventions offered by psychologists at Outlook, the first government-funded disfigurement support unit in the United Kingdom, have shown improvements for a large proportion of attendees after one session, and for others with more complex difficulties after six to eight sessions of individual treatment. Changes include reductions in social anxiety and appearance-related distress and increased utilization of effective coping strategies. In response to the difficulties experienced by many children with visible differences when transferring from primary to secondary school, Outlook offers a one-day group intervention before entering secondary school, with a half-day follow-up during the first midterm break at the new school. Although well received by participants, numbers are currently too small to draw definitive conclusions regarding the efficacy of these interventions.

Changing Faces, a charitable foundation based in the United Kingdom, has considerable experience offering advice and relevant literature to self-referred individuals and families. Kish and Lansdown have described Changing Face's program for children and adolescents with visible differences, which provides emotional support (e.g., encouragement to express feelings), cognitive strategies (e.g., to promote positive self-image), and behavioral change (e.g., social interaction skills). Clarke describes the Changing Faces approach for adults.

A variety of self-help groups exist for individuals with congenital abnormalities and their families. Some are organized by affected people or their families, some are run by charitable foundations, and others are led by health-care professionals. The "jury is still out" regarding the most appropriate aims and structure of self-help groups, though benefits are experienced by many participants. However, others prefer not to define themselves as members of a stigmatized group and find other peoples' disfigurements more difficult to tolerate than their own. Patient-led groups may too often focus on reporting negative experiences, but they can be a powerful source of emotional and social support when a positive focus is maintained. Professionals can offer structured guidance for the group's activities. However, members may feel that an unaffected person is unable to appreciate the realities of the difficulties involved.

It is generally accepted that adjustment problems for people with visible differences would ease if society were less obsessed with appearance and if the public were better educated concerning the causes of disfigurement and the problems experienced by affected people. In recent years there have been many helpful television documentaries, books, and sympathetic films designed to promote acceptance of diversity and a focus on the value of inner qualities rather than outward appearance alone.

Changing Faces offers resources (including booklets, videos, and ideas for classroom-based activities) to schools concerned with the well-being of pupils with visible differences. The resources promote inclusive attitudes and positive ideas concerning diversity. Having discovered high levels of appearance-related distress and negative body image in nondisfigured secondary school adolescents, Lovegrove recognized the compelling need to provide support for affected adolescents. She developed a classroom-based intervention that educates participants about the causes of disfigurement, challenges appearance-related myths, and generates strategies that participants use to tackle their own social difficulties. Initial results show significant improvements in body image, self-esteem, and social confidence compared with nonintervention controls.

Educative approaches are also being developed for health-care professionals and employers. A survey by Changing Faces indicated that nurses caring for people with disfiguring conditions are aware of the psychosocial problems experienced by their patients yet feel they lack the skills to deliver appropriate support. In response, Changing Faces developed condition-specific information packets and one-day training courses for nurses. Initial results indicate their increased levels of confidence in offering support, with resultant patient benefits. Changing Faces also offers workshops and literature for employers to encourage staff to treat customers and/or job applicants equally, regardless of their appearance.

HOW EFFECTIVE ARE THE INTERVENTIONS?

Surgery and prosthetics can contribute to a patient's sense of "normality" by making a condition less noticeable. However, complete eradication of a congenital abnormality is rare; there is usually some residual deformity. Hughes reviewed studies of patients who have undergone surgical intervention for congenital deformities. The findings are not clear-cut; however, the majority report enhanced self-esteem, more positive appearance ratings, and/or improvements in social confidence following the surgery. Kalick examined outcomes for patients with port wine stains who had received laser treatment and found that psychosocial adjustment was highly correlated with treatment outcome, with little role played by personality traits. Sarwer and colleagues found that long-term follow-up of patients with congenital craniofacial disfigurement revealed greater body image dissatisfaction, lower self-esteem, and poorer quality of life more often (though not invariably) than in an age- and gender-matched control group.

The early reports of the outcomes of SIST and cognitive-behavioral interventions are promising. Despite many indicators of the efficacy of both surgical and psychosocial interventions however, conclusions should be viewed cautiously. The methodological difficulties that hamper assessments of outcome are considerable, including small numbers of people with particular conditions, a high proportion of operations occurring in infancy and early childhood, the lack of longitudinal research, the difficulties in choosing appropriate control groups, and confusion over choices of the most appropriate outcome measures. Additionally, satisfaction with outcome may change with age. Some (but by no means all) personal accounts describe the benefits of increasing maturity and the accompanying reduction in the importance of physical appearance to body image and self-esteem.

HOW SHOULD OUTCOMES BE MEASURED?

Demand is currently increasing for the use of relevant and sensitive measures of change in medical outcome research (see Pruzinsky and Cash's chapter in Part III). To date, assessment of surgical intervention has relied largely on measures of appearance and function (e.g., nasal symmetry and quality of speech in cleft care). These measures facilitate comparisons of physical outcomes between treatment teams, but they are not good predictors of patient adjustment (see Rumsey's chapter in Part IV), and are usually completed by care providers rather than patients. Whose expectations and judgments of outcome should be used as the definitive benchmark? Carr argues that intervention effectiveness depends on the extent to which it meets the person's needs. A thorough assessment of these needs is therefore desirable prior to intervention.

In the course of treatment, patients experience emotional, behavioral, cognitive, and physical changes. Arguably, it is inappropriate to measure one aspect, such as physical appearance or body image, in isolation. Yet it is rarely feasible to capture all potential variables. Which constructs are critical to adjustment? The "usual suspects" include self-esteem, social anxiety, body image, and quality of life; however, the results of studies using these measures are inconsistent. Perhaps this inconsistency is due to confusion over definition and measurement, or, alternatively, these may not be the most appropriate constructs to measure.

Even if these issues were resolved, decisions concerning the most appropriate method of data collection remain. Quantitative measures (including standardized scales) offer the benefits of statistical rigor and ease of comparison, but they may bear little relevance for a particular individual. Qualitative approaches are more patient-centered, but these make comparisons between individuals and groups difficult. Despite the lack of straightforward answers to these questions, it is generally agreed that outcome measures should include patient-oriented psychosocial measures in addition to provider-centered treatment variables.

CLINICAL IMPLICATIONS AND THE PROVISION OF CARE

Several shifts in approaching the care of people with visible differences are currently desirable. For example, given the multifactorial nature of adjustment, the prevailing biomedical model should be expanded to offer psychosocial support and intervention as routine adjuncts or alternatives to appearance-enhancing treatment. Many options for delivering psychosocial support exist, including developing a nurse specialist role and providing referral routes for expert support and intervention. Choices in the type and timing of treatments should be offered, whenever possible, to address individual preferences.

Another welcome shift in the attitudes of care providers would be to view the individual with a congenital condition as a "normal" person who happens to have been born with a visible abnormality, in contrast to the often implicit search for psychopathology. A broad focus on developing a range of coping skills should be adopted, and the affected person should be discouraged from putting his or her life "on hold" until surgery produces the "miracle cure."

Although, as noted, congenital disfigurements allow for extensive planning regarding surgical interventions, slavish adherence to fixed protocols of care should be avoided. Care providers may need to curb their enthusiasm to intervene, given that differences in psychological reactions to a congenital disfigurement are considerable, and enduring difficulties do not necessarily result. Surgery may refocus concern on the abnormality and detract from other more normal aspects of life. Prospective patients need to feel free to decline treatment. Personal accounts testify to feelings of relief and release when the decision not to have any more surgery is made.

Patient involvement in treatment decisions and in the assessment of outcome should be encouraged at every stage of treatment. Careful preparation for surgery is crucial, and realistic expectations of outcome should be encouraged at all times. Patients and families may have unrealistic expectations of the potential for change and may be disappointed by a result that is considered good by the clinician (see Storry's account in Lansdown and others). Reactions to correcting an abnormality are not universally positive. People born with a visible difference tend to incorporate this difference into their self-image. Even if they long to have the disfigurement removed, some—especially those undergoing changes to facial appearance—describe the shock felt when catching sight of the new self in reflective surfaces, together with an overwhelming feeling that "this is no longer the real me."

ADDITIONAL RESEARCH QUESTIONS

Research in this area offers many challenges. In addition to the complexities of methodology and measurement discussed earlier, thorny questions remain. How do the various forms of intervention compare and for whom are they most effective? Which components of the interventions produce the most change? How do the needs of people from differing cultural backgrounds vary? How might these needs be met? Endriga and Kapp-Simon highlight the multiple domains of risk and protection in cleft and craniofacial conditions, including cognitive, social and temperamental variables in the affected person, family environment and treatment variables. We are only just beginning to understand the range and complex interplay of factors that affect each individual's psychosocial need, motivation to seek treatment, and adjustment following intervention.

CONCLUSIONS

A visible difference resulting from a congenital abnormality increases the risk of negative effects on body image, self-esteem, and other factors contributing to psychological well-being. The prevailing biomedical approach to interventions can offer improvements, but these, in isolation, are unlikely to maximize body image functioning and quality of life. Greater and more enduring benefit may result from a biopsychosocial approach that integrates surgical/medical treatments with interventions (such as SIST and CBT) designed to promote psychosocial adjustment and resilience. Macgregor stresses that the burden of adjustment falls most often on the disfigured person; we must attempt to provide him or her with effective tools to facilitate this adjustment. It is also imperative that, despite the tidal wave of concern with appearance that threatens to engulf even the most reasonable and measured among us, efforts to tackle appearance-related discrimination by educating the public, changing the messages promulgated by the media, and influencing societal ideals continue.

INFORMATIVE READINGS

Carr, T. (1997). Assessment and measurement in clinical practice. In R. Lansdown, N. Rumsey, E. Bradbury, T. Carr, & J. Partridge (Eds.), *Visibly different: Coping with disfigurement* (pp. 131–147). Oxford: Butterworth-Heinemann.—A review of the advantages and disadvantages of a range of assessment methods for adults and children with visible disfigurements.

Clarke, A. (1999). Psychosocial aspects of facial disfigurement: Problems, management and the role of a lay-led organization. *Psychology, Health and Medicine, 4*, 128–141.—A review of relevant research and description of the model of care provided for adults with visible disfigurement by the charitable foundation, Changing Faces.

Endriga, M., & Kapp-Simon, K. A. (1999). Psychological issues in craniofacial care: State of the art. *Cleft Palate Craniofacial Journal, 36*, 3–11.—A review of the psychological literature on cleft lip and palate and other craniofacial conditions.

Harter, S. (1999). *The construction of the self: A developmental perspective.* New York: Guilford Press.—A synthesis of theory and research on constructions of the self across the lifespan.

Hughes, M. J. (1998). *The social consequences of facial disfigurement.* Aldershot, England: Ashgate.—Review of research and report of an empirical inquiry into the social consequences of surgery for facial cancer.

Kalick, S. M. (1983). Laser treatment of port wine stains: Observations concerning psychological outcome. In K. Arndt, J. Noe, & S. Rosen (Eds.), *Cutaneous laser therapy: Principles and methods* (pp. 215–229). New York: Wiley.—A chapter describing a study examining the psychological factors related to patient satisfaction with laser treatment for port wine stains.

Kapp-Simon, K. (1995). Psychological interventions for the adolescent with cleft lip and palate. *Cleft Palate Craniofacial Journal, 32*(2), 104–108. An overview of developmental tasks in adolescence, the impact of a cleft on adolescents, and a discussion of appropriate interventions.

Kish, V., & Lansdown, R. (2000). Meeting the psychosocial impact of facial disfigurement: Developing a clinical service for children and families. *Clinical Child Psychology and Psychiatry, 5*, 497–512.—Describes the model of care used by Changing Faces for children, adolescents, and families affected by facial disfigurement.

Lansdown, R., Rumsey, N., Bradbury, E., Carr, T., & Partridge, J. (Eds.). (1997). *Visibly different: Coping with disfigurement.* Oxford: Butterworth-Heinemann.—Aimed at health-care professionals and people affected by disfigurement, and includes personal accounts, a summary of research, and recommendations for the provision of care.

Lovegrove, E. (2002). *Adolescence: Appearance and anti-bullying strategies.* Unpublished PhD thesis, University of the West of England, Bristol, England.—Research program exploring the psychosocial concerns of adolescents and strategies to address them.

Macgregor, F. C. (1974). *Transformation and identity: The face and plastic surgery.* New York: New York Times Book.—Examines the social significance of the face, the impact of societal reactions, and patients' adjustment following plastic surgery.

Robinson, E., Rumsey, N., & Partridge, J. (1996). An evaluation of the impact of social interaction skills training for facially disfigured people. *British Journal of Plastic Surgery, 49*, 281–289.—An article highlighting the gains in psychosocial well-being in a sample of 64 adults undergoing social interaction skills workshops.

Sarwer, D. B., Bartlett, S. P., Whitaker, L. A., Paige, K. T., Pertschuk, M. J., & Wadden, T. (1999). Adult psychological functioning of individuals born with craniofacial anomalies. *Plastic and Reconstructive Surgery, 103,* 412–418.—Empirical evaluation of long-term body image and other psychosocial outcomes in patients with congenital facial disfigurements.

Thompson, J. K., Heinberg, L. J., Altabe, M., & Tantleff-Dunn, S. (1999). *Exacting beauty: Theory, assessment, and treatment of body image disturbance.* Washington, DC: American Psychological Association.—An account of the history, theory, research, and clinical applications of body image disturbance.

Body Image Adaptation to Reconstructive Surgery for Acquired Disfigurement

THOMAS PRUZINSKY

This chapter focuses on how individuals respond to reconstructive surgery after having acquired a disfigurement. The physical and psychosocial variables influencing individual adaptation to surgical reconstruction are numerous and complexly interrelated. This brief chapter describes those factors particularly relevant to the process of adapting to reconstructive surgery at five specific time periods: predisfigurement, acquiring disfigurement, initial surgical reconstruction, subsequent reconstructive surgeries, and final surgical outcome. The clinical and empirical literature on patients' response to reconstructive surgery for facial trauma and breast disfigurement is used to exemplify this adaptation process.

PREDISFIGUREMENT BODY IMAGE AND PSYCHOSOCIAL FUNCTIONING

Body image adaptation to reconstructive surgery must be understood in terms of the individual's predisfigurement body image and psychosocial functioning. Body image formation is, of course, subject to many influences, including the objective appearance of the individual (including the face and/or breasts). Particularly relevant variables include the individual's degree of appearance investment, appearance evaluation, overall psychological functioning, social skills, sexual functioning, and social support. (See

Cash's chapter reviewing the cognitive-behavioral perspective on body image.)

A consistent clinical observation has been that individuals who are very invested in their appearance prior to their disfigurement are at significantly greater risk for developing body image problems postdisfigurement. Similarly, individuals who have had poor psychological functioning and deficits in social support, social skills, and sexual functioning prior to acquiring disfigurement are more likely to be negatively affected.

Unfortunately, despite these clinical convictions, there has been limited empirical research in the facial trauma and breast reconstruction literatures on the effect of these variables on body image functioning. Heinberg and colleagues found that interpersonal distress (including poorer adjustment in family, social, and sexual relationships) was an important predictor of deciding to undergo reconstructive surgery. Similarly, Yurek and colleagues documented the role of sexual schemas in patients prior to breast cancer on postoperative sexual and body image functioning.

FACTORS RELATED TO ACQUIRING DISFIGUREMENT

Physical factors related to acquiring disfigurement that can influence body image adaptation to reconstructive surgery include the cause of as well as the location and degree of the disfigurement. Many psychosocial variables and developmental factors also influence the affected person's response to incurring a disfigurement.

Cause of Disfigurement

Body image adaptation to surgical reconstruction of disfiguring conditions acquired after birth is assumed to be more psychologically challenging than adapting to surgical reconstruction of disfiguring congenital conditions (see chapters by Rumsey). Although empirical documentation for this assumption is limited, there is no question that the "path" (or trajectory) of body image change for individuals with acquired disfigurement differs from those with congenital conditions. Starting life with a disfiguring condition rather than an intact body dramatically influences one's body experience.

Furthermore, disfigurement from an injury may have body image implications that are different from those of disfigurement acquired from disease. For example, disfigurement caused by an automobile accident is sudden, unexpected, and definitive. In contrast, disfigurement caused by breast cancer may occur over time (e.g., lumpectomy followed by mastectomy), may be somewhat anticipated, and may or may not progress (e.g., from one breast to the second). Rybarzck and Behel (in this volume) note that in the rehabilitation population, the response to acquiring a disability varies as a function of whether it results from life-saving interventions (e.g., cancer treatment) or as result of apparent "random" or unnecessary actions (e.g., accidents).

Facial trauma is invariably the result of "unnecessary events" (e.g., accidents, assaults), whereas other forms of acquired facial disfigurement (e.g., from head and neck cancer) stem from life-saving interventions. However, there is a dearth of research documenting the effects of such differences in causation on body image functioning.

Most but not all acquired breast disfigurement is the result of life-saving (or cancer-preventing) surgical interventions. There may be different responses to breast reconstruction as a function of the proximal cause of breast disfigurement. That is, evidence affirms that satisfaction rates of breast reconstruction patients postmastectomy are higher than for reconstruction done after removal of breast implants or as a result of surgery done to reduce the future risk of cancer occurrence (e.g., in prophylactic mastectomy).

Location of Disfigurement

It is clinically and intuitively understood that hidden disfigurement (e.g., breast disfigurement) is very likely to be easier to adjust to than disfigurement exposed in everyday social interaction (e.g., the face or hand). Macgregor has documented the profound social and psychological challenges of the facially disfigured. However, as Rumsey notes in her chapter on congenital disfigurement, there are unique body image implications of "hidden" disfigurements; many such individuals report experiencing anxiety or shame associated with "hiding" flaws that may be "exposed" later. Alan Breslau, the founder of the Phoenix Society for Burn Survivors, has argued that the person with "hidden burns" has enduring challenges related to concealment and exposure. Interestingly, Heinberg and colleagues found that the location of the burn injury did not predict which patients chose to undergo reconstructive surgery. There appear to be no studies comparing the relative body image effects of hidden versus visible disfigurements or changes in these effects due to reconstructive surgery.

Degree of Disfigurement

Because body image is fundamentally subjective, we assume that, for any particular individual, there is no necessary correlation between extent of disfigurement and degree of body image distress. However, an empirical counterpoint to this general axiom is the consistent documentation of the psychological and body image advantages of lumpectomy (breast conservation surgery) versus mastectomy. That is, smaller disfigurement is very reliably associated with less psychological distress, including less body image distress. However, Rowland notes that these differences may not maintain over time, underscoring the need to evaluate longitudinal changes in body image and perception of disfigurement.

There are no data currently available on the relative impact of larger versus smaller facial disfigurements. Both Rumsey (this volume) and Macgregor make the counterintuitive observation that larger facial disfigurements are easier to cope with socially than more moderate deformities. Perhaps larger deformities allow the disfigured person to reliably predict and adjust to the nature of the social response to his or her disfigurement, whereas more moderate disfigurements are far less predictable; a markedly negative social response may be followed by a nonplussed one.

Developmental Considerations

Body image adaptation must be understood in terms of patient-specific developmental contexts. Acquiring a disfigurement and undergoing reconstruction has different ramifications for children, adolescents, and adults. Patients' developmental stage influences their ability to cope with the losses inherent in acquiring disfigurement and to formulate realistic expectations about surgical reconstruction. Although these observations seem obvious, little developmental research exists for them. Pruzinsky and Doctor offer qualitative descriptions of how the patient's age when acquiring traumatic disfigurement and undergoing surgical reconstruction can influence body image.

Schain noted that because older women undergoing mastectomy may not be as invested in their breasts as younger women, they might have different motivations for, and experiences of, surgical reconstruction. In contrast, Rowland notes that "attractiveness is not primarily a concern of younger women; older women may react as strongly as younger women to breast loss" (p. 302). While the issue of age and motivation for breast reconstruction is not yet empirically resolved, intuitively and clinically it seems obvious that the potential body image implications of breast cancer and reconstruction are different for a 20-year-old woman than a 60-year old woman. That is, a 60-year-old woman has lived most of her life with intact breasts. Her experiences of her sexuality, pregnancy, breastfeeding, clothing/bathing suit/intimate attire choices, and breast change across the lifespan are all different from a woman 40 years younger.

Psychosocial Variables

Psychosocial variables influencing the response to acquired disfigurement have been discussed in detail elsewhere. Rowland, for example, provides a concise overview of the breast cancer literature. With respect to facial trauma, my colleagues and I at Yale University conducted one of the few empirical investigations of the body image consequences of facial trauma (non-burn-related). We found that relative to age- and gender-matched controls, individuals sustaining a facial trauma were statistically more likely to report less overall satisfaction with life, greater levels of depression, posttraumatic stress symptoms, problems with alcohol, as well as greater body image distress. These findings illustrate the wide range of variables to consider when evaluating the psychological responses to acquired facial disfigurement—in particular, the effects of posttraumatic stress symptoms.

INITIAL SURGICAL RECONSTRUCTION

Everyone involved usually approaches initial surgical reconstruction with great hope and anticipation. However, it is rarely possible for surgical reconstruction to return the patient to his or her predisfigurement appearance. The patient's preoperative cognitions, beliefs, and assumptions related to expectations regarding surgical reconstruction will influence body image adaptation. Unrealistically high expectations or insufficient understanding of surgical risks (e.g., surgical complications) can obviously influence patient adaptation to surgical outcomes. Postsurgically, there is invariably a significant period of healing before an outcome is ascertained and a new body image can be integrated. There is often significant volatility in patients' perceptions of surgical outcomes, as they attempt to adapt to the appearance changes and physical sensations associated with healing.

Surgical Reconstruction of Facial Trauma

The empirical literature on the psychological adaptation of facial trauma patients to reconstructive surgery is surprisingly sparse, given the substantial prevalence of acquired facial disfigurement due to burn injuries, cancer, and accidents. Fortunately, we have Frances Macgregor's 1979 book, *After Plastic Surgery: Adaptation and Adjustment*, summarizing her long-term qualitative investigation of the social and psychological experiences of individuals with facial disfigurement. One of her patients describes the body image volatility she experienced at this point in the adaptation process:

> With a long series of reconstructive stages, there is a kaleidoscopic transformation in actual appearance, hence in body image. The memory of the previous concept of one's physical self, however dimly preserved, impinges on the fragile reality of the transient faces. The difficulty is compounded at times by a seeming regression in the course of the operations, when the appearance actually becomes more distorted and more rejection-provoking, as in the case of forehead flaps or pedicle grafts, donor sites and scars. Under such circumstances the integration of the body image becomes temporarily, at least, an impossibility. (p. 23)

It is hoped that future research on the postoperative experiences of patients undergoing facial reconstruction will elucidate these initial struggles as well as the longer-term challenges in body image adaptation so commonly observed clinically. Such data do not exist, despite clinically consistent reports of continued profound negative effects due to facial disfigurement even after the surgical healing has occurred. While many patients who have undergone reconstructive surgery for facial trauma demonstrate remarkable resilience, others report a dramatic reduction in quality of life and often suffer in silence with little recognition of their plight from society or the medical community. Macgregor described the experience as one of "social death" for some of these individuals.

Breast Reconstruction

Breast reconstruction is currently the fastest growing and fourth most common reconstructive surgery procedure performed by board-certified plastic surgeons. The American Society of Plastic Surgeons reported 78,832 such reconstructions conducted in 2000. Research on the psychological effects of breast reconstruction consistently documents postsurgical body image improvement. However, Rowland and colleagues recently reported that body image experience for breast reconstruction patients was similar to patients without reconstruction. Similarly, Yurek and colleagues documented "no reduction in body change stress" for mastectomy patients undergoing reconstruction when compared to mastectomy patients without reconstruction in the early postoperative period.

The effects of breast reconstruction or the decision to forgo reconstruction, therefore, are not clearly understood. Nevertheless, it is hard to question the clinical and empirical findings that many women benefit from breast reconstruction. Fortunately, the empirical research on psychological adaptation to breast reconstruction has become increasingly sophisticated, addressing such issues as who declines to undergo this surgery, whether immediate or delayed breast reconstruction has differential body image effects, and whether women adapt more readily to breast implants or to use of their own tissue.

Choosing or Refusing Breast Reconstruction

Currently, there is no clear evidence of specific psychological or body image factors differentiating woman undergoing breast reconstruction from the significant proportion that forego the procedure. Rowland reports that most women choosing reconstruction are psychologically healthy and benefit from surgery when they seek to satisfy "internal" motivations (e.g., to achieve personal goals) versus "external" motivations (e.g., to please or change someone else). However, it is not known, for example, if women declining reconstruction have more resilient body images or more well developed body image defenses (e.g., denial) or if they are less invested in their appearance. Rowland does note that patients forgoing reconstruction appear to be "at increased risk for subsequent emotional or surgical disappointment after reconstructive procedures may select themselves out at the time of consultation [for reconstruction]" (p. 302). It is also not clear how breast prostheses influence body image adaptation for women who decide against reconstruction.

Immediate versus Delayed Reconstruction

Regarding the timing of breast reconstruction, research usually supports the efficacy of immediate reconstruction over delayed reconstruction. However, Rowland and colleagues documented that women are more likely to benefit from reconstruction the longer the time since the mastectomy. Mock found no difference between immediate and delayed reconstruction on body image functioning. Salient questions regarding the most efficacious timing for breast reconstruction surgery appear to remain unanswered.

The clinical rationale for immediate reconstruction is, in part, to spare women the experience of (1) living with mastectomy scars, (2) wearing breast prostheses, and (3) undergoing a second operation. However, a question repeatedly posed in the scientific and clinical literature is: Does immediate breast reconstruction circumvent the "mourning" process "necessary" for adapting to breast loss? While Schain reports that adjustment to breast loss is not negatively influenced by immediate reconstruction, Rowland notes that "clinicians have reported this as a problem in long-term follow-up of these patients" (p. 303). These are important and as yet unresolved body image issues.

One possible influence on a woman's evaluation of breast reconstruction relates to the standards by which comparisons are made. That is, women undergoing immediate versus delayed breast reconstruction are more likely to compare the reconstructive outcome to their premastectomy breast appearance. In contrast, women who have been living with disfigurement brought about by mastectomy for months or years who then undergo reconstruction are more likely to judge the quality of their reconstructed breast(s) relative to their mastectomy scars.

Implants versus Autologous Tissue

Currently, more women have breast reconstruction using their own tissue (autologous reconstruction). In earlier eras women were more likely to choose reconstruction using breast implants. Using the patient's own tissue eliminates concerns regarding potential health risks associated with breast implants. However, autologous techniques entail longer surgical procedures, higher risk of surgical morbidity, and secondary scarring at the sites from where tissue is taken in order to reconstruct the individual's breast(s).

Psychological research comparing autologous versus implant reconstruction is relatively new. A recent prospective study by Wilkins and colleagues compared the outcomes of using tissue/expander implant procedures versus autologous (TRAM flap) procedures and also addressed the relative efficacy of immediate versus delayed reconstruction. They found that autologous procedures "produced significantly greater improvements in body image for women receiving delayed reconstruction" (p. 1023); however, women undergoing delayed reconstruction also started with comparatively lower levels of body image function.

ADDITIONAL SURGICAL REFINEMENT

Reconstructive surgery often involves multiple stages because incremental improvements in, for example, facial appearance can often be achieved through further surgical intervention. However, it is not at all clear to what degree these surgical changes facilitate body image change. Similarly, in breast reconstruction there is mixed evidence regarding the psychological value of nipple/areola complex reconstruction and/or surgical revisions of the breast mound. The body image effects of further surgery for improving the symmetry of the breasts (e.g., by reducing the size of a noncancerous breast) are also unclear.

At this point in the process, the individual needs to accommodate his or her body image hopes and expectations to what is surgically possible. Patient-perceived discrepancies (e.g., between past and present body image or between ideal and actual reconstruction) are likely to be most salient in influencing perceived quality of life. Patients and surgeons must decide the most appropriate surgical endpoint. Does more surgery necessarily result in greater body image improvement and enhanced quality of life? Currently, we do not know the answer to this question.

RECONSTRUCTION ENDPOINT

The decision not to pursue additional surgery initiates another stage in body image adaptation. We do not know how or why patients reach this decision or whether it is influenced by body image considerations. In her chapter (in this volume) on facilitating body image change in congenitally disfigured patients, Rumsey notes: "Personal accounts testify to feelings of relief and release when the decision not to have any more surgery is made" (p. 436). Clearly, it is only at the end of surgical reconstruction that we can truly assess long-term body image outcomes for patients undergoing facial or breast reconstruction. Data regarding this stage of body image adjustment are sorely needed.

SUMMARY AND CONCLUSIONS

Body image adaptation to surgical reconstruction for an acquired disfigurement is a complex process involving a myriad of constantly evolving physical, psychological, and social variables. There is much we do not understand about this process. However, it is clearly evident that for many but not all individuals, there is tremendous psychological suffering associated with these changes that must be specified and treated. In the future, we should evaluate to what degree patients' quality of life can be improved through surgical intervention, and we must assess the efficacy of psychosocial interventions (e.g., body image therapies) in facilitating the highest possible quality of life.

INFORMATIVE READINGS

Fauerbach, J. A., Heinberg, L. J., Lawrence, J. W., Munster, A. M., Palombo, D. A., Richter, D., Spence, R. J., Stevens, S. S., Ware, L., & Muehlberger, T. (2000). Effect of early body image dissatisfaction on subsequent psychological and physical adjustment after disfiguring injury. *Psychosomatic Medicine, 62*, 576–582.—Demonstrates progress made in measuring body image concerns in specific populations and provides clearer elucidation of the process of adjusting to disfigurement.

Heinberg, L. J., Fauerbach, J. A., Spence, R. J., & Hackerman, F. (1997). Psychologic factors involved in the decision to undergo reconstructive surgery after burn injury. *Journal of Burn Care and Rehabilitation, 18*, 374–380.—Documents how subjective perception of appearance influences decisions to undergo reconstructive surgery.

Macgregor, F. C. (1977). *After plastic surgery: Adaptation and adjustment.* Westport, CT: Praeger.—A very informative review of the social and psychological factors influencing adaptation to congenital and acquired facial disfigurement.

Mock, V. (1993). Body image in women treated for breast cancer. *Nursing Research, 42*, 153–157.—Frequently cited study on body image and breast reconstruction.

Pruzinsky, T., & Doctor, M. (1994). Body images and pediatric burn injury. In K. Tarnowski (Ed.), *Behavioral aspects of pediatric burns* (pp. 169–191). New York: Plenum Press.—Reviews a broad range of body image issues in pediatric adjustment to burn injury.

Roberts, C., Wells, K. E., & Daniels, S. (1997). Outcome study of the psychological changes after silicone breast implant removal. *Plastic and Reconstructive Surgery, 100*, 595–599.—Considers body image and other psychological issues in breast explantation patients.

Rowland, J. H. (1998). Psychological impact of treatments for cancer. In S. L. Spear (Ed.), *Surgery of the breast: Principles and art* (pp. 295–313). Philadelphia: Lippincott-Raven.—Reviews numerous psychological issues related to breast cancer, with a concise yet thorough review of breast reconstruction.

Rowland, J. H., Desmond, K. A., Meyerowitz, B. E., Belin, T. R., Wyatt, G. E., & Ganz, P. A.

(2000). Role of breast reconstructive surgery in physical and emotional outcomes among breast cancer survivors. *Journal of the National Cancer Institute, 92,* 1422–1429.—Methodologically sophisticated study by highly experienced researchers.

Schain, W. S. (1991). Breast reconstruction: Update of psychosocial and pragmatic concerns. *Cancer, 68,* 1170–1175.—Albeit somewhat dated, nonetheless clearly addresses critical issues still requiring close consideration.

Wilkins, E. G., Cederna, P. S., Lowery, J. C., Davis, J. A., Kim, H. M., Roth, R. S., Goldfarb, S., Izenberg, P. H., Houin, H. P., & Shaheen, K. W. (2000). Prospective analysis of psychosocial outcomes in breast reconstruction: One year postoperative results from the Michigan Breast Reconstruction Outcome Study. *Plastic and Reconstructive Surgery, 106,* 1014–1025.—Comparison of the psychosocial outcomes (including body image and sexual functioning) for over 250 women undergoing varied reconstruction techniques (autologous tissue vs. breast implants) at different times (immediate vs. delayed) by 23 surgeons.

Yurek, D., Farrar, W., & Andersen, B. L. (2000). Breast cancer surgery: Comparing surgical groups and determining individual differences in postoperative sexuality and body change stress. *Journal of Consulting and Clinical Psychology, 68,* 697–709.—Methodologically sophisticated study of breast reconstruction.

51

Psychopharmacological Treatments for Body Image Disturbances

ANDREA ALLEN
ERIC HOLLANDER

Disturbed body image is a central feature of body dysmorphic disorder (BDD) and eating disorders. Patients suffering from these disorders often experience two distinct forms of body image disturbance: perceptual distortion and body dissatisfaction. Perceptual distortion is the more dramatic disturbance, as exemplified by emaciated patients with eating disorders who perceive themselves as fat, or clear-skinned patients with BDD who see themselves as disfigured by acne scarring. Body dissatisfaction seems to be the more frequent disturbance; although it is assumed to stem from the imaginary imperfection, body dissatisfaction is only modestly, if at all, correlated with perceptual distortion.

Important similarities between BDD and eating disorders extend beyond body image disturbance. Because these disorders all have prominent obsessive and compulsive features, it can be valuable to view them as part of an obsessive–compulsive spectrum. (See discussion of this spectrum in Hollander, 1996.) The obsessions of patients with eating disorders include fear of fatness, as well as preoccupation with the focus of their body dissatisfaction (weight and body shape) and worry about managing their perceived flaw (e.g., via exercise, diet, food preparation and consumption, or purging). They also retain obsessive and compulsive traits after substantial remission of their anorexia nervosa or bulimia nervosa symptoms. The obsessive thoughts of patients with BDD focused on their body dissatisfaction (most often, skin, facial features, or hair, but can be any body part) and worry about managing this perceived defect (e.g., changing or concealing it, worrying about how they appear to others, and how others will react to them). In eating-disordered patients, compulsive behaviors typically involve rituals for eating and exercise or purging. In BDD, compulsive behaviors may include mirror checking, comparing one's appearance with others, and seeking reassurance excessively.

Patients' levels of insight or delusionality are critical to treatment and may be evident in either the misperception of their own body or their exaggerated beliefs about the importance of attractiveness, including the belief that others take special notice of their physical imperfection. Delusionality in BDD, particularly related to perceptual distortion, has been a major focus of research and discussion. It was once thought that two distinct disorders existed, one of which was delusional, but current opinion is that there is one disorder with a range of possible insight. (See extended discussion of this topic in the chapter by Pruzinsky on body image disturbances in psychotic disorders.) The term "body dysmorphic disorder" is used to refer to the entire range, but the distinction remains in that, in the DSM-IV, those with poor insight can receive the additional diagnosis of delusional disorder, somatic type. About half of patients with BDD would qualify as delusional at any point in time, but it is now clear that for many of these patients, insight varies from day to day.

THE PHARMACOLOGY OF BODY DYSMORPHIC DISORDER

Historically, research on pharmacological treatment of BDD does not usually specify the extent of change in patients' body image distortion or dissatisfaction. Outcome success is based on ratings of overall severity and on assessment of BDD-specific symptoms using the Yale–Brown Obsessive–Compulsive Scale (modified for BDD [BDD-YBOCS]). The BDD-YBOCS is used to measure different aspects of BDD-related obsessive thoughts and compulsive behaviors (time occupied, interference with functioning, distress, resistance, and degree of control are rated in relation to obsessions and compulsions separately) as well as degree of insight and avoidance. No specific assessment of degree of perceptual distortion or level of dissatisfaction is made; however, standardized ratings of delusionality are now in use. No standardized assessment of the specific body parts that are the focus of dissatisfaction or the degree of distress associated with them is routinely used in BDD pharmacotherapy research. Likewise, specific behavioral rituals are not catalogued.

Not surprisingly, because BDD was recognized as a distinct disorder only a dozen or so years ago, controlled research on pharmacological treatment of the disorder is still very limited. Only two studies have been completed to date. With our colleagues at Mt. Sinai, we conducted a double-blind crossover trial comparing the effectiveness of the tricyclic antidepressants clomipramine and desipramine in adults with BDD. Clomipramine, a potent serotonin reuptake inhibitor (SRI), was superior to desipramine, a norepinephrine reuptake inhibitor, in acute treatment of BDD. Greater improvement on clomipramine was observed in ratings of overall BDD severity and of specific symptoms such as obsessive ruminations, behavioral rituals, and social functioning. Overall, based on the criterion of 25% or greater reduction in BDD-YBOCS score, 65% of patients positively responded to clomipramine and 35% to desipramine. An important finding was that clomipramine was as, or more, effective in treating delusional than non-delusional patients; this outcome confirmed findings from open-label studies and indicated that antipsychotic medications may not be necessary in treating delusional patients. This study demonstrated that serotonergic activity is the key to treatment efficacy in BDD; both BDD symptoms and comorbid depression responded more positively to clomipramine than desipramine. In addition, the study demonstrated that delusional symptoms appear to be secondary to obsessive preoccupation in BDD.

The second double-blind controlled trial was recently completed by Phillips and her colleagues (personal communication), which found that fluoxetine was superior to placebo in treating obsessions and compulsions in adults with BDD. Fluoxetine was also equally effective in delusional and nondelusional patients.

In general, improvement in overall severity of BDD is correlated with a decrease in compulsive behaviors and obsessions and an increase in insight. The extent to which either body image distortion or dissatisfaction is ameliorated by pharmacotherapy is not known. In clinical practice, it is clear that patients with BDD can experience a dramatically improved quality of life and still believe their appearance is very flawed; just as individuals without BDD can be quite happy and function well despite a flawed appearance. Patients with BDD may accomplish their improved functioning, despite an ongoing body image disturbance, by placing less importance on their appearance, or they may simply be better able to keep the thoughts out of their mind, indicating a decrease in obsessive thinking. Some patients do report that one or more of their flaws are no longer present or are not as noticeable as they had previously believed.

Thus two controlled studies support preliminary reports that BDD responds to SRIs. Case reports, chart reviews, open-label studies, and clinical practice suggest that the other currently available SRIs, fluvoxamine, sertraline, paroxetine, citalopram, and venlafaxine, are also effective. It is important to note that higher doses of SRIs are required to treat BDD than are needed for depression. There have been no dosing studies in BDD to date, but available research and clinical practice suggest that guidelines developed from OCD research can be used for BDD. As with depression, it often takes several weeks for improvement to occur. One-third or more of patients will not have a clinically meaningful response to any one adequate SRI trial; if such is the case, a trial with another SRI should be undertaken. The majority of responders experience only a partial reduction in symptoms, and symptoms generally recur if medication is discontinued.

Case reports, open-label studies, and clinical experience suggest that neuroleptics, antidepressants with less potent serotonin uptake inhibition (e.g., tricyclics other than clomipramine, serotonin and norepinephrine reuptake inhibitors other than venlafaxine, and trazodone), benzodiazapines, lithium, and anticonvulsants are ineffective or much less beneficial as monotreatments in BDD. However, if a patient with BDD has only a partial response to an SRI, augmentation with other agents may be helpful. The most promising are buspirone augmentation of an SRI and clomipramine combined with one of the other SRIs. Low doses of atypical antipsychotics, such as risperidone or pimozide, are also used to augment SRIs. Benzodiazapines can be useful in addition to SRI treatment for patients with severe anxiety, although buspirone and clonazepam would be the initial choices for treatment.

In selecting a psychotropic medication, special note should be taken of appearance-related side effects because patients often refuse to take medications that can exacerbate the disturbing aspect of their appearance, even if the effect is very rare. The most common appearance-related side effects are hair loss or growth, weight gain or loss, and acne or rashes. SRIs are generally well tolerated with manageable side effects (e.g., drowsiness, stomach or intestinal discomfort, dry mouth, headache). However, particularly at the higher doses needed for BDD, a notable minority of patients find the side effects intolerable and thus discontinue treatment or lower the dose below recommended levels. Side effects can be minimized by raising the dosage slowly, and some side effects diminish or even disappear over time. Clomipramine generally has more side effects than newer SRIs and is therefore not the first treatment choice for most patients.

Cognitive-behavioral treatment (CBT) appears to be effective in BDD, and the common recommendation is to combine CBT with SRI treatment. Unfortunately, there has been no controlled research on the comparative or combined efficacy of these modalities. If BDD responds to treatment similar to other obsessive–compulsive spectrum disorders, then cognitive-behavioral therapy could also help in preventing relapse.

The most common comorbid disorders, social phobia, depression, and obsessive–compulsive disorder, are also successfully treated with SRIs. Personality disorders, which are generally more resistant to treatment, are frequently seen in patients with BDD. All comorbid disorders complicate treatment and indicate a poorer prognosis for patients with BDD.

PHARMACOLOGY OF EATING DISORDERS

Pharmacotherapy has a long history of treating eating disorders. Early research focused on its efficacy in aiding weight gain or loss. In time, psychotropic medications were also used to treat comorbid conditions such as depression. Aided by the discovery that, in some circumstances, antidepressants had an independent effect on symptoms of eating disorders, research came to focus increasingly on the role of psychotropic treatment for the disorders. To date, however, research on their efficacy in treating body image disturbance is extremely limited; body dissatisfaction has been measured in only a minority of treatment studies, and body distortion in none.

The priority in treating eating disorders is on weight restoration, if necessary, and modifying the compulsive eating behaviors rather than on body image disturbance. However, changing the body image may be the most difficult aspect of recovery and may be of particular importance because the severity of body image disturbance is related to treatment resistance, and persistence of body image disturbance after treatment has been shown to predict relapse.

Bulimia Nervosa

Antidepressant medications have an established role in treating bulimia nervosa (BN) because they reduce the frequency of core compulsive behaviors, such as bingeing and purging. All classes of antidepressants are effective, including tricyclics, monoamine oxidase inhibitors (MAOIs), and SRIs; fluoxetine has an FDA indication for BN. This beneficial effect on BN compulsions is independent of the antidepressant's effect on depression. Psychological treatment (CBT or interpersonal therapy) is also effective in treating BN. Overall, CBT is the most effective monotherapy; the combination of CBT and medication may be more effective than either alone, but the research on this is not definitive.

In a thorough review of controlled treatment trials using eating-disordered patients, Rosen evaluated the extent to which body image disturbances were assessed, treated specifically, and ameliorated by treatment. He identified studies that used pure measures of body dissatisfaction (e.g., Eating Disorders Inventory Body Dissatisfaction Scale, Eating Disorder Examination Shape and Weight Concern Scales, and Body Shape Questionnaire), rather than measures that confounded body image with attitudes toward eating or with behavioral reports (e.g., Eating Attitudes Test). Rosen found only seven pharmacotherapy trials in BN that assessed change in body image dissatisfaction. Five of these studies showed no changes in body image disturbance that were attributable to medication. One of three studies of desipramine showed body image improvement, as did one of two fluoxetine trials. Eight controlled pharmacotherapy trials that reported specific scales measuring body dissatisfaction have been published since Rosen's review. Five were trials of fluoxetine, and three of these found some indications of improvement in body image dissatisfaction. Thus fluoxetine may have modest efficacy in treating body dissatisfaction in BN; however, it seems to be less effective than CBT.

There are differences between the more compulsive and more impulsive disorders on the obsessive–compulsive spectrum in terms of latency to response and maintenance of response. Patients with BN are more impulsive and therefore may have a more rapid response to SRIs, but there is evidence that relapse may occur, as would be expected in some cases, despite continuing pharmacotherapy. Experience with other impulsive disorders suggests that augmentation with a mood stabilizer or perhaps low doses of atypical neuroleptics might help maintain the effect in these patients. Switching to another SRI may also be helpful. In almost all cases, some symptoms remain, and symptoms usually worsen when medication is discontinued.

Anorexia Nervosa

The efficacy of psychopharmacological treatment in anorexia nervosa (AN) is unclear. Indeed, psychotropic agents are not indicated in treating acute AN because they are ineffective in severely underweight patients with AN. That is, these medications are not only ineffective in helping to increase weight, but they do not demonstrate even their expected efficacy for depressive or obsessive–compulsive features. Research on the pharmacotherapy of AN has not assessed body image disturbance.

In AN treatment, weight gain is easier to obtain than weight maintenance, and the majority of patients relapse within 1 year. Thus recent research on using psychotropic medication for patients with AN has focused on its efficacy in preventing relapse (weight loss) when taken after weight restoration. Kaye and his colleagues provide preliminary evidence that fluoxetine may be effective not only in helping individuals with AN maintain weight but also with containing AN-related obsessions and compulsions. This outcome is consistent with the finding that SRIs reduce appearance-related obsessions and compulsions in patients with BDD, as measured by an instrument similar to the BDD-YBOCS. However, the specific effect on body dissatisfaction is unknown. In addition, no measures of delusionality or body distortion were included. Thus the efficacy of fluoxetine in treating body image disturbance in AN remains unclear.

In general, research findings emphasize the importance of combining treatment modalities when working with patients who have AN. Patients with acute AN are most successfully treated in a structured inpatient or partial hospitalization setting that combines medical and nutritional rehabilitation with psychosocial treatment. Determining whether and when to use a psychotropic medication should be made on an individual basis. The clearest role for psychopharmacological intervention is the use of SRIs to treat remaining obsessive–compulsive symptoms or depression after the medical and nutritional condition of the patient has been stabilized and weight has been regained.

In clinical practice, pharmacotherapy for patients with AN who are at an acceptable weight is similar to that provided to individuals with BDD. Higher doses of SRIs may be necessary along with an extended treatment trial period; likewise, SRI treatment may be augmented with low doses of atypical neuroleptics and/or anxiolytics. Note that patients with AN, unlike those with BDD, may benefit from olanzapine augmentation because of its tendency to cause rapid weight gain and its otherwise favorable side effect profile. The use of other antidepressants, such as tricyclics and monoamine oxidase inhibiters, is generally not advised because of less favorable side effect profiles, greater danger in overdose or misuse, and lower efficacy in treating obsessive–compulsive features in other disorders. In refractory cases, synthetic forms of tetrahydrocannabinol (THC) and oral opiates (i.e., morphine) might be helpful for patients with AN, whereas opiate antagonists (i.e., naltrexone) might be helpful for those with BN.

DISCUSSION

SRIs have been shown to be helpful in reducing body image disturbance in BDD and BN. SRIs appear to be effective in reducing the time devoted to, and the distress associated with, obsessions and compulsions and in making it easier for patients to stop these intrusive symptoms. These specific improvements could account for the overall reduction in distress and increase in functioning. In addition, SRIs reduce delusionality (often a sign of body distortion) in patients with BDD. Research has not been conducted on the efficacy of pharmacotherapy in ameliorating body image disturbances in AN. Although it is unlikely that SRIs or any other pharmacotherapy would be helpful for severely underweight patients with AN, research on the efficacy of SRIs in reducing body image disturbance during the maintenance phase of treatment should be conducted with this population.

The important aspects of body image dissatisfaction are not being measured clearly in current treatment research: body distortion; body dissatisfaction; the importance of attractiveness to the individual's self-esteem; belief in the importance of attractiveness to achieving success and happiness in life; the degree of delusionality; and the intensity of preoccupation regarding these beliefs. Eating disorder research has developed measures of body distortion (though these have not been used in pharmacology research) and body dissatisfaction; more recently, measures of preoccupation have been developed. BDD research regularly uses measures of preoccupation and delusionality. Each area of research could benefit from developing valid and reliable ways to assess those aspects of body image disturbance that they currently do not address.

INFORMATIVE READINGS

Allen, A., & Hollander, E. (2000). Body dysmorphic disorder. *Psychiatric Clinics of North America, 23*, 617–628.—Overview of body dysmorphic disorder, including its clinical characteristics and treatment.

American Psychiatric Association Work Group on Eating Disorders. (2000). Practice guideline for the treatment of eating disorders (revised). *American Journal of Psychiatry, 157*(Suppl.), 1–39.—Current practice guideline for eating disorders; covers the clinical features, course, epidemiology, and the full range of treatment modalities to be considered, including nutritional rehabilitation, psychosocial interventions, and medication.

Hollander, E. (1996). Obsessive–compulsive disorder-related disorders: The role of selective serotonin reuptake inhibitors. *International Clinical Psychopharmacology, 11*, 75–87.—Discusses the shared features, comorbidities, and role of serotonin reuptake inhibitors in treating obsessive–compulsive spectrum disorders, including body dysmorphic disorder and eating disorders.

Hollander, E., Allen, A., Kwon, J., Aronowitz, B. R., Schmeidler, J., Wong, C., & Simeon, D. (1999). Clomipramine vs. desipramine crossover trial in body dysmorphic disorder: Selective efficacy of a serotonin reuptake inhibitor in imagined ugliness. *Archives of General Psychiatry, 56*, 1033–1039.—First controlled medication trial with patients who have body dysmorphic disorder.

Kaye, W. H. (2001). Anorexia and bulimia nervosa. *Annual Review of Medicine, 51*, 299–313.—Reviews the phenomenology, course, treatment, and biological influences of anorexia nervosa and bulimia nervosa.

Kaye, W. H., Nagata, T., Weltzin, T. E., Hsu, K., Sokol, M. S., McConaha, C., Plotnicov, K. H., Weise, J., & Deep, D. (2001). Double-blind placebo-controlled administration of fluoxetine in restricting- and restricting-purging-type anorexia nervosa. *Biological Psychiatry, 49*, 644–652.—Reports a study of the efficacy of fluoxetine in reducing the rate of relapse among patients with anorexia nervosa, when prescribed after weight restoration.

Phillips, K. A., Albertini, R. S., Siniscalchi, J., Khan, A., & Robinson, M. (2001). Effectiveness of pharmacotherapy for body dysmorphic disorder: A chart-review study. *Journal of Clinical Psychiatry, 62*, 721–727.—Reports a chart review study of 90 outpatients with body dysmorphic disorder covering over 200 pharmacotherapy trials with outcome data based on standardized assessment measures.

Phillips, K. A., Kin, J. M., & Hudson, J. L. (1995). Body image disturbance in body dysmorphic disorder and eating disorders: Obsessions or delusions? *Psychiatric Clinics of North America, 18*, 317–324.—Reviews the issues involved in the body image distortion found in body dysmorphic disorder and eating disorders; includes a historical review.

Rosen, J. (1996). Body image assessment and treatment in controlled studies of eating disorders. *International Journal of Eating Disorders, 20*, 331–343.—Reviews psychological and pharmacological treatment trials studying eating disorders; focuses on the extent of body image disturbance treatment and assessment and the efficacy of the programs in effecting changes in body image.

Walsh, B. T., Wilson, G. T., Loeb, K. L., Devlin, M. J., Pike, K. M., Roose, S. P., Fleiss, J., & Waternaux, C. (1997). Medication and psychotherapy in the treatment of bulimia nervosa. *American Journal of Psychiatry, 154*, 523–531.—Report of a randomized placebo-controlled treatment trial that compared the efficacy of cognitive-behavioral therapy, supportive therapy, and fluoxetine for treating patients with bulimia nervosa; it included measures of behavioral and attitudinal change.

VIII

Changing Body Images: Psychosocial Interventions

Psychodynamic Approaches to Changing Body Image

DAVID W. KRUEGER

Body image is integral to the sense of self and self-organization. The self and its emotional processes are inherently embodied, cocreated within a relationship, and continuously revised. There is no realm of thought, feeling, or action that can be conceived without bodily engagement and expression. As noted in my earlier chapter in this volume, "Psychodynamic Perspectives on Body Image," the extent to which an individual experiences affects as mental states (i.e., as feelings) rather than solely as body sensations depends on how well primary caregivers facilitated and correctly identified and labeled affective and somatic experiences for the infant and growing child. A preverbal sense of having a boundary between the self and the world (of being within one's skin) and the experience of a solidified sense of self are established through interaction with attuned others. As a cohesive sense of self evolves, the boundary between mind and body dissolves. In the absence of empathic attunement by primary caregivers, the child continues to experience feelings internally, as a body state or experience, or registered only when embedded within an action sequence, but not differentiated and distinguished as feelings within a mental state.

Empathic attunement and accurate labeling of physical and emotional states teach the child how to (1) identify, differentiate, and desomatize affect, (2) develop an emotional literacy, and (3) experience self-efficacy and mastery. A caregiver's failure to attune empathically to the child leads to unawareness of feeling in the child or to the development of psychosomatic symptoms to bridge an unintegrated mind and body. These acquired limitations in articulating and communicating feeling compromise the child's ability to self-reflect and regulate affect, as well as to distinguish between and communicate feelings and bodily experiences. The rift between the mind and body, psyche and soma, can often be traced to its roots in a child's relationship to the mother's body. For example, the mother's disconnection from her own body and subsequent attachment pattern with the child can create a corresponding failure in the association/integration of mind and body in her child.

Those individuals who have not consolidated a distinct, accurate and cohesive sense of body self engage in concrete thinking that is self-referential but not self-reflective. Their capacity for abstraction and representation of their body and feelings is partially undeveloped. Though perhaps quite articulate about, and accomplished in matters of the world, these individuals may feel lost, without a language, when focusing internally on their feelings. Unmetabolized experiences, spoken for the first time by the body and not by words, can be brought into awareness as more than just a somatic state of sensation only when they come alive within the therapeutic dyad; perhaps only the therapist can give them words. Often these experiences are perceived, in a sensing or visceral way, by the therapist, who then reflects them back to the patient for further shaping and refining.

Lacking an ability to distinguish among the nuances of emotional experiences, and without a cohesive body image, these individuals elicit body or self-awareness and regulate affect via the felt experiences of their own bodies. Their representation of self must emerge from immediate experience of the body self, not from a stable symbolic representation (image) of the body and psychological self. Lacking a cohesive sense of body self or image, it must be evoked by, for example, self-stimulation, self-harm, or any action symptom, such as excessive consumption of food by an eating-disordered patient. Action symptoms have both a restitutive function of creating an awareness of the body, and defensive function of regulating affect via action. These patients are not primarily denying awareness of their body and feelings, for they have not learned how to desomatize and differentiate affect and bodily sensation in order to deny them; they have not as yet integrated mind and body enough to split them defensively. At the time of a current emotional insult, they may feel lost and disorganized and attempt regulation by turning their organizing focus onto the body.

TRUE BODY SELF AND FALSE BODY SELF

The term "false self" describes the defensive self-organization/concept/representation formed by an individual as a result of inadequate caretaking and failures in empathy. Under these conditions, the infant is forced to accommodate to the conscious and unconscious needs of the caretaker on whom he or she is dependent. The false self begins to emerge as the infant's own needs are subjugated and continues to function and diversify as developmental needs are omitted or annexed to a parent.

A false body self may be a component of the false self. A false body self is created by inaccurate, inconsistent mirroring responses by original caretakers, who fail to resonate empathically with and accurately label the child's full contingent of body self experiences. A funhouse mirror or a mirror with parts blackened out produces an inauthentic image. Empathic nonresponse, distorted feedback, compromised sensory stimulation, or shaming responses regarding the interior or surface of the body self in early development may result in persistent feelings of shame, ugliness, or inadequacy. Body image can also become distorted by early traumatic experiences involving bodily invasion and disruption of bodily integrity. The body image may become a target for enactment of pathogenic conflicts—the Rorschach onto which the lack of such cohesiveness is projected. Shame may reflect core fantasies about the self that manifest in body image distortion. The results of unmet developmental needs and core organizing assumptions of inadequacy and defectiveness may be woven into body image as a component of the false self, forming a false body self.

Individuals who have a false body self typically describe the sense of never having lived in their own bodies, of never authentically inhabiting them. Their bodies never seem to be their own; their bodies do not become integrated as a seamless aspect of the self. In some instances eating, exercise, or other self-stimulating physical activities are attempts to create a sensory bridge to feeling and inhabiting one's body. A false body self is nonetheless an organization of a semicoherent, often fluctuating body self and image, yet inaccurate and distorted, such as being obese or misshapen, even when not so in reality. Often the actual body is constructed to fit with the false body self, such as literally becoming obese. Not being at ideal body weight is not the same as a false body self, though the two can coexist. Various forms of self-harm or severe images of ugliness (body dysmorphic disorder) can become a concretized expression of self-hatred and self-disgust.

The meaning of the body self and its image, and the psychological significance of aspects of the body acquire their most dominant properties, perceptions, and subjective experience from the early relational patterns with others. The physical body and the psychic structure of body self are interwoven and organized into body and self-representations that coalesce in the icon of body image. With normal development, body self and image are integrated and in synchrony. Body images are the representations of experienced bodily perceptions and sensations, the amalgamation of specific, physical feeling states. In disrupted development, body image can fluctuate markedly with state of mind and affect change over the course of a single day (as can be demonstrated in sequential body image drawings). Body image is the mental representation of the physical self and becomes inseparable from the psychological self-representation, including self-image and self-concept.

As certainly as deficits and conflicts can coalesce into a false self, these same deficits can be focused on the core ego organizer of body self. A body image can be accurate (e.g., when the person is obese) and still be a carrier and container of shame and humiliation.

Coming to know and talk about one's body in emotional detail in a treatment process allows a patient to focus on the distinction between true and false body self and image. The painful odyssey of recognizing and reclaiming the body self requires specific internal sensory and affective foci, somatic attunement, and the alignment of physical characteristics to match true body self with its corresponding body image. The more fully that the actual (real) body and true body self are experienced, the greater the distinction from false body self.

CLINICAL OVERVIEW

The dilemma for patients who have not yet fully integrated body self and psychological self is that they are unaware of what they do not feel and cannot find a way to express this state of not knowing. In the process of treatment, interpreting unconscious processes, symbolism, or underlying fantasies may not be useful until a core foundation has been established within the patient's internal experience. To recognize basic sensations and states of mind and to approximate an articulation of these, a patient must have an internal point of reference. Basic sensations and feelings must be identified and differentiated. At certain moments the most important function that we perform as therapists is to register the patient's affective experience and put into words this acknowledgment of what may be an unformulated subjective experience. In this regard, at times empathy may require an act of our imagination of how our patients would feel if they *could* feel—thereby offering some point of reference for experiences as yet unimaginable by the patient.

In psychotherapy the embodiment of these preverbal, undifferentiated, or unsymbolized experiences may manifest in body-based transferences and countertransferences. Implicit memories of processes, experiences, and associative links (as distinguished from explicit memory of facts and events) that are not paired with conscious awareness or verbal narrative are experienced in the bodies of both patient and therapist. Often unrecognized and unformulated, implicit (procedural) memories manifest as nonverbal transference/countertransference embodiments such as restlessness, bodily stimulation, gestures, and movements. These embodiments and enactments can be addressed as fundamental and necessary experiences of the clinical exchange in forming a cohesive developmental foundation for the patient.

Body-based transferences and countertransferences manifest in the language of the patient's immediate felt experience. Examples include the felt experience or expression of pushing away, holding, touching, turning away, hitting home, striking out, fending off, being fed up, emptiness, fullness, or paralysis. The patient's implicit (procedural and associative) memory activated in therapy (which we call transference) may include experiences and metaphors of the body: dichotomies of inside and outside, engulfment and expulsion, and awareness of each of the senses. Other forms of somatic communication may be observed as the patient creates sensory experiences by touching certain parts of his or her body, by tensing and relaxing certain muscle groups, as well as movements and gestures of stroking the wall, couch, or fabric, and an endless number of facial expressions. Corresponding fantasies of movements, various actions, and various interactions between patient and therapist, as well as somatic and psychic memories of developmental experiences from the patient's past—all form part of the somatic transference (the body's procedural memory) of bodily experience. The mutual and collaborative focus on facilitating the patient's awareness of both mind and body directly activates and incorporates fundamental experiences, transferences, and countertransferences.

A patient may have to speak in action language ("I felt like running/ smoking/drinking") or somatic language ("I felt my stomach rumbling") before being able to differentiate feelings. For some individuals, affect may be undifferentiated as well as unformulated, accessible only through action and action language. This part of the process cannot be bypassed, because patients engaged in action and action symptoms may not be able to answer the question, "How do you feel?" They do not know how they feel as they engage in action sequences; the subsequent awareness and differentiation of feelings is a stepwise process.

In this developmental hierarchy, emotion is not just "desomatized"; it is a developmental evolution with specific phases of recognition and differentiation. The inability to articulate a feeling prior to an action symptom may not be purely a defensive response but a developmental nonattainment that has to be addressed as a prequel to experiencing and articulating pure feeling. The patient's first step is to move from an external to an internal point of reference, to *inhabit* experience; in this regard, evolving from action to action language is a developmental step. Experience is registered from an internal perspective allowing somatic and emotional components to be distinguished. A differentiation of feeling into the subjective awareness can then be formulated, mastered, and communicated.

"LISTENING" FOR NONVERBAL MATERIAL

In the beginning, developmentally, there are no words. Words are not necessary for the original self, the body self, or early communication. Before language exists, we communicate at a nonverbal, affective level: facially, posturally, gesturally, affectively, and by sensing, touching, and holding. Verbal language is a relatively late acquisition ontogenetically and phylogenetically. Even in the adult, nonverbal communication accompanies every word; in treatment, nonverbal information emerges steadily from the patient. Posture, gesture, body rumblings, voice changes and quality, as well as silence are all means of expression available to the apparently immobile patient.

The simplest explanation deserves consideration first: that nonverbal behavior is communication with a significant nonverbal implication. As we learn more about the patient's early preverbal and nonverbal developmental needs, we must also remain alert to his or her affective and autonomic communication. Nonverbal behaviors are rich in meaning and history and are indicators of motivation, fantasy, and psychodynamics. Gesture and movement predate speech and reveal basic and powerful affect. In fact, gestures and movements can be scrutinized for the following characteristics:

- Unity of movement and affect.
- Position of the body and interrelationships of body parts (position of hands, arms, feet, and legs in relation to the rest of the body).
- Coordination of verbal and nonverbal movement in regard to timing, intensity, and change over time.
- Patient's associations to movements and gestures.
- Kinesthetic patterning and meanings in terms of the transference.
- Symbolic content.
- Symbolic reenactments (movements that recreate a primary attachment relationship).

To decode various actions and movements that embody unarticulated and unsymbolized experience requires exploration and discovery through the therapeutic relationship, leaving no detail to the imagination. The body has its own dialects, its own channels of memory. The body of memory, the body of fantasy, the body we create, and our actual body each may be different, with issues initially outside awareness of the body, actual and perceived.

Fundamental emotions may remain embodied, with perceptions communicated in concrete, physical terms such as heaviness, weighted down, dullness, deadness, lightness, buoyancy, floating, lifted up. This somatic language is often a counterpart to using the body in action symptoms, with its corresponding action language.

The therapeutic setting contains attributes that are symbolic equivalents of an optimum caretaker–child relationship: consistency, reliability, empathic attunement, specific and defined boundaries, focus on the patient, acceptance of what is otherwise alienating, and a holding environment. These attributes are important in the treatment of all patients, even those with more organized and developmentally advanced internal structure. The body self as well as psychological self must be integrated in the developmental foundation and structure of self-awareness and evolving cohesiveness.

One function of the therapist is to help the patient develop an internal point of reference by accurately recognizing and assisting him or her to articulate affective states. The patient's experience of affect evolves from one of pure somatic experience to one of differing types of affect, and then to making verbalizations about them. Verbalizing not only provides a sense of mastery by articulating feelings but also, more importantly, facilitates the accurate perception of (1) body self and image and (2) psychological self and their synthesis. The blending of affect and cognition of bodily and psychic self, consolidates a sense of self. In the clinical exchange, both patient and therapist must stay attuned to and grounded in the rich bodily experiences and imagery the patient experiences from moment to moment. Somatic and sensory experience bridge right-brain feeling and left-brain thinking.

Nonverbal communication can activate response patterns in the patient that include cognitive, behavioral, and affective components. For example, a stranger's staring can sometimes activate aggression. Patients who cannot verbalize feeling could be asked, "How does that staring make you feel like acting?" This kind of attunement to nonverbal cues is not only a component of mother–infant and therapist–patient interactions but also of healthy adult interactions.

The therapist's empathic immersion, resonance, and response provide a new framework of experience in which the patient can develop an internal point of reference wherein he or she is able to subjectively register feelings and differentiate among them. This experience of effectiveness and empathic attunement can then become internalized by the patient as self-empathy. Ultimately, the individual integrates the entire therapeutic process and achieves self-regulation from the newly developed internal center of initiative, affects, and esteem. In this manner, the healthy development of body self and image as well as psychological self can resume.

INFORMATIVE READINGS

Aron, L., & Anderson, F. (Eds.). (1998). *Relational perspectives on the body.* Hillsdale, NJ: Analytic Press.—A compilation of clinically useful chapters on psychopathology and treatment related to the body self.

Dimen, M. (2000). The body as Rorschach. *Studies in Gender and Sexuality 9*, 39–47.—The body seen as a screen onto which are projected various self-referential fantasies or concepts that affect body image.

Fonagy, P. (1998). Moments of change in psychoanalytic theory: Discussion of a new theory of psychic change. *Infant Mental Health Journal, 19*, 346–353.—One of several related papers describing the development of mentalization.

Goodwin, J., & Attias, R. (1999) *Splintered reflections: Images of the body in trauma.* New York: Basic Books.—Various aspects of trauma that impact the body image and body self require attunement in the clinical setting and the impact of empathic attunement to body and mind.

Krueger, D. (2002). *Creating a new story: Toward a psychoanalytic integration of body self and psychological self*. New York: Brunner/Routledge.—A clinically oriented exploration of developmental disruption of body self and psychological self, and the cocreation of a new understanding and experience in treatment.

Wyre, H., & Welles, J. (1994). *The narration of desire: Erotic transferences and counter-transferences*. Hillsdale, NJ: Analytic Press.—Vivid clinical exploration of the importance of preverbal/nonverbal mother–child bodily interactions as manifest in the transference and countertransference.

Experiential Approaches to Changing Body Image

JUDITH RUSKAY RABINOR
MARION A. BILICH

This chapter describes the various forms of experiential therapy aimed at facilitating personal growth and change in body image. The experiential perspective assumes that body image is multidimensional and includes mental representations (thoughts, feelings, and images) as well as sensory (auditory, visual, and kinesthetic) and somatic components. Therefore, if the goal is to change an individual's thoughts, feelings, sensations, and perceptions related to body image, then verbal intervention alone is limited. Direct work with sensory and somatic experiences must be included in a comprehensive treatment approach. Since the formation of body image begins at a preverbal developmental stage, techniques designed to encourage nonverbal exploration and expression will be effective at creating change at that level. This level of intervention may be particularly important for clients whose body image disturbances stem from early childhood experience.

Experiential techniques can be categorized in relation to their primary orientation to the mind/body. Table 53.1 provides a representative, though not exhaustive, listing of experiential forms of psychotherapy and personal growth that foster change in body image. As with any attempt at categorization, there is much overlap among the various approaches.

TABLE 53.1. Experiential Forms of Psychotherapy and Personal Growth for Body Image Change

Mental representation approaches

   Imagery
      Client-generated imagery (nondirected)
      Guided body image techniques
   Hypnosis
   Journal writing
   Metaphor and poetry therapy
   Affirmations

Somatic techniques

   Breathing exercises
   Relaxation exercises
   Body awareness exercises
   Massage therapy
   Rolfing
   Alexander technique
   Feldenkrais methods

Sensory techniques

   Music therapy
   Dance/movement therapy
   Art therapy
   Massage and self-touch

Integrated approaches

   Psychodrama
   Bioenergetics
   Body Talk
   Family sculpting
   Focusing (Eugene Gendlin)
   Gestalt therapy
   Somatic experiencing (Peter Levine)
   Synergy (Ilana Rubenfeld)

BASIC ASSUMPTIONS

Experiential approaches to psychotherapy all share an emphasis on the interrelatedness of mind and body; they all assume that the body impacts thoughts and feelings, and vice versa. Experiential approaches also share the following assumptions.

- *Assumption 1. Experiential approaches emphasize* present *experience.* These techniques have as their goal *insight through attention to the here-and-now.* Hornyak and Baker emphasize that this focus is often facilitated by methods that involve the client in either physical or imagined action (each of which is addressed later).
- *Assumption 2. Experiential approaches emphasize working directly with the body.* Because experiential techniques *are based on the assumption that the earliest sense of self is rooted in the body,* they target the somatic domain. As early as 1923 Freud stated, "The ego is first and foremost a body ego." Before we have the capacity for language, we use the physical body to explore, understand, experience, and master the world.
- *Assumption 3. Experiential approaches facilitate nonverbal expression.* In *Relational Perspectives on the Body,* Dimen states that conflicts and concerns related to the body are so profoundly significant that they often cannot be verbalized. Body image serves as a nonverbal metaphor that provides a psychological "home" for the displacement and projection of intrapsychic and

interpersonal conflicts by clients who lack the ability to put emotional conflicts into words. (See chapters in this volume by Krueger.)

• *Assumption 4. Experiential approaches are a "backdoor" to the unconscious.* St. John explains that physical sensations provide access to affective states, and that both verbal and nonverbal explorations of these sensations can uncover previously suppressed, repressed, or denied elements of experience. Therefore, when working directly with the body, it is possible to access unconscious as well as preconscious memories and emotions not readily accessible by verbal interaction alone.

CLINICAL CONSIDERATIONS

The unique characteristics of experiential techniques, which are always integrated into ongoing psychotherapy, require special consideration. First, it is important to be aware that experiential therapies can unleash powerful affective states and memories. Therefore, before any experiential technique is utilized, a climate of safety and trust must be established within the therapy relationship. The therapist, of course, must also consider the client's capacity to tolerate possibly intense levels of affect. Similarly, the therapist must be adequately trained in these techniques and have the temperament as well as the skill to take be active and directive in treatment—a role not suited to all therapists. If a referral to an experiential therapist is needed, the primary provider must consider the effects such a referral will have on treatment.

TECHNIQUES

The following section describes some of the techniques listed in Table 53.1. This is not a comprehensive guide but rather a sampling of those techniques that illustrate how and why experiential approaches are useful in changing body image.

Mental Representation Approaches

These therapies focus on changing internal mental representations of the body self. Clinicians working with diverse populations have reported success using guided imagery, a particularly powerful approach because body image is an *image* amenable to change. In using this approach, the therapist guides the client to focus on past situations that elicit sensory and affective material and "watch" what unfolds in the mind's eye. Often, deeply repressed material that manifests itself in a negative body image is evoked and can then be addressed constructively.

Kearney-Cooke describes the use of theme-centered guided imagery that helps clients trace their psychosocial development and identify and re-work past experiences of familial and nonfamilial trauma. Kearney-Cooke has created specific imagery techniques that help clients explore the roots of their feelings about their bodies at different developmental stages. In this way, the origins of negatively laden body parts are identified. This neg-ativity can also be uncovered during writing exercises in which the patient composes a letter to his or her body or body part.

Hutchinson developed a group approach to changing body image that included guided imagery and journal writing. She developed a 7-week pro-gram wherein participants supplemented imagery and journal writing with audiotaped homework exercises. She found statistically significant improve-ment in body image and self-image. Subsequently, she expanded her proto-col to 12-week group meetings lasting 2½ hours each and found that this ap-proach significantly affected women's relationships to their bodies and, by extension, to themselves.

Somatic Approaches

The somatic approaches change body image by helping the client reconnect to the body in a very concrete manner. These approaches are based on the idea that what we observe in the world depends on our capacity for obser-vation and awareness; expanding our awareness of the body facilitates the capacity to observe and experience life. Techniques such as deep breathing, massage, and yoga, which bring attention back into the body, are especially useful for clients whose body image problems include a sense of being dis-connected or alienated from body experience. For example, individuals with schizophrenia especially benefit from somatic techniques that focus their at-tention on their bodies in a nonthreatening way.

Our culture emphasizes the body as a source of beauty and fitness but ignores and discourages awareness of the body as a source of relaxation, comfort, and emotional wisdom. Becoming aware of the "lived experience" of our bodies, which is central to the somatic approach, is a way of tapping into these positive states. A variety of techniques facilitate self-monitoring of body awareness and focus as a way of perceiving sensations and feelings in a nonthreatening way.

Basic to many experiential and somatic techniques are breathing and relaxation exercises. Breathing exercises focus attention on *present* bodily experience simply by focusing on one's breathing pattern. Another technique, Jacobson's progressive relaxation method, involves progressing through the body, tensing and releasing each muscle group before moving to the adjacent area. The objective is to facilitate awareness of internal sen-sations, a prerequisite to feeling one's emotions. *Body scanning* offers the opportunity to explore the external manifestations of the body through the use of one's hands or in one's imagination. *Emotional body scanning* locates the somatic roots of emotions and helps clients "ground" themselves in their bodies.

Levine's *Waking the Tiger: Healing Trauma,* one of the newer approaches, is particularly useful in healing trauma held in the body. In a series of graded exercises, participants learn to identify the *felt sense,* the somatic components assumed to be associated with trauma, including hyperarousal, constriction, dissociation and freezing. According to Eugene Gendlin, who coined the term in his book *Focusing,* a felt sense is a "bodily awareness, an internal aura that encompasses all you feel and know about a subject" (p. 35). By learning how to let go of the habituated trauma-based bodily responses and replacing them with a more expanded somatic response (for example, learning to feel sad instead of numb), a healing process is initiated.

Sensory Approaches

Sensory-oriented techniques include dance and movement, art, and music therapy. These approaches engage the body's senses—visual, kinesthetic, and auditory—to change body image. Like other experiential techniques, they initially bypass verbal modes of functioning, thereby reaching a deeper level of consciousness.

Because these approaches reconnect the individual to the body through the senses, they are especially useful for those in whom the felt sense is distorted, rigid, or traumatized. This population includes people with schizophrenia, eating-disordered individuals, those who have lost a limb or body part to illness or accident, and those who have been sexually or physically abused. Like the somatic techniques described above, these techniques are particularly useful in grounding clients in their bodies.

Dance therapy focuses on the kinesthetic aspects of body experience through a series of structured and nonstructured movement exercises that increase the patient's sensory awareness. In the early 1970s, studies found that moving to music was particularly effective in increasing positive body image and awareness of the body's spatial characteristics. In 2000, Dibbell-Hope published a study of women with breast cancer that found that dance therapy promoted a marked improvement in body image and self-esteem.

Improvisational movement and directed movement exercises provide clients with awareness of how long-held emotions are stored in the body and offer new patterns for being in the world. These exercises require one to open to the unknown, the unexpected, the unfamiliar—and, often, the undesired. When one improvises, one accepts as the norm a state of being "lost." Improvisation often uncovers issues relegated to the unconscious. When we allow ourselves to experience our spontaneous impulses, we are cut loose from familiar reference points and become grounded in our bodies.

Art therapy aimed at changing a person's body image can include activities such as clay sculpting or drawings of the body and the creation of masks and collages. These techniques are especially suited to working with children whose body images have been impaired by severe, chronic illness or by trauma. Children naturally choose art as a means of self-expression and are more comfortable exploring and expressing feelings about their bodies through this medium than verbally.

Music therapy is used less frequently in therapies that address body image, but it has been successful with individuals who tend to intellectualize. In a music therapy session that is focused on body image, rhythm, melody, and harmony are used to evoke feelings about the body. Receptive activities, such as listening to music, as well as expressive activities, such as music and song writing or playing instruments, may occur. Receptive activities *evoke* memories and associations in the body, whereas expressive activities facilitate nonverbal *expression* of those memories and associations.

Integrated Approaches

The approaches described above are often integrated into comprehensive treatment programs aimed at changing body image. For example, most use some form of imagery, and even those based in nonverbal expression, such as art and dance therapies, usually have a verbal component in which clients are encouraged to articulate their newfound awareness.

One of the newer integrative approaches, initially developed to treat posttraumatic stress disorder, is eye movement desensitization and reprocessing (EMDR). It was developed by Francine Shapiro, who discovered, while treating trauma survivors, that moving the eyes back and forth decreased the intensity of distressing memories. She hypothesized that in traumatic conditions, the normal patterns of information processing are disrupted and, as a result, the information about the trauma is stored differently from ordinary information. She developed a comprehensive and integrative set of protocols to address and reprocess this dysfunctionally stored information. A recent article applauded EMDR for its utilization of auditory, visual, kinesthetic, and olfactory descriptors of imagery and sensations. In 2000, Sobanski and Schmidt reported research demonstrating the effectiveness of EMDR with seven clients who had body dysmorphic disorder, five of whom had complete symptom resolution. In another 2000 article, Dziegielewski and Wolfe reported clinical improvement in a 26-year-old woman using EMDR concurrently with a Body Satisfaction Log, which records body image satisfaction moment to moment.

Another integrative approach, Body Talk, was developed by movement educator Anna Halprin in 1989 for HIV-positive women (see St. John reference in the Informative Readings list). This group approach combines movement exercises with psychodynamic exploration to create interventions that operate simultaneously at the verbal and nonverbal levels. Through movement improvisations, these participants grappled with the unknown aspects of their self- and body images, allowing their physical vulnerability and fear of death to coexist with the bodily pleasure and engagement of the unrestricted movement. Body Talk is particularly useful for individuals confronting severe, chronic, and life-threatening illnesses that bring with them physical changes and shame that adversely affect body image.

Family sculpting and psychodrama have also proven useful in supporting traditional verbal therapy for family-of-origin work with patients who are bulimic. These techniques circumvent the family's well-practiced defenses of minimization, rationalization, and intellectualization and offer a corrective experience of living in one's body.

SUMMARY AND CONCLUSIONS

Body image is a multidimensional experience comprised of sensations and feelings that may not have verbal counterparts. Traditional talk therapy does not allow access to the sensory and nonverbal aspects of body image. Experiential approaches initially bypass the verbal arena, allowing for a deeper, richer experience of the body. Each experiential approach is a different manifestation of the principle that therapists can produce change in the client's relationship to his or her body and self-image by intervening somatically.

A modest number of clinical reports describe experiential approaches to changing body image. These often focus on clients with eating disorders. However, body image problems occur in a large segment of the population, including people with birth defects, those confronting life-threatening illnesses, accident survivors, those who suffer from body dysmorphic disorder or schizophrenia. Additionally, nonclinical populations—such as adolescents of both genders, balding men, and women at all stages in the life cycle—experience body dissatisfaction and could benefit from experiential approaches.

Unfortunately, there is a scarcity of well-designed research studies investigating the effectiveness of experiential approaches to changing body image. Many of the existing studies lacked randomized controls and employed too few subjects to draw conclusions. In addition, it is difficult to evaluate the techniques individually, since they are often used as adjunctive therapies or as components of more comprehensive treatment approaches. However, future research studies will hopefully address which experiential approaches are most effective with which populations.

INFORMATIVE READINGS

Arnold, S. C. (1994). Transforming body image through women's wilderness experiences. *Women and Therapy, 15*(3–4), 43–54.—Explores how activities such as climbing, rafting, and hiking offer women opportunities to experience a sense of body mastery.

Dibbell-Hope, S. (2000). The use of dance/movement therapy in psychological adaptation to breast cancer. *Arts in Psychotherapy, 27*(1), 51–68.—A research study that found marked improvement in body image and self-esteem in women with breast cancer who participated in dance therapy.

Dimen, M. (1998). Polyglot bodies: Sinking through the relational. In L. Aron & F. Sommer (Eds.), *Relational perspectives on the body* (pp. 65–93). Hillsdale, NJ: Analytic Press.—A good psychoanalytic perspective on body image.

Dziegielewski, S. & Wolfe, P. (2000). Eye movement desensitization and reprocessing (EMDR) as a time-limited treatment intervention for body image disturbance and self-esteem: A single subject case study design. *Journal of Psychotherapy in Independent Practice, 13*, 1–16.—Self-esteem and body image avoidance showed clinical improvement and authors suggest that EMDR is a promising time-limited treatment.

Feldendenkrais, M. (1991). *Awareness through movement: Health exercises for personal growth.* San Francisco: Harper San Francisco.—Though this book does not directly address body image change, provides practical guidelines for implementing the technique.

Gendlin, E. T. (1982). *Focusing.* New York: Bantam Books.—Helpful for teaching clients to unlock body wisdom; this technique is the basis of many experiential approaches to changing body image.

Hornyak, L. M., & Baker, E. K. (Eds.). (1989). *Experiential therapies for eating disorders.* New York: Guilford Press.—A collection of experiential approaches to treating eating disorders, in which each chapter highlights a different approach.

Hutchinson, M. D. (1988). *Transforming body image: Learning to love the body you have.* Watsonville, CA: Crossing Press.—Offers an 8-week program for effecting change in women's body image.

Jacobson, E. (1974). *Progressive relaxation* (3rd ed.). Chicago: University of Chicago Press.—The classic text on progressive relaxation, originally published in 1938.

Kearney-Cooke, A. (1989). Reclaiming the body: Using guided imagery in the treatment of body image disturbance among bulimic women. In L. M. Hornyak & E. K. Baker (Eds.), *Experiential therapies for eating disorders* (pp. 11–33). New York: Guilford Press.—Gives excellent case material on use of imagery toward changing body image in women with eating disorders.

Levine, P. (1997). *Waking the tiger: Healing trauma.* Berkeley, CA: North Atlantic Books.—Examines how trauma is held in the nervous system and is based on the concept that the body has an innate capacity to heal from trauma.

Newman, L. (1992). *SomeBody to love: A guide to loving the body you have.* Chicago, IL: Third Side Press.—Guided imagery and writing exercises aimed at exploring women's issues about their body and eating.

Probst, M., Van Coppenolle, H., & Vandereycken, W. (1995). Body experience in anorexia nervosa patients: An overview of therapeutic approaches. *Eating Disorders: The Journal of Treatment and Prevention, 3*(2), 145–157.—Good review of experiential approaches for a hard-to-reach population.

Pruzinsky, T. (1990). Somatopsychic approaches to psychotherapy and personal growth.

In T. F. Cash & T. Pruzinsky (Eds.), *Body images: Development, deviance, and change* (pp. 296–315). New York: Guilford Press.—Comprehensive overview of experiential approaches to changing body image.

Shapiro, F. (2001). *Eye movement desensitization and reprocessing: Basic principles, protocols, and procedures* (2nd ed.). New York: Guilford Press.—Both a practical text and a review of theoretical and research issues from the creator of EMDR.

Sobanski, E., & Schmidt, M. (2000). Body dysmorphic disorder: A review of current knowledge. *Child Psychology and Psychiatry Review, 5*(1), 17–24.—Excellent review of treatment approaches to BDD and includes a good review of assessment tools.

St. John, M. (1992). Anti-body already: Body oriented interventions in clinical work with HIV positive women. *Women and Therapy, 13*(4), 5–25.—Describes Halprin's "Body Talk" program, an experiential approach to correcting body image problems associated with the stigma of HIV diagnoses.

Cognitive-Behavioral Approaches to Changing Body Image

THOMAS F. CASH
MELISSA D. STRACHAN

HISTORICAL AND CONCEPTUAL FOUNDATIONS

During the past 40 years, the cognitive or cognitive-behavioral paradigm emerged as a "fourth force" in psychotherapy, on the heels of psychoanalytic, strictly behavioristic, and humanistic approaches. Although cognitive-behavioral therapies (CBT) do not derive from a singular perspective, the shared tenets and values of CBT proponents often include (1) either a rational or a constructivist emphasis on individuals' learned views of their environment, their life events, and themselves; (2) the related proposition that cognition mediates behavior and behavioral change as well as emotion and emotional change; (3) a belief that cognitive contents and processes can be accessed and altered; and (4) a valuing of psychological science for understanding, preventing, and treating problems in living.

The scientific allegiance of CBT has afforded it a central position among empirically supported treatments of psychological disorders. CBT's proponents believe that, through carefully executed clinical trials, effective treatment based on specifiable interventions is demonstrable. Such data encourage application of CBT to different problems and different populations. In this manner, CBT has evolved as a treatment of choice for many disorders, including body image dysfunctions. To appreciate the conceptual bases of CBT approaches to changing body image, see two chapters in Part I of this volume: Cash presents a detailed cognitive-behavioral model, and Williamson and his colleagues discuss a cognitive information-processing perspective.

This chapter addresses three questions:

1. Is body image CBT an empirically validated treatment for body image dysfunction?
2. What are the elements of this treatment?
3. In what directions must we move to apply and expand our knowledge of the utility of body image CBT?

THE EFFICACY OF BODY IMAGE CBT

Therapist-Directed CBT with Body-Dissatisfied Women

The systematic application of CBT to body image disturbances largely began in 1987, when Butters and Cash published a report on their randomized, controlled study of body image CBT. Fifteen women dissatisfied with their bodies were treated individually for 6 weeks. Participants learned the skills of self-monitoring, relaxation, imaginal desensitization, rational responding to cognitive distortions, and relapse-prevention strategies. Sixteen wait-list controls subsequently received a 3-week cognitive variant of the program. Multiple therapists followed a manualized protocol. Assessments included an array of measures testing body image and psychosocial functioning. Women in the treatment condition improved significantly, compared to their own pretest functioning and to the control group. They became more satisfied with their appearance, evaluated their looks more favorably, and experienced less affective discomfort when viewing their reflection in a mirror. In addition, CBT participants reported reduced appearance investment, fewer dysfunctional appearance-related beliefs, and improved psychosocial adjustment. All gains had been maintained at a 2-month follow-up. The control group treated with cognitive but not behavioral elements of the program, experienced comparable improvements in body image and adjustment.

In a 1987 study by Dworkin and Kerr, 79 body-dissatisfied women were randomly assigned to one of three therapy conditions or a wait-list control group. All therapy conditions consisted of three individual sessions. Women in the cognitive therapy condition were taught to recognize and alter negative body image self-statements. Those in the CBT condition used these cognitive strategies plus self-reinforcement and guided imagery. A reflective therapy condition entailed exploring body image experiences. Although all participants, even untreated controls, reported significant improvements in body image and self-esteem, the three treatments produced greater change. Cognitive therapy showed the best therapeutic effectiveness. The authors speculated that elements of the CBT regimen (e.g., guided imagery of becoming fat) might have attenuated its effectiveness relative to cognitive therapy alone. No follow-up data were collected.

In 1989 Rosen, Saltzberg, and Srebnik treated 13 body-dissatisfied women with a six-session trial of group CBT. For control comparison, 10 women attended group sessions offering education and support but minimal treatment. Both conditions included information about, and discussion of, size perception, maladaptive body image beliefs, and negative body image behaviors; only the CBT condition involved structured cognitive and behavioral interventions. The results confirmed that CBT was superior to the minimal treatment condition in producing significant improvements in accurately estimating body size, in body appearance and shape dissatisfaction, and behavioral avoidance related to body image. Changes had been maintained at a 6-week follow-up.

In 1990, Rosen and his collaborators extended these findings by including training in size perception for the group CBT protocol. Twenty-seven body-dissatisfied women were randomly assigned to CBT alone or CBT plus perception training. Both groups improved significantly and equally, exhibiting less body size distortion, body image dissatisfaction, weight preoccupation, fat anxiety, drive for thinness, physical self-consciousness, and behavioral avoidance. Thus training to enhance the accuracy of perceptual body image did not add to treatment efficacy. All outcomes had been maintained 3 months later.

In 1994, Fisher and Thompson compared group body image CBT with a combined anaerobic/aerobic exercise program. These 6-week interventions were compared to an untreated control condition. All three groups of body-dissatisfied women showed equivalent improvements in perceptual body image and behavioral avoidance. However, relative to controls, CBT and exercise therapy produced comparably superior changes in weight-related anxiety and body dissatisfaction. Attrition at follow-up precluded conclusions about maintenance of treatment gains.

Therapist-Assisted and Self-Directed Body Image CBT

A series of studies have evaluated body image CBT in formats involving varying degrees of face-to-face contact with a therapist. In 1995, Grant and Cash compared two modalities of body image CBT, based on Cash's 1991 audiocassette program. One modality used a therapist-led group therapy format; the other was primarily self-directed, with only modest "therapist" contact. Twenty-three body-dissatisfied women were treated for 11 weeks. Results indicated that the two treatment conditions had equivalent success. Clients evaluated their appearance more favorably and reported reductions in body image dysphoria, weight-related concerns, cognitive distortions in body image, and less avoidance and anxious self-focus during sexual relations. Both conditions also led to less social anxiety, better social self-esteem, and fewer symptoms of eating disturbance and depression. Changes had been sustained as of 2 months later. These results support the efficacy of body image CBT, even when largely self-directed.

Cash and Lavallee extended these findings to a modality with even less therapist involvement. They assigned the self-help book *What Do You See When You Look in the Mirror?* (Cash, 1995), which is similar to the 1991 audiocassette program. The 12 body-dissatisfied women who completed the program became significantly less invested in, and more satisfied with, their appearance and reported decreased body image dysphoria. They also evinced reductions in depressive symptoms and eating disturbances. Albeit based on a small sample size, outcomes were statistically comparable to those found by Grant and Cash. No follow-up data were collected.

Lavallee and Cash subsequently compared a purely self-directed body image CBT program with a self-esteem CBT intervention that did not focus on body image. Thirty-seven body-dissatisfied individuals (mostly women) were randomly assigned to one of two 9-week bibliotherapy conditions: reading the Cash (1995) self-help book on improving body image, or a CBT book on self-esteem by McKay and Fanning. Both conditions led to significant positive changes in body image evaluation, investment, and affect. However, compared to the self-esteem program, body image CBT recipients evaluated their body image problems after treatment as differentially less severe, and most effect sizes for body image change were larger for the body image CBT condition. Clinical significance analyses indicated higher "functional recovery" rates with body image CBT than self-esteem CBT (i.e., 74% vs. 39%). Furthermore, body image CBT participants evinced fewer maladaptive eating behaviors and better social self-esteem. Thus, although self-esteem CBT can improve a negative body image, a CBT program that targets body image is more effective in reducing the clinical severity of the body dissatisfaction.

Recently we (Strachan and Cash) compared the efficacy of psychoeducational versus additional cognitive-change components provided by Cash's 1997 *Body Image Workbook* version of body image CBT. Both conditions were administered in a self-help modality. Eighty-nine body-dissatisfied volunteers (mostly women) were randomly assigned to one of two 6-week self-directed conditions: (1) psychoeducation plus self-monitoring, or (2) this treatment combined with procedures to identify and alter dysfunctional body image cognitions. Both conditions produced statistically and clinically significant improvements in body image evaluation, investment, and affect among program completers. Accompanying improvements in social self-esteem, social anxiety, and depression were evident, whereas changes in eating pathology were weaker. Results were confirmed in the more conservative intent-to-treat analyses. Follow-up assessments were not conducted. The lack of differential effectiveness between the two self-help conditions was likely due to program attrition and lower compliance with the cognitive-change components. A comparison of these results with those studies that included at least modest therapist contact suggests better compliance and outcomes for the latter. Clinicians who use a self-directed program as an adjunct to therapy would be well advised to monitor and reinforce clients' program adherence and progress.

Body Image CBT with Other Populations

As other authors in this volume attest, both obesity and body dysmorphic disorder (BDD) involve substantial body image dysfunctions. In 1995 James Rosen and colleagues employed body image CBT with these two populations. Rosen, Orosan, and Reiter recruited 51 obese women with severe body dissatisfaction and a frustrating history of dieting and weight loss attempts. One group of women received group body image CBT that targeted body image issues especially pertinent to obesity; a control condition offered no treatment. Treatment consisted of seven group sessions that included psychoeducation, self-monitoring, cognitive restructuring, and behavioral exposure. The CBT-treated women showed differentially significant improvements on all body image measures, and their self-esteem also improved. Furthermore, they felt more in control of their eating, and the rate of binge eating fell significantly. Except for eating restraint, all improvements had been sustained at a 4.5-month follow-up.

Rosen, Reiter, and Orosan also investigated body image CBT using 54 women who met DSM-III-R criteria for BDD. Relative to an untreated control condition, eight sessions of group body image CBT successfully enhanced appearance satisfaction, reduced the severity of cognitive and behavioral BDD symptoms, and improved self-esteem. Results revealed that 81% of treated participants had significant BDD improvements at posttest, with a 77% improvement rate at a 4.5-month follow-up. In her chapter in this volume, Phillips further discusses the effectiveness of CBT in the treatment of BDD.

COMPONENTS OF A BODY IMAGE CBT PROGRAM

As indicated above, Cash's CBT program for changing a negative body image has been periodically revised. The most current refinement is *The Body Image Workbook: An 8-Step Program for Learning to Like Your Looks*, which contains over 40 "Self-Discovery Helpsheets" and "Helpsheets for Change." The *Workbook* may be self-administered by people without clinically severe disorders, or may be used by therapists to provide body image treatment to patients. The elements of this version of the program are summarized as follows:

- The *Workbook*'s introduction describes body image problems and summarizes the program, including its empirical foundations.
- *Step 1* takes baseline assessments using scientific measures of key facets of body image. Using interpretations of their assessment profile, program participants set specific goals for change.
- *Step 2* teaches individuals how developmental and historical events, including the inculcation of body image attitudes via familial, cultural, and social experiences, serve to predispose them to later difficulties. They learn how these vulnerabilities are activated by and pervade day-to-day thoughts, emotions, and behaviors that may become self-perpetuating. The self-discovery process includes mirror-exposure activities and the construction of an autobiography of body image development. Completing a structured "Body Image Diary," participants learn to monitor current body image experiences by attending to and recording the precipitants of distress and how this distress affects their thoughts, emotions, and behaviors. This diary is used systematically throughout the program (see Cash's Chapter 19 in this volume).
- *Step 3* teaches "Body and Mind Relaxation" by integrating muscle relaxation, diaphragmatic breathing, mental imagery, and positive self-talk to promote skills for managing emotions in response to a dysphoric body image. These skills are applied in desensitization exercises that foster body image comfort and control in relation to distress-provoking stimuli.
- *Step 4* identifies dysfunctional "appearance assumptions"— beliefs or schemas that mediate daily body image experiences. Examples include:

> "If I could look just as I wish, my life would be much happier."
> "Physically attractive people have it all."
> "The only way I could ever like my looks would be to change them."

Program participants learn to become aware of the influence of these assumptions in everyday life and to question and even refute them.
- *Step 5* teaches individuals to identify particular cognitive distortions in their "Private Body Talk"—their body-related thought processes—and offers strategies for modifying them. Such distortions include comparing one's appearance to that of more attractive people, thinking of one's looks in dichotomous extremes (e.g., as ugly or good-looking, fat or thin), or arbitrarily blaming one's appearance for life's difficulties or disappointments. Clients extend their diary keeping to incorporate cognitive restructuring exercises for correcting these distortions and discovering the emotional and behavioral consequences of cognitive changes.
- *Step 6* teaches workbook participants specific behavioral strategies for altering avoidant behaviors related to body image. These behaviors might include avoiding particular activities (e.g., exercising, going without makeup, or having sex), situations (e.g., the beach or gym), or people (e.g., attractive individuals) that might engender self-consciousness and body image

distress. Participants also target and modify "appearance preoccupied ritu-als," such as repeated mirror checking or excessive grooming regimens. These self-tailored strategies typically include interventions of graduated exposure and response prevention.

• *Step 7* uses the metaphor of satisfaction with one's interpersonal rela-tionships (i.e., a good marriage or friendship) to promote a proactive, posi-tive relationship with one's body. Program participants engage in prescribed exercises for "body image affirmation" and "body image enhancement"—for example, by reinforcing activities that pertain to physical fitness and health, sensate enjoyment, and grooming for pleasure rather than for con-cealment or reparation of perceived flaws. This step emphasizes engaging in body-related activities through positive reinforcement by creating experi-ences of mastery and pleasure.

• *Step 8* has participants retake body image assessments, score them to receive feedback about attained changes, and then set goals for further-needed changes. A review of relapse-prevention strategies helps them iden-tify and prepare for future situations (e.g., difficult interpersonal situations) that might induce body image dysphoria.

FUTURE DIRECTIONS FOR RESEARCH AND CLINICAL PRACTICE

The reviewed studies clearly affirm the efficacy of body image CBT for a range of body image problems. These positive outcomes extend to related aspects of psychosocial adjustment, such as self-esteem, social and emo-tional well-being, and eating behaviors. As discussed in the two chapters on prevention that follow, innovative applications of the principles and proce-dures of body image CBT hold promise for preventing problems related to body image. Longer-term follow-up studies that evaluate the comparative efficacy of specific treatment components are clearly needed.

Given the importance of body image in both psychological and physical disorders, it is surprising that scientific evaluation of body image CBT has not expanded to more diverse populations. Many "comprehensive" treat-ment programs for eating disorders include brief information addressing body image issues. However, in view of evidence that body image change is predictive of more favorable outcomes in eating disorder treatment, we should isolate and study the inclusion of more extensive body image CBT in these programs. Because research has focused principally on body dissatis-fied college women, we must study body image CBT applied appropriately for men, older adults, adolescents, and children. Moreover, we might well ask: Can body image CBT help people disfigured by congenital conditions, disease, or trauma? What is the value of body image CBT as alternative or adjunctive assistance to people who seek cosmetic surgery? Much remains to be learned about the utility of CBT in preventing and treating body image difficulties.

INFORMATIVE READINGS

Butters, J. W., & Cash, T. F. (1987). Cognitive-behavioral treatment of women's body-image dissatisfaction. *Journal of Consulting and Clinical Psychology, 55,* 889–897.—One of the first controlled investigations of body image CBT.

Cash, T. F. (1991). *Body-image therapy: A program for self-directed change.* New York: Guilford Press.—Audiocassette series with a short client workbook and a clinician's manual.

Cash, T. F. (1995). *What do you see when you look in the mirror?: Helping yourself to a positive body image.* New York: Bantam Books.—The author's first self-help version of his body image CBT program (now out of print).

Cash, T. F. (1997). *The body image workbook: An 8-step program for learning to like your looks.* Oakland, CA: New Harbinger.—The most recent version of the author's body image CBT program.

Cash, T. F., & Grant, J. R. (1996). The cognitive-behavioral treatment of body-image disturbances. In V. Van Hasselt & M. Hersen (Eds.), *Sourcebook of psychological treatment manuals for adult disorders* (pp. 567–614). New York: Plenum Press.—Reviews the causes and consequences of body image dysfunctions and details specific body image CBT techniques and interventions.

Cash, T. F., & Lavallee, D. M. (1997). Cognitive-behavioral body-image therapy: Further evidence of the efficacy of a self-directed program. *Journal of Rational-Emotive and Cognitive-Behavior Therapy, 15,* 281–294.—Examines body image CBT as self-help with minimal professional contact.

Cash, T. F., & Strachan, M. D. (1999). Body images, eating disorders, and beyond. In R. Lemberg (Ed.), *Eating disorders: A reference sourcebook* (pp. 27–36). Phoenix, AZ: Oryx Press.—An overview of the author's (T. F. C.) body image CBT program for body dissatisfaction, including the implications for its use in treating eating disorders.

Dobson, K. S. (Ed.). (2001). *Handbook of cognitive-behavioral therapies* (2nd ed.). New York: Guilford Press.—A comprehensive and contemporary volume that describes the historical, theoretical, and empirical foundations of CBT, as well as its clinically rich application to a range of problems and disorders.

Dworkin, S. H., & Kerr, B. A. (1987). Comparison of interventions for women experiencing body image problems. *Journal of Counseling Psychology, 34,* 136–140.—One of the earliest controlled studies to establish body image CBT as efficacious.

Fisher, E., & Thompson, J. K. (1994). A comparative evaluation of cognitive-behavioral therapy (CBT) versus exercise therapy (ET) for the treatment of body image disturbance. *Behavior Modification, 18,* 171–185.—Provides further evidence of the efficacy of body image CBT and suggests the potential value of exercise value.

Grant, J. R., & Cash, T. F. (1995). Cognitive-behavioral body-image therapy: Comparative efficacy of group and modest-contact treatments. *Behavior Therapy, 26,* 69–84.—A study confirming the effectiveness of body image CBT both in a therapist-directed modality and in a largely self-directed format.

Lavallee, D. M., & Cash, T. F. (1997, November). *The comparative efficacy of two cognitive-behavioral self-help programs for a negative body image.* Poster presented at the convention of the Association for Advancement of Behavior Therapy, Miami Beach, FL.—Provides further support for the effectiveness of body image CBT in a self-help format.

Rosen, J. C. (1997). Cognitive-behavioral body image therapy. In D. M. Garner & P. E. Garfinkel (Eds.), *Handbook of treatment for eating disorders* (2nd ed., pp. 188–201). New York: Guilford Press.—Describes the tenets and techniques of CBT for treating body image cognitions, behaviors, and emotions associated with disordered eating.

Rosen, J. C., Cado, S., Silberg, N. T., Srebnik, D., & Wendt, S. (1990). Cognitive behavior therapy with and without size perception training for women with body image disturbance. *Behavior Therapy, 21*, 481–498.—Supports the efficacy of body image CBT and indicates that training to correct perceptual distortions does not enhance efficacy.

Rosen, J. C., Orosan, P., & Reiter, J. (1995). Cognitive behavior therapy for negative body image in obese women. *Behavior Therapy, 26*, 25–42.—A controlled study confirming the efficacy of body image CBT, independent of weight loss, among obese women.

Rosen, J. C., Reiter, J., & Orosan, P. (1995). Cognitive-behavioral body image therapy for body dysmorphic disorder. *Journal of Consulting and Clinical Psychology, 63*, 263–269.—Establishes the efficacy of body image CBT for patients with this disorder.

Rosen, J. C., Saltzberg, E., & Srebnik, D. (1989). Cognitive behavior therapy for negative body image. *Behavior Therapy, 20*, 393–404.—Finds body image CBT to be more effective than an education-and-support treatment.

Strachan, M. D., & Cash, T. F. (2002). Self-help for a negative body image: A comparison of components of a cognitive-behavioral program. *Behavior Therapy, 33*, 235–251.—Evaluates the effectiveness of psychoeducational and cognitive elements of body image CBT.

Psychoeducational Approaches to the Prevention and Change of Negative Body Image

ANDREW J. WINZELBERG
LIANA ABASCAL
C. BARR TAYLOR

In this chapter we present an overview of the conceptual and empirical rationale for psychoeducational approaches to enhancing body image, describe the components typically found in these programs, review the evidence of their effectiveness, outline their advantages and limitations, and discuss the issues still to be addressed.

THE NATURE OF PSYCHOEDUCATION

Psychoeducational programs address psychological issues that may not require the interventions of a psychotherapist. By psychoeducational programs, we mean educational material that is provided through various media—print, audiotapes, videotapes, computer software, or "live" lectures. These materials can be presented either individually (e.g., reading a workbook) or in groups (e.g., school-based programs). Information is typically structured in a manner that gives participants a framework with which to understand the nature of their problem, identify and change the undesired behaviors and attitudes, and become aware of possible consequences for not changing the undesired behavior. The focus of the education is rarely insight

alone. Rather the goal is to teach specific strategies for changing participants' social and personal environments, thoughts, attitudes, and behaviors.
Several reviews of self-directed media-based psychoeducational programs
(e.g., workbooks, audiotapes, and videotapes), including several meta-
analyses, find that these programs are moderately effective, with effect sizes
that range from .50 to .75. However, the overall effectiveness of psychoeducational programs remains unknown because no comprehensive review of
all types of psychoeducational programs (including programs that employ
the assistance of a helping professional) has been undertaken to date.

The causes of body image problems can be presented from a variety of
theoretical perspectives: psychodynamic, cognitive-behavioral, sociocultural, and feminist. Psychoeducational programs focused on improving body
image typically include informational and behavioral components designed
to unfold in a structured manner. Although many men experience body image dissatisfaction, body image enhancement programs historically have
been developed for and used by women or girls. Most of these programs
take a sociocognitive learning approach in which participants are helped to
understand their environment and cognitions and are offered specific steps
for change. Problematic behaviors and attitudes are typically defined as
learned—which means that they can be *un*learned. Participants are usually
responsible for maintaining their own motivation and adherence to the program protocol.

TYPICAL FEATURES OF PSYCHOEDUCATIONAL
BODY IMAGE PROGRAMS

The primary mode of delivery for body image programs has been through
bibliotherapy (e.g., books, workbooks, or magazine articles) and lectures.
Lectures, including workshops, seminars, and discussion groups, have been
developed for general audiences (e.g., presentations to college students) as
well as for targeted groups with known body image concerns (e.g., part of
an eating disorder treatment program). Recently, the Internet has provided a
mode of delivery that has the potential to reach a still wider audience.

Body image psychoeducation typically begins with a description of the
social construction of beauty, its narrow definition within Western culture,
and the effects of socialization on the development of body image. Body dissatisfaction is normalized and its possible consequences identified, such as
lowered self-esteem, eating disorders, and social discomfort or isolation.
Throughout the program a sense of hope and optimism is offered, as participants are encouraged to follow the specific steps and strategies outlined in
the intervention.

A fundamental part of most programs is teaching participants to self-
monitor the external and internal triggers of their body dissatisfaction. They

are encouraged to challenge negative self-statements and to change any self-defeating personal and social environments (e.g., exposure to media encouraging unhealthy standards of beauty, or friends who make critical comments) as a way to promote experiences that foster body acceptance. Participants are also taught various problem-solving strategies and ancillary coping strategies, such as relaxation training and stress management techniques. Some programs encourage the active engagement of social support (e.g., soliciting feedback from significant others) during the learning process (and thereafter).

THE EFFECTIVENESS OF PSYCHOEDUCATIONAL APPROACHES TO BODY IMAGE ENHANCEMENT

Given the ubiquitous media attention on body image discontentment and the plethora of self-help books on the topic (over 130 books available in 2001), it is surprising how few well-controlled studies of psychoeducational approaches to body image enhancement exist. Studies of psychoeducational interventions can be divided into three categories: (1) interventions for enhancing body image only, (2) prevention interventions for negative body image and eating disorders, and (3) those for body image enhancement and eating disorders/chronic dieting. Body image and eating disorder treatments are often combined because excessive weight concern has been found to be a factor in the development and maintenance of eating disorders. Table 55.1 lists intervention studies in each category; studies were selected for this table based on the level of control in the experimental design and the representation of each category.

To our knowledge, Thomas Cash's body image enhancement program is the only psychoeducational program that focuses exclusively on body image and has been evaluated in randomized clinical trials. Described in Cash and Strachan's chapter in this volume, this program is currently available as *The Body Image Workbook: An 8-Step Program for Learning to Like Your Looks.* Cash and his colleagues have demonstrated that a self-directed body image enhancement program, based on the same principles Cash employs in his cognitive-behavioral therapy of patients with body image disturbances, is effective in helping women increase their level of body satisfaction. In one study, Cash and Lavallee found that over 80% of participants experienced significant improvement in their body image. Cash found similar results when the self-directed intervention was augmented with either weekly face-to-face or telephone contact with an assistant who reviewed assignments, answered questions, and reinforced adherence to the treatment. Subsequently, Strachan and Cash found statistically and clinically significant improvements in body image for selected psychoeducational aspects of the program when purely self-administered.

TABLE 55.1. Studies of Psychoeducational Body Image Interventions

Author and title/name of program	Description	Target population (female)	Body image measures	Results for body image measures (with effect sizes)
Body image programs				
Cash & Lavallee (1997) "What Do You See When You Look in the Mirror" [previous version: "Body-Image Therapy: A Program for Self-Directed Change"]	Three conditions varying levels of therapist contact: minimal, modest, and group Varied 8–20 weeks No control condition	Negative body image	Multiple measures (e.g., SIBID)	Modest/group contact (combined): 1.1^a Minimal contact: 1.2^a No group differences
Strachan & Cash (2000) *The Body Image Workbook*	Two purely self-help conditions Psychoeducation with and without specific cognitive components 6 weeks	Negative body image	Multiple measures (e.g., BASS subscale of MBSRQ)	Psychoeducation with cognitive restructuring: 0.4^a Psychoeducation without cognitive restructuring: 0.8^a No group differences
Body image and eating disorder prevention programs				
Kaminski & McNamara (1996) Psychoeducational program for high-risk college women	Lecture, group discussion, and assignments facilitated by graduate students 8-week 90-minute sessions	High risk for bulimia	EBQ—Weight Dissatisfaction EDI—Body Dissatisfaction Body Esteem Scale	1.5 2.8 1.8
Springer, Winzelberg, Perkins, & Taylor (1999) Body Traps	Lecture, group discussion, and assignments Class taught by graduate student 10 2-hour classes	Negative body image	BSQ EDE-Q/W EDE-Q/S	0.4 0.2 0.4
Winzelberg, Eppstein, Eldridge, Wilfley, Dasmahapatra, Dev, & Taylor (2000) Student Bodies	Student Bodies and wait-list condition Online discussion group moderated by graduate student Eight sessions	High weight and shape concerns	BSQ EDE-Q/W EDE-Q/S	0.5 0.4 0.5
Celio, Winzelberg, Wilfley, Eppstein-Herald, Springer, Dev, & Taylor (2000) Student Bodies	Comparison of Student Bodies (8-week online program) with Body Traps (eight 2-hour classroom meetings) and wait-list condition	High weight and shape concerns	BSQ EDE-Q/WS	Body Traps: 0.1 Student Bodies: 0.3 Body Traps: 0.1 Student Bodies: 0.5

TABLE 55.1. *(continued)*

Author and title/name of program	Description	Target population (female)	Body image measures	Results for body image measures (with effect sizes)
Eating disorder and chronic dieting treatment programs				
Higgins & Gray (1998) Freedom from Dieting	Class lecture, group discussion, and assignments Six 2-hour classes plus intro and review meeting; run by health educators Wait-list condition	Chronic dieters	BSQ	2.4
Davis, Olmsted, & Rockert (1990) Brief Group Psychoeducation for Bulimia Nervosa	Lectures and readings; five 90-minute sessions over 4 weeks Therapist led Wait-list condition	Bulimia nervosa	EDI—Body Dissatisfaction	0.5 Pre–post effect size could only be calculated on treatment group with published data
Olmsted, Davis, Rockert, Irvine, Eagle, & Garner (1991) Brief Group Psychoeducation for Bulimia Nervosa	Comparison of individual cognitive-behavioral therapy (19 1-hour sessions over 18 weeks) and psychoeducational group (five 90-minute sessions over 4 weeks) Therapist led No control condition	Bulimia nervosa	EDI—Body Dissatisfaction	No significant findings
Phelps, Sapia, Nathanson, & Nelson (2000) Eating Disorder Prevention Program	Interactive lessons and group discussion; three studies: middle school, high school, and college participants Six sessions—4 weeks All studies included comparison conditions/classes	Middle and high school—part of academic curriculum College—sorority members	EDI—Body Dissatisfaction	Middle school and high school: no significant findings College: significance of $p < .05$ but effect size could not be calculated from published data

Note. BASS, Body Areas Satisfaction Scale; BSQ, Body Shape Questionnaire; EDI, Eating Disorders Inventory; EDE-Q/W, Eating Disorders Examination–Questionnaire, weight concern subscale; EDE-Q/S, Eating Disorders Examination–Questionnaire, shape concern subscale; EDE-Q/WS, Eating Disorders Examination–Questionnaire, weight and shape concern subscales combined; EBQ, Eating Behaviors Questionnaire; MBSRQ, Multidimensional Body-Self Relations Questionnaire; SIBID, Situational Inventory of Body Image Dysphoria.

[a]Due to lack of control group, effect size (ES) calculated using treatment condition only. Formula used with control group ES = $\Delta\overline{X}_T - \Delta\overline{X}_C)/SD_C$. Formula used without control group ES = $(\overline{X}_{Tpst} - \overline{X}_{Tpre})/SD_{pre}$. In general, effects in the 0.3 range or below are considered weak, and those of 0.7 or above are considered strong.

A number of combined body image dissatisfaction and eating disorder prevention programs have been developed and delivered to adolescents and young adults. Kaminski and McNamara's psychoeducational program targets a population at high risk for developing bulimia. They found that participants significantly improved their body image and followed healthier behaviors in comparison with a control group. Another such program, developed at the Stanford University Behavioral Medicine Media Laboratory, has been successfully delivered through the Internet. Named "Student Bodies," the Stanford program targets young women with weight and shape concerns, as well as unhealthy eating attitudes and behaviors. Four iterations of the program have been evaluated thus far, using a wait-list control group for comparison and a 3- or 4-month follow-up. In each trial, participants improved their overall body image, reduced their weight and shape concerns, and adopted healthier eating attitudes and behaviors.

Some programs that focus on the treatment of eating disorders or chronic dieting also incorporate body image components. In a 1996 review of clinically controlled eating disorder treatments, James Rosen found that about one-third of the studied treatments addressed body image, although few included behavioral interventions and self-monitoring assignments for improvement in this area. Only three studies that Rosen reviewed were psychoeducational interventions. One program, developed by Davis and colleagues for bulimia nervosa, combines lectures and readings. The results of their studies have been equivocal. All have found an improvement in dietary practices, but body image results have been mixed. For chronic dieters, Higgins and Gray found that a 6-week program that combined lectures, group discussion, and homework assignments helped participants improve their body image relative to a wait-list group.

ADVANTAGES AND DISADVANTAGES OF BODY IMAGE PSYCHOEDUCATIONAL PROGRAMS

Psychoeducational programs offer a number of advantages to both participants and providers. For participants, they offer greater privacy and convenience, which may be of particular importance for individuals who are uncomfortable about publicly acknowledging body image concerns. Self-directed interventions are likely to reach people who might be unwilling to seek face-to-face interventions. Moreover, such programs are not costly and may appeal to those who have limited financial resources.

For health-care providers, psychoeducational programs are inexpensive to deliver, easy to disseminate, and flexibly self-paced. As part of a stepped care regimen, self-directed psychoeducational approaches can be used as the first step. Participants who fail to improve sufficiently from self-care would then receive psychotherapy. This approach could enhance the cost–benefit ratio of stepped care programs. Internet-delivered approaches also have the potential to assess participants on an ongoing basis; these convenient programs can provide both participants and health-care providers with information on progress and can alert both to problems that may require additional efforts.

Psychoeducational approaches are by no means a panacea, however. Text-based interventions may require high levels of reading comprehension and motivation. Although this reliance on literacy is less likely to be a problem with programs designed for college-educated participants, it may be more difficult for programs designed for the public at large. Most programs require a willingness to persistently self-monitor and the ability to generalize the self-monitoring experiences from one area of life to another.

Psychoeducational approaches also require significant motivation in participants throughout the intervention. In the "Student Bodies" program, we have found that adherence decreases over time. Strachan and Cash made similar observations in their research with the *Body Image Workbook*. This decrease is disturbing because overall adherence predicts more positive outcomes. The self-directed and prestructured format of psychoeducational programs may be ineffective for participants who need or want more interactive or personalized formats.

Finally, psychoeducational interventions do little to change society's norms on body image and beauty. In Chapter 56, Levine and Smolak identify a range of ecological and activist approaches in the prevention of body image problems.

PSYCHOEDUCATIONAL PROGRAMS FOR BOYS AND MEN

As noted, most body image enhancement programs have been developed for, and used by, women. Although the underlying principles are probably applicable to males, it is likely that many of the programs would require significant modification for boys or men to find them acceptable. Examples addressing the body image concerns that men face, such as the pressure to achieve a well-muscled body, would need to be incorporated. Cash's *Body Image Workbook* was purposefully written in this manner to appeal to both men and women. Still, because women clearly use body image enhancement programs more frequently, our understanding of how to construct and maximize the effectiveness of such programs (e.g., content, tone, and pace of program) is based on these gendered experiences.

RESEARCH QUESTIONS

Many important research questions regarding psychoeducational approaches to body image improvement remain unanswered. Most programs have been led or assisted by professionals or paraprofessionals. It is unknown how this factor affects outcomes. Too few studies have examined purely self-directed psychoeducational interventions or the use of a layperson as a group leader or moderator. It is uncertain which participant characteristics predict the best outcomes of psychoeducational approaches. Studies that dismantle intervention components are needed to determine which features are most important and effective. In particular, little is known about the specific knowledge that may be required of participants in order to make attitudinal and behavioral changes. Maintaining participants' motivation is crucial to the success of psychoeducational approaches, yet few studies have examined adherence. How often do which participants read or apply the program materials? We need to discover how self-contained and self-directed approaches can maintain motivation and enhance adherence to the psychoeducational protocol.

Finally, we need to understand how participants' lack of success in a psychoeducational program affects their willingness to seek other assistance. If psychoeducational interventions are to contribute to a stepped care approach, it is essential that program failure not discourage people from seeking additional assistance.

Notwithstanding these limitations and issues, we are optimistic about the efficacy of psychoeducational interventions for body image enhancement. Our scientific and clinical understanding of the factors that produce compliance and improvement and enhance compliance must grow. Our ability to integrate self-directed approaches into a comprehensive treatment system must improve. With these advances, psychoeducational approaches can become the first choice in the treatment of body image problems.

INFORMATIVE READINGS

Cash, T. F. (1997). *The body image workbook: An 8–step program for learning to like your looks.* Oakland, CA: New Harbinger.—A structured cognitive- behavioral approach to improving body image in a self-directed workbook format, used as the basis of Cash's psychoeducational intervention studies.

Cash, T. F., & Lavallee, D. M. (1997). Cognitive-behavioral body-image therapy: Extended evidence of the efficacy of a self-directed program. *Journal of Rational-Emotive and Cognitive Behavior Therapy, 15*(4), 281–294.—Cash's (1995) CBT self-help treatment was administered with minimal professional contact. The results of the study demonstrated outcomes and levels of compliance that were equivalent to those previously found under conditions involving greater degrees of professional contact.

Celio, A., Winzelberg, A., Wilfley, D., Eppstein-Herald, D., Springer, E., Dev, P., & Taylor, C. B. (2000). Reducing risk factors for eating disorders: Comparison of an Internet- and a classroom-delivered psychoeducational program. *Journal of Consulting and Clinical Psychology, 68*(4), 650–657.—Compares Internet-delivered (Student Bodies) and classroom-delivered ("Body Traps") psychoeducational interventions for the reduction of body dissatisfaction in a college student sample.

Davis, R., Olmsted, M.P., & Rockert, W. (1990). Brief group psychoeducation for bulimia nervosa: Assessing the clinical significance of change. *Journal of Consulting and Clinical Psychology, 58*(6), 882–885.—This study documents the diversity of outcomes that individuals reported following their participation in a brief psychoeducational intervention that was designed to promote bulimia nervosa symptom management.

Davis, R., Olmsted, M.P., & Rockert, W. (1992). Brief group psychoeducation for bulimia nervosa: II. Prediction of clinical outcome. *International Journal of Eating Disorders 11*(3), 205–211.—Davis and colleagues found that greater self-reported depression, higher frequency of vomiting, and a history of low adult body weight were strongly associated with poor outcome in a brief psychoeducational intervention designed to promote bulimia nervosa symptom management.

Gould, R. A., & Clum, G. A. (1993). A meta-analysis of self-help treatment approaches. *Clinical Psychology Review, 13,* 169–186.—Reviews 41 studies evaluating various self-help formats, length of treatment, and adherence.

Higgins, L. C., & Gray, W. (1998). Changing the body image concern and eating behaviour of chronic dieters: The effects of a psychoeducational intervention. *Psychology and Health, 13*(6), 1045–1060.—This study evaluated a psychoeducational program designed to improve body image and normalize eating in female chronic dieters. One year after the completion of the program most participants had stopped dieting and were engaging in natural eating.

Kaminski, P. L., & McNamara, K. (1996). A treatment for college women at risk for bulimia: A controlled evaluation. *Journal of Counseling and Development, 74*(3), 288–294.—College women who received McNamara's 8-week psychoeducational program reported significantly improved levels of self-esteem and body satisfaction, as well as reduction in the reliance on potentially dangerous methods of weight management compared to controls at post-test and follow-up.

Olmsted, M. P., Davis, R., Rockert, W., Irvine, M. J., Eagle, M., & Garner, D. M. (1991). Efficacy of a brief group psychoeducational intervention for bulimia nervosa. *Behaviour Research and Therapy, 29*(1), 71–83.—Compares a psychoeductional intervention and cognitive-behavioral therapy for bulimia nervosa.

The Perfect Body (video and user guide). Copyright 1993 by The Regents of the University of California and distributed by Intermedia, Inc., 1700 Westlake Avenue North, Suite 724, Seattle, WA 98109–3068, (800) 553–8336.—The video explores cultural messages and personal pressures women feel to look "perfect"; four college women share their struggles with body image and discuss the pressures they have felt from media, men, each other, and the thin-obsessed culture.

Phelps, L., Sapia, J., Nathanson, D., & Nelson, L. (2000). An empirically supported eating disorder prevention program. *Psychology in the Schools, 37*(5), 443–452.—Evaluates a school-based eating disorder prevention program with female middle, high school, and college students.

Rosen, J. C. (1996). Body image assessment and treatment in controlled studies of eating disorders. *International Journal of Eating Disorders 20*(4), 331–343.—A literature review of experimentally controlled studies of eating disorder treatment programs that assess body image found that cognitive-behavioral eating disorder programs for bulimia nervosa result in modest body image improvement. Rosen found that although cognitive restructuring is widely used, behavioral interventions and self-monitoring techniques that target body image have not been reported by most eating disorder programs.

Springer, E. A., Winzelberg, A. J., Perkins, R., & Taylor, C. B. (1999). Effects of a body image curriculum for college students on improved body image. *International Journal of Eating Disorders, 26*(1), 13–20.—This study evaluated the eating and body image attitude and behavior changes that occurred in female students who completed a college level course on the biology and psychology of eating and body image disorders. The results of this uncontrolled study showed that students significantly improved their body image and eating behavior and attitudes.

Stanford University Behavioral Medicine Media Laboratory: *http://bml.stanford.edu/multimedia_lab/.*—This website describes the work of the Behavioral Medicine Media Laboratory, within the Laboratory for the Study of Behavioral Medicine, in the Department of Psychiatry and Behavioral Sciences at Stanford University Medical Center.

Strachan, M. D., & Cash, T. F. (2002). Self-help for a negative body image: A comparison of components of a cognitive-behavioral program. *Behavior Therapy, 33,* 235–251.—This study compared two 6-week long, self-help body image improvement programs: (1) psychoeducation plus self-monitoring, or (2) treatment combined with procedures to identify and alter dysfunctional body-image cognitions. Both interventions were found to produce clinically significant improvements in multiple facets of body image and psychosocial functioning.

Taylor, C. B., Winzelberg, A., & Celio, A. (2001). Use of interactive media to prevent eating disorders. In R. Striegel-Moore & L. Smolak (Eds.), *Eating disorders: New directions for research and practice.* Washington, DC: American Psychological Association.—An overview of the use of interactive technology to reduce the incidence of eating disorders and a summary of the results from several trials of the Student Bodies intervention.

Winzelberg, A. J., Eppstein, D., Eldredge, K. L., Wilfley, D., Dasmahapatra, R., Dev, P., & Taylor, C. B. (2000). Effectiveness of an Internet-based program for reducing risk factors for eating disorders. *Journal of Consulting and Clinical Psychology, 68*(2), 346–350.—This study evaluated a web-based body image enhancement program with college-age women in a randomized clinical trial. Participants of the intervention were found to improve their body image and eating attitudes and behavior.

www.something-fishy.org.—This website offers a comprehensive list of online body image resources on the Internet. (Note that authors' and sponsors' biases are not always clearly stated on web pages. One should be cautious in following any health recommendations offered on Internet websites.)

56

Ecological and Activism Approaches to the Prevention of Body Image Problems

MICHAEL P. LEVINE
LINDA SMOLAK

Social and cultural factors help create negative body image and disordered eating in females and males. Consequently, social learning theory (SLT) and cognitive-behavioral theory (CBT) have guided development of universal (primary) prevention programs for children and adolescents. These interventions, typically lasting 6–12 weeks, are implemented in schools by psychologists or teachers using direct instruction, symbolic modeling, role playing, and homework assignments. Our review of 42 published and unpublished outcome studies indicates that this approach is not consistently effective, and that when positive findings concerning body esteem and eating behaviors do emerge, they tend to be *short-term* effects. Given that prevention is the only viable solution to the widespread problems of negative body image and disordered eating in females, this chapter considers viable alternatives or supplements to psychoeducation.

AN ECOLOGICAL PERSPECTIVE

SLT and CBT emphasize the role of reciprocal determinism among individual factors, behavior, and environment, including sociocultural influences in shaping negative body image and disordered eating. Given this perspective, it is perplexing that prevention programs have focused on students as individuals and not on changing the physical and social environments that frame negative body image. Changes in peer norms, school policies, teacher behavior, and community practices have long been an established part of SLT-driven prevention programs for substance abuse and cardiovascular health. Moreover, community psychologists have shown that disease and suffering are nonspecific products of an imbalance between too much stress and socioeconomic exploitation versus too little social support, too few coping skills, and too little hope. Community psychology and a more comprehensive social learning model agree that prevention programs should strive to create healthier environments, role models, and opportunities for girls and boys. The U.S. government has taken a small but positive step in this direction by creating the BodyWise program for middle school educators (*www.health.org/gpower/adultswhocare2/resources/pubs/bodywise.htm*).

THE RELATIONAL EMPOWERMENT MODEL

Feminist Theory

An ecological perspective is a crucial component of the relational empowerment model that is derived from feminist theories of female development. Females are extraordinarily more likely than males to suffer from negative body image and disordered eating (with the possible exceptions of binge eating disorder and body dysmorphic disorder). Fundamental aspects of negative body image and disordered eating (e.g., anxiety, self-consciousness, and self-effacing silence, as well as helplessness and internalized anger) are directly linked to patriarchal social influences on female developmental transitions (e.g., early adolescence). Negative body image, the dieting mentality, and disordered eating are intensely personal and personally unhealthy. However, they are understandable adaptations to patriarchal society, in general, and to the many contexts in which female bodies are objectified and devalued. These contexts include prejudice against fat women, weight-related teasing, sexual harassment, sexual violence, and the ubiquitous media venues in which slender women are glorified as objects of male lust and female envy. Thus the deeply personal feelings that constitute negative body image are necessarily contextual and political. This means that psychoeducation about slender beauty ideals and individual resistance skills will be insufficient to foster critical understanding of the body-in-context and to effect healthy changes in relationships, norms, values, and relationships.

Piran's Work

Niva Piran's relational empowerment model of prevention differs radically from SLT and CBT approaches. Drawing from feminist theory and participatory models of health promotion, it begins not with a "program" or "curriculum" designed by experts, but with dialogues between herself and stakeholders (e.g., students, teachers) in a system (e.g., a school). These discussions construct and affirm knowledge about specific contextual factors that shape participants' body image feelings and actions. These participants, not SLT or any other theory, are positioned as the ultimate authorities on, and over, their own bodies. Program goals are derived from dialogue within the group, not from quantitative research generated by experts seeking to apply general psychosocial principles.

The active processes of describing and then critically evaluating "lived experiences" of racism, harassment, and gender inequity help participants transform the private feelings of shame, concealment, and frustration inherent in body dissatisfaction into a shared, public understanding. Permitting girls to voice the truths in their own lives sets the stage for the construction of alternative, healthier norms and practices within the group, and from there to individual and group actions that change environments outside the group. This process reconnects girls with the body as a site for constructive social action and self-expression, not for shame and isolating self-consciousness. A female mental health professional serves as a group facilitator and a forceful advocate for systemic change, in part through coordination of dialogue between students, educators, and parents. She reinforces the links between analysis, voice, and action by also "speaking up" and "speaking out" to ensure that influential adults understand the need for contextual changes.

For over 15 years, Piran has used this approach within a very high-risk setting: an elite, residential ballet company. Dialogues guided by the students (girls and boys in separate groups, ages 10–18) focused on sexual harassment, lack of privacy, sexism, racism, and other forms of disrespect toward the developing female body. Piran helped students articulate what they knew to be best for their development, to create healthy group norms, and to work toward changes in school policies, the school ethos, and, in a few instances, staff. Across three different sets of students at three different time periods (1987, 1991, and 1996), Piran found that the prevalence of eating disorders among the girls was reduced from 10% to just 1% in the case of anorexia nervosa, and there were no cases of bulimia nervosa. There were also significant reductions in the percentage of students who binged and relied on unhealthy forms of weight management (e.g., self-induced vomiting).

Media Literacy

Piran's approach provides multiple opportunities for girls as a collective to critically evaluate contextual influences on body image. Several prevention programs have applied this type of "literacy" (consciousness raising) and activism to mass media. These programs, however, follow the SLT–CBT model in that educational activities ("lessons") are scripted by mental health professionals. Groups of adolescent girls examine the content (including what is left out) and impact of mass media "stories" about the body told via programs, articles, and advertisements, and the application of computer technology and other tricks to construct images of the female body that sell fantasies and products. Invariably, the girls construct and affirm a shared sense of outrage over some of the media's themes and practices. The group facilitator helps them voice their protest and create new media with healthier messages. The goal is critical thinking and constructive social action, not cynicism or blanket rejection of mass media. To borrow a metaphor from Erica Austin of Washington State University (personal communication, June 30, 1998), mass media are necessary tools in democratic societies, so media literacy skills can be thought of as "safety glasses."

To date, there are six short-term evaluations of media literacy programs in existence for adolescent girls and young women. These programs tend to reduce internalization of the slender beauty ideal, to increase self-acceptance and self-efficacy directed toward social change, and to improve life skills. Although such results are promising, current media literacy work needs to be augmented in order to have a meaningful impact on body image.

Combining Psychoeducation, Literacy, and Activism

The most successful SLT prevention program, developed by Dianne Neumark-Sztainer at the University of Minnesota, combined psychoeducation with opportunities for girls to change norms and values at their high school. "Full of Ourselves," created by Catherine Steiner-Adair and colleagues at the Harvard Eating Disorder Center (*www.hedc.org*), extends this integrated approach by incorporating aspects of the relational empowerment model. The Harvard program's 70 activities, delivered in eight 45- to 90-minute units across 8–15 weeks, help girls ages 12–14 improve their body image, refrain from dieting, and distinguish hunger for food from emotional needs. Together, the girls learn about weightism as a prejudice, developing bodies versus the culture of thinness, the politics of body image, and assertion, leadership, and activism. Participants work closely with each other and with trained adult mentors, and the girls serve as mentors themselves for younger girls (ages 9–11). In a recent large-scale, controlled evaluation with a 6-month follow-up, the program was shown to improve body esteem and reduce both negative self-talk about the body and internalization of the slender beauty ideal; however, weight management behavior was unaffected. As is the case for media literacy, more work is necessary.

HEALTH-PROMOTING SCHOOLS

Theory

Except for Piran's intervention, current prevention programs do not coordinate their efforts with social structures. Further, programs to date have not focused on peer relationships, parents, teachers, and other adults. Schools are a logical setting for examination and transformation of various social influences on body image and disordered eating. The concept of a "health-promoting school" was developed by the World Health Organization in the 1980s. It is now being implemented by the European Network of Health-Promoting Schools (*www.who.dk/enhps*) and the Australian Health Promoting Schools Association (*www.hlth.qut.edu.au/ph/ahpsa*).

Health-promoting schools create student–staff–community partnerships whose aim is to make schools and the community healthier and safer. Learning and development are facilitated by good health, which is much more likely in environments that are safe, responsive, and caring. Such environments apply democratic principles of participation and equity, including equal access to empowerment for students and staff, as well as freedom from teasing, harassment, fear, and oppression. Students, staff, parents, and community resources share the responsibility for constructing healthier school environments and for evaluating their impact. The foundation for clarifying problems and deciding on solutions is comprised of discussion, relationship building, and critical thinking—not bureaucratic power. This democratic approach ensures that changes in individual behavior, teacher training, teaching styles, school policies, school norms, etc., are sustainable.

Although its perspective is explicitly holistic, the theory of health-promoting schools divides the focus of prevention and intervention into three categories:

- School organization, ethos, and environment
- Curriculum, teaching, and learning
- School–community partnerships

School Organization, Ethos, and Environment

Schools should designate and train a resource person (probably a counselor, social worker, or psychologist) to assume responsibility for overseeing the project. The first task involves facilitating discussions among stakeholders (e.g., students, teachers, parents, community professionals) to clarify school goals concerning health promotion, including body image, nutrition, and physical activity. Specific areas for discussion include what happens at school that makes students feel good or bad about their bodies, food service and student behavior in the cafeteria, and opportunities that girls have for experiencing success unrelated to their physical appearance. Guiding principles include:

1. No one is to blame for negative body image and disordered eating, but everyone (male and female alike) is responsible for prevention and health promotion.
2. Because stigmatization of overweight people and glorification of di-

eting are unhealthy, educators should never dispense weight loss advice, regardless of the child's size.

3. Because racism limits opportunities to be something other than a voiceless body, multiethnic teams are important for modeling and teaching respect for diversity in ethnicity as well as in weight and shape.

The resource person also helps the school system and students survey school policies and practices that influence body image and eating. Are there contests or participation requirements that focus on weight and shape? Do textbooks and classroom posters show a diversity of weights and shapes among females and males? Do the hallways feature posters that objectify women? School environments are fluid, so assessment of policies, practices, and the physical setting is an ongoing process. The resource person should be a "sounding board" or advocate for both students and staff.

Teasing and harassment by peers and adults contribute to negative body image and disordered eating. Unfortunately, by age 10 or 11, girls feel that teachers, principals, and other important adults have quit taking their complaints seriously. Their concerns are minimized by advice to "just ignore" boys who are teasing them, or to "just avoid" uncomfortable situations. It is essential for schools to have a clearly stated and well-publicized policy that champions equity, fairness, and respect by prohibiting body-related teasing. Students and staff need to learn that comments or touching in regard to weight, breast size, and body shape are as taboo as comments about race or disability. Students must know to whom they should report incidents. Staff and community must take these reports seriously. The resource person can help the school system publicize its policies to the community, train staff and students in dealing with violations, and monitor the effectiveness of these efforts.

SLT, CBT, and relational empowerment theories all agree that classroom "lessons" should be modeled by the positive attitudes and behaviors of teachers, coaches, and other staff. These attitudes and behaviors include refraining from "fat jokes"; dressing with style and individual expression, regardless of shape and weight; refusing to avoid healthy and fun activities because of body image issues; and enjoying a variety of nutritious and, in moderation, not particularly nutritious foods.

Curriculum, Teaching, and Learning

Another important level of intervention is curriculum development, including teacher training. Teachers should convey to students that classrooms are safe and respectful places, that cultural literacy training is valuable, and that, in addition to facts (e.g., genetic influences on weight and shape), students should learn life skills, such as problem solving and assertion.

Teachers across the curriculum should also encourage student involvement in community service projects, creative arts, and daily physical activities.

A health-promoting curriculum is integrated vertically and developmentally across the grades. For example, elementary school lessons might concentrate on nutrition for strength and stamina, physical activities for fun, and the unfairness and unacceptability of weight-and-shape prejudice. In late elementary school and early middle school, topics might shift to fat deposition in healthy pubertal development and the nutritional needs of older children and young adolescents involved in sports and dancing. The curriculum is also integrated horizontally, lessons elaborated in mathematics, research methodology, biology, social studies, history, and art. For example, in the eighth grade (ages 13–14), each of these classes might address appropriate aspects of the clash between the natural diversity of weights and shapes and the narrow cultural values about femininity, beauty, and restraint.

School–Community Partnerships

The resource person ensures that parents and mental health professionals participate in conversations with stakeholders about health-promoting strategies for their community. These discussions should help everyone appreciate how negative body image is connected to other parental concerns: low self-esteem, depression, eating disorders, obesity, poor coping skills, cigarette smoking, and lowered ambitions. The resource person also facilitates the establishment of a system for identifying, referring, and treating students who have an eating disorder or warning signs of the disorder.

Parents are particularly important in school–community partnerships. Student homework assignments should encourage dialogues with parents. Parents can work with school staff and local business and media to help students construct community activism and education projects. In this process, parents need accurate information about pubertal development, media literacy, and physical fitness. They must know how to respond to questions such as "Mommy, am I fat?" or "Does this dress makes me look fat?" The resource person can forge broader ties by connecting staff and parents to organizations such as the National Eating Disorders Association (*www.nationaleatingdisorders.org*).

CONCLUSIONS AND FUTURE DIRECTIONS

Jennifer O'Dea and Danielle Maloney reported promising results from their limited application of the health-promoting schools approach to a high school in Australia. Their work supports the value of continued development of the relational empowerment and ecological approaches. Because ignorance and prejudice nurture negative body image and disordered eating, there is an important role for psychoeducation by adult experts. But prevention also requires that students, teachers, parents, and other stakeholders in the community have the opportunity to clarify body image issues and use this information to improve their social and physical environments.

This review has focused on girls because currently they are disproportionately affected by negative body image and its consequences. But boys are part of the school environment, so their perspectives, especially on teasing, need to be understood if change is to be effective and equitable. In addition, research suggests the growth of a new cultural ideal for boys' bodies, a muscular ideal that is taught and enforced in the manner of the thin ideal for girls. This standard of male attractiveness and power has dangerous consequences, including steroid abuse. Ecological programs need to be aware of, and responsive to, male body image issues.

Another challenge for health-promoting schools is achieving a balance between student, educator, and parental input. Elementary school is the most important period for *preventing* negative body image, but it is unclear to what extent girls and boys ages 6–11 could or should participate in clarifying and changing unhealthy contextual factors. Nevertheless, we believe that the health-promoting schools concept offers an excellent opportunity to combine the best features of the SLT, CBT, and relational empowerment approaches in an emphasis on the 4 C's of prevention: consciousness raising, competencies, connections with others, and change in community norms and values.

INFORMATIVE READINGS

Friedman, S. S. (2000). *Nurturing GirlPower: Integrating eating disorder prevention/intervention skills in your practice.* Salal Books. Available from Salal Communications, Ltd., 101-1184 Denman St. #309, Vancouver, BC V6G 2M9 Canada, (604) 689-8399.—Applies the feminist empowerment model to middle school girls and provides specific exercises to help adults become healthier role models and create positive settings for adolescents.

Levine, M. P., & Piran, N. (2001). The prevention of eating disorders: Towards a participatory ecology of knowledge, action, and advocacy. In R. Striegel-Moore & L. Smolak (Eds.), *Eating disorders: New directions for research and practice* (pp. 233–253). Washington, DC: American Psychological Association.—Reviews current prevention research and proposes ways to engage individuals and groups in creating environments conducive to positive body image and healthier eating and exercising.

Levine, M. P., & Smolak, L. (2001). Primary prevention of body image disturbances and disordered eating in childhood and early adolescence. In J. K. Thompson & L. Smolak (Eds.), *Body image, eating disorders, and obesity in youth: Assessment, prevention, and treatment* (pp. 237–260). Washington, DC: American Psychological Association.—Detailed review of prevention studies with children ages 8–13 that discusses developmental principles and important contexts in children's lives.

Neumark-Sztainer, D. (1996). School-based programs for preventing eating disturbances. *Journal of School Health, 66,* 64–71.—Offers a model for integrating different components of the curriculum, teacher training, and the school environment toward promotion of positive body image and healthy eating.

Neumark-Sztainer, D., Butler, R., & Palti, H. (1995). Eating disturbances among adolescent girls: Evaluation of a school-based primary prevention program. *Journal of Nutrition Education, 27,* 24–30.—Evaluates a promising prevention approach in Israel that uses social learning theory to train teachers, educate girls, and encourage them to be social activists in their high school.

O'Dea, J., & Maloney, D. (2000). Preventing eating and body image problems in children and adolescents using the Health Promoting Schools Framework. *Journal of School Health, 70,* 18–21.—Outlines the general theory of health-promoting schools, considers its potential for prevention of negative body image, and briefly describes an application in an Australian high school.

Perry, C. L. (1999). *Creating health behavior change: How to develop community-wide programs for youth.* Thousand Oaks, CA: Sage.—A handbook for applying social learning theory to development of health promotion at community, school, curricular, and family levels.

Piran, N., Levine, M. P., & Steiner-Adair, C. (Eds.). (1999). *Preventing eating disorders: A handbook of interventions and special challenges.* Philadelphia: Brunner/Mazel.—Includes several chapters by Piran on the relational empowerment model, as well as chapters on media literacy and other forms of social activism.

Steiner-Adair, C., Sjostrom, L., Franko, D. L., Pai, S., Tucker, R., Becker, A. E., & Herzog, D. B. (in press). Primary prevention of eating disorders in adolescent girls: Learning from practice. *International Journal of Eating Disorders.*—Evaluates a promising prevention program in the United States that applies the relational empowerment model to young adolescent girls. The program uses lessons, adult mentors, and mentoring opportunities for the girls themselves. The focus is on educating the girls about body image while involving them in the development of life skills, leadership, and social activism.

IX

Conclusions and Directions

Future Challenges
for Body Image Theory, Research,
and Clinical Practice

THOMAS F. CASH
THOMAS PRUZINSKY

In this concluding chapter we take a "step back" to gain perspective on the many important ideas our contributors have made regarding how the field of body image can move forward—conceptually, scientifically, and clinically. Our goal here is not merely to summarize the key conclusions of our contributors. Rather, building from the previous 56 chapters, we articulate epigrammatic statements regarding our beliefs about the most important future directions for understanding body image functioning.

In order to organize these views about the future of body image theory, research, and clinical practice, we revisit the organization of the book and specify how progress can be made in understanding and applying this complex construct with respect to (1) conceptual foundations; (2) developmental perspectives; (3) assessment; (4) individual and cultural differences; (5) body image dysfunctions and disorders; (6) changing the body through medical, surgical, and other interventions; and (7) changing body image through psychosocial interventions.

Although we organize our discussion around these distinct areas, we also encourage recognition of the interconnections among them. It is evident that the preponderance of our recommendations pertains to elucidating conceptual foundations. Clearly, comprehensive elaboration and refinement of the boundaries and referents of the body image construct is a necessary prerequisite to progress in understanding body image development, assessment, dysfunction, and change.

BODY IMAGE CONCEPTUAL FOUNDATIONS

• Despite considerable historical interest in defining body image as a more far-reaching construct, contemporary usage has come to mean our experiences of our physical appearance. We must recognize that embodiment entails more than self-perceived aesthetics. It includes experiences of the body's functioning (e.g., perception and experience of all forms of sensation; how we experience the aging process) and level of competence (e.g., kinesthetics, physical fitness, athleticism). The human experience of embodiment is complex and varied. However, most contemporary conceptualizations of body image functioning fail to capture this richness.

• Body image must be conceptualized and studied in ways that transcend eating disorders, or else our understanding of the meanings of human embodiment will be distorted by our single-pointed focus on eating disorders. The body image concept is very broad; weight-related and appearance-related concerns comprise only a limited portion of the total applicability.

• We must give greater attention to the dimension of body image investment, which is the degree of cognitive and behavioral importance that people assign to their body and the extent to which the body's appearance defines their sense of self (i.e., self-schemas, self-objectification, etc.). Greater precision in understanding and evaluating body image investment can serve to clarify a fundamental axiom of body image functioning—objective appearance is not necessarily indicative of the subjective experience of appearance. Any progress in understanding body image development, dysfunction, or change must be based on a fundamental understanding of the nature of body image investment.

• Body image is often conceived and assessed exclusively as a trait-like construct. We must better recognize and consider the roles of situational and emotional contexts in the fluid and dynamic experience of body image in daily life. Thus we must study body image fluctuations within individuals and seek to understand how such variation relates to individual psychological attributes and actual physical characteristics.

• Despite the enormous scientific literature on the psychosocial influences of physical attractiveness, body image researchers seldom incorporate such "objective" appearance variables (other than body mass) into their studies. The inclusion of these variables could help us ascertain the significance of body image independent of, and in interaction with, veridical parameters of physical appearance.

• It would be informative to put more of the *body* back into the study of body image by gaining a more informed understanding of the physiological and neurophysiological substrates of body image experience (e.g., sensitivity to touch, awareness of physiological arousal). Developing this knowledge may influence our understanding of individual differences as well as point us toward the most efficacious approaches for prevention and treatment.

• The causal and consequential roles of body image must be better examined in close interpersonal contexts—in families, friendships, and romantic relationships. We must enhance our understanding of how body image affects and is affected by processes of social attachment and social functioning.

• The behavioral aspects of body image have been largely neglected. We must improve our understanding of how people create and manage their own body image via appearance-managing behaviors in everyday life.

• We must learn more about both adaptive and maladaptive coping strategies that people use in response to the challenges to body image functioning that occur in everyday life (e.g., exposure to media messages and "ideals"; situations and events that accentuate one's looks; the effects of aging; the experience of common illness and injury; mood-related changes in appearance perception, etc.).

• Further research on hypotheses derived from an information-processing model of body image would facilitate our understanding of how cognitive or distortions influence body image experiences in varying contexts.

• Reflecting the pathology-driven paradigm of psychology and allied disciplines, most body image research focuses on dissatisfaction and dysfunction. A "paradigm shift" that recognizes and studies the development and experience of a "positive body image" is imperative. This shift would include investigations of the role of resilience and protective factors in life experiences as well as dimensions of personality that shape adaptive, healthy responses.

DEVELOPMENTAL PERSPECTIVES

• Body image research tends to focus on adolescents and young adults, mostly college students. We must expand our knowledge of body image to include children and midlife and later-life adults.

• We have surprisingly little understanding of the longitudinal development of body image. For example, does the objectively unattractive child who develops a negative body image continue to experience such negative self-evaluations during adulthood? Does the young adult with a positive body image experience the process of aging with greater equanimity than the young adult with persistently negative body image?

• Integration of the body image construct into current comprehensive theories of development may prove useful—for example, the specification of body image variables in attachment or "identity process theory" models.

• Most research attempts to capture body image experiences at different ages or developmental periods by cross-sectionally comparing cohorts. Prospective research on body image is crucial. Such studies are also needed to elucidate the influences of various sociocultural (e.g., media exposure) and interpersonal (e.g., appearance teasing/criticism) variables.

BODY IMAGE ASSESSMENT

• Despite the widespread acknowledgment that body image is a multidimensional construct, too many researchers define the construct with a singular measure (e.g., body satisfaction). This singularity is partially a result of limited conceptualization of the body image construct—which, in turn, limits measurement. Limited measurement results, at best, in an incomplete understanding of body image. At worst, limited measurement distorts our understanding of body image functioning.

• The available body image assessments for adolescents and adults are myriad; those for children are few. The development and validation of multidimensional body image assessments for children is an important and very challenging endeavor. Constructing a more precise understanding of body image developmental variables will lead to clearer understanding of the etiology of both negative and positive body image, which in turn will directly influence the content of prevention and treatment programs. There is, perhaps, no single more pressing challenge for body image researchers and clinicians than to further develop and refine body image measurement of children.

• Recent advances in the assessment of perceptual body image reflect the utility of psychophysical methods, which now need to be examined in relation to other facets of the body image construct. The use of these methods, as well as computer-based morphing technologies, is promising and should be explored beyond the perception of body size.

• The important historical contribution of projective techniques, although currently out of vogue, to our understanding of body image should not be relegated to the empirical "dust bin." Similarly, future understanding of body image very likely can benefit from an improved appreciation of the psychometric and clinical strengths and weaknesses of projective techniques.

• We should begin to consider the development of "standardized" body image assessment modules. We need to move toward an era in which each new researcher does not need to "reinvent the wheel" of body image assessment. Similar to the development of practice guidelines for providing psychotherapy, we should begin to move toward defining clearly efficacious methods of body image assessment for specific purposes and contexts.

• Progress needs to be made in balancing the needs of clinicians and researchers for context-specific body image assessments and assessments that evaluate generalized, dispositional dimensions of body image (e.g., appearance evaluation and investment).

• Greatly needed are large-scale, multi-site, demographically representative studies of the multiple facets of body image. Such a collaborative venture among scientists would provide a descriptively informative database for the most commonly used or promising assessments.

INDIVIDUAL AND CULTURAL DIFFERENCES

• Comparative cross-cultural studies of body image are crucial to enhance our understanding of the diversity of body images and the influence of culture on body image development, dysfunction, and change.

• We need more gender balance in our research, despite progress in this area over the past decade. The data that exist clearly point to important gender differences, for example, in the nature of weight-related concerns, emphasis on muscularity, and body image schematic themes. Body image functioning is highly relevant to the quality of life for males as well as females.

• A clear understanding of diversity in body image functioning requires studying the influences of national, racial, and ethnic differences, as well as sexual orientation. A precise understanding of the role of culture in body image formation and experience must consider individual differences in cultural assimilation and identity. Thus we must not seek only to discern differences between certain groups; we must also understand the heterogeneity of body image experiences within these groups.

• We need a much clearer understanding of body image diversity among individuals with congenital medical conditions (e.g., craniofacial disfigurement, short stature, dental deformity). Because the ultimate goal of many researchers and clinicians is to prevent or treat negative body image development, we can learn much from those individuals who adapt, whether well or poorly, to such physical conditions.

BODY IMAGE DYSFUNCTIONS AND DISORDERS

• Compared to the literature on eating disorders, other disorders related to body image (e.g., body dysmorphic disorder, gender identity disorder, somatic delusional disorder) have received little investigation and clearly warrant greater attention.

• "Negative body image" is a poorly defined term and reflects a condition whose prevalence is unclear. We must develop a consensual meaning of this concept that recognizes the impact of body image on individuals' quality of life. There is an implicitly recognized, albeit not fully articulated, continuum of body image dysfunction. A dimensional approach to the "classification" of body image problems should be developed as a complement to the dominant prototypical approach taken by the current DSM.

• Greatly needed are prospective investigations and causal modeling studies of body image variables as predisposing causes ("diatheses") of various psychopathologies or problems in living. For example, we need to better understand the role of body image in the development of social phobia, depression, and sexual dysfunctions.

• Similarly, we need to examine how body image processes may function to maintain such psychosocial problems and increase the likelihood of relapse following treatment for these problems.

PHYSICAL INTERVENTIONS AND CHANGES IN BODY IMAGE

• We need more evidence on the durability of changes in body image via bodily change (e.g., weight loss, cosmetic surgery, medical treatments of appearance-altering conditions, etc.). What social and psychological variables influence the process of assimilating a new body image? We also need a great deal more understanding of the "trajectories" of body image change. For example, how are the body image effects of surgical interventions that reconstruct congenital facial disfigurement different from the body image effects of facial reconstruction for acquired disfigurement?

• Researchers should evaluate whether changes in the body brought about by "external" interventions (e.g., gastric stapling surgery resulting in weight loss) are experienced as qualitatively different from changes in the body brought about through one's own actions (e.g., dieting or exercise leading to weight loss).

• We must expand our examination of the significance of body image in specific medical contexts. Despite the astronomical number of people with congenital physical problems, dermatological disorders, dental deformities, cancer, urological or endocrinological conditions, or HIV/AIDS, we know *very little* about how the body image consequences influence their quality of life. The number of people affected by eating disorders is minute in comparison to the number of people coping with these body-altering conditions. Yet few professionals have devoted themselves to understanding the ways in which physical diseases and disabilities challenge how people experience their body, how they vary so dramatically in response to their physical problems, or how we can assist those who are suffering. This is a salient shortcoming for future body image researchers and clinicians to address.

• Body part transplantation represents an important new scientific and clinical domain. From a body image perspective, what is it like to live with transplanted body parts? What factors predict positive body image adaptation to transplantation? New forms of transplantation, including hand and full-face transplantation, are now being developed and will clearly have profound implications for recipients' body image.

- Physical exercise is a two-edged phenomenon, sometimes promoting a positive body image and other times having deleterious effects. A more precise understanding of the complex effects of physical activity is essential.
- What are the motivations for and responses to the now common body modification practices of tattooing and body piercing? What social, personality, and body image variables predict such behavior? Do these "body adornments" affect recipients' body image experiences?

PSYCHOSOCIAL INTERVENTIONS AND BODY IMAGE CHANGE

- Documenting the efficacy of currently available psychosocial interventions more accurately will serve the critical purpose of providing the empirical basis for greater dissemination of these interventions and third-party support for their use. Stated simply, empirical verification of intervention efficacy will lead to more people being helped.
- We need to continue our evaluations of cognitive-behavioral body image therapy as an empirically supported treatment with more diverse populations, especially children and men. We clearly need longer follow-ups to determine whether its favorable outcomes are maintained.
- We must specify more precisely those components of body image interventions that contribute to the effectiveness of programs for treating and preventing eating disorders. What are the most essential ingredients and how should they be delivered to maximize outcomes?
- Controlled clinical trials must be conducted to examine the efficacy of contemporary psychodynamic approaches (especially interpersonal therapy) and experientially based treatments of body image problems. Are there aspects of these approaches that could be integrated with extant cognitive-behavioral strategies to provide more comprehensive and effective programs?
- Expanding research on preventing negative body image is crucial to determine creative ways to enhance the efficacy of psychoeducation as well as ecological/activist interventions. How can we use technology, media, and institutions most effectively to promote body acceptance among children, adolescents, and adults?
- It is crucial that we evaluate the role and contribution of body image psychoeducation and psychotherapy as adjunctive interventions for people receiving medical/surgical treatments (e.g., in cosmetic and reconstructive surgeries). Further development and validation of these interventions are particularly pressing, because some of these individuals have ongoing body image concerns that can profoundly compromise their quality of life.

A FINAL CHALLENGE

The future of science and practice related to body image greatly depends on our willingness to question the adequacy of our assumptions and knowledge. The greatest promise for the field is for it to become more interdisciplinary. All too often body image has "belonged" to psychology, even more to a subset of clinical psychologists with professional interests in eating disorders. While body image research that has focused on women and eating disorders has certainly been of great benefit and has advanced the field tremendously, it has also narrowed our thought and inquiry. We hope that this volume has helped expand readers' appreciation of the complexity and applicability of the phenomenology and conceptualization of body image. In addition, we hope that our contributors' wisdom will serve as a catalyst for new ideas, more productive research, more effective interventions, and further-reaching applications. After all, as we have come to appreciate more fully, the experience of embodiment is central to the quality of human life.

Index

517